RUNNING INJURIES

GARY N. GUTEN, MD

Assistant Clinical Professor
Department of Orthopaedics
Medical College of Wisconsin
Milwaukee, Wisconsin

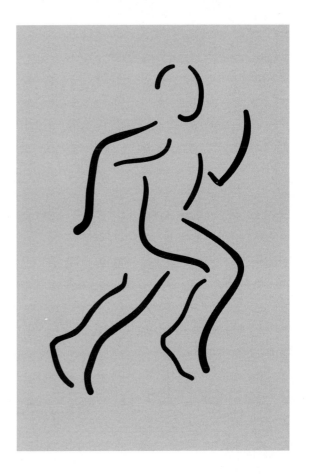

RUNNING
INJURIES

W.B. SAUNDERS COMPANY
A Division of Harcourt Brace & Company
Philadelphia London Toronto Montreal Sydney Tokyo

W.B. SAUNDERS COMPANY
A Division of Harcourt Brace & Company

The Curtis Center
Independence Square West
Philadelphia, Pennsylvania 19106

Library of Congress Cataloging-in-Publication Data

Running injuries / [edited by] Gary N. Guten.

p.   cm.

ISBN 0–7216–6843–7

1. Running injuries—Treatment.   I. Guten, Gary N.
  [DNLM: 1. Running—injuries.   2. Athletic Injuries—therapy.
  3. Orthopedics.   4. Pain—etiology.   QT 260.5.R9 R943 1997]

RC1220.R8R86 1997   617.1′027—dc20

DNLM/DLC   96–27149

RUNNING INJURIES   ISBN 0–7216–6843–7

Printed in the United States of America.

Last digit is the print number: 9   8   7   6   5   4   3   2   1

Marvin M. Adner, MD

Associate Chief of Medicine, Metrowest Medical Center, Framingham, Massachusetts
Medical Syndromes in Runners

Judith F. Baumhauer, MD

Assistant Professor and Chief of Division of Foot and Ankle Surgery, University of Rochester Medical Center, Rochester, New York
Ankle Pain in Runners

Stuart Berger, MD

Associate Professor of Pediatrics, Medical College of Wisconsin; Medical Director, Children's Heart Center and Children's Hospital of Wisconsin, Milwaukee, Wisconsin
The Cardiopulmonary Effects and Consequences of Running in Children—Good or Bad?

Brian E. Black, MD

Medical Director, Center for Children's Orthopedics, and Medical Director, Spinal Performance Center, St. Francis Hospital, Milwaukee, Wisconsin
The Adolescent Runner

William G. Clancy, Jr., MD

Clinical Professor of Orthopedic Surgery, University of Alabama, Birmingham; Staff Orthopedic Surgeon, Alabama Sports Medicine and Orthopedic Center, Birmingham, Alabama
Strengthening and Flexibility Concepts for Runners

Ellen J. Coleman, MA, MPH, RD

Nutrition Consultant, The Sport Clinic, Riverside, California
Nutrition and Running

Gregg R. Foos, MD

Associate Professor, Department of Orthopedic Surgery, Monmouth Medical Center, Long Branch, New Jersey
Arthroscopy of the Knee in Runners

Carl Foster, PhD

Professor of Medicine (CHS), University of Wisconsin Medical School, Madison, Wisconsin; Director, Department of Clinical Physiology, Milwaukee Heart Institute, Milwaukee, Wisconsin
Overtraining Syndrome

James M. Fox, MD

Southern California Orthopedic Institute
Arthroscopy of the Knee in Runners

Charles J. Gatt, Jr., MD

Clinical Assistant Professor of Surgery, Division of Orthopedic Surgery, University of Medicine and Dentistry of New Jersey, Robert Wood Johnson Medical School, New Brunswick, New Jersey
Back Pain in Running

John S. Gould, MD

Clinical Professor of Orthopaedic Surgery, University of Virginia; Alabama Sports Medicine and Orthopaedic Center, and Health South Medical Center, Birmingham, Alabama
Ankle Pain in Runners

Gary N. Guten, MD

Assistant Clinical Professor, Department of Orthopaedics, Medical College of Wisconsin; Medical Director of Sports Medicine Performance Center, St. Francis Hospital, Milwaukee, Wisconsin
Overview of Leg Injuries in Running

Frank W. Jobe, MD

Clinical Professor, Department of Orthopaedics, University of Southern California School of Medicine, Los Angeles, California; President, Kerlan-Jobe Orthopaedic Clinic; Medical Director, Biomechanics Laboratory, Centinela Hospital Medical Center; Orthopedic Consultant, Los Angeles Dodgers, PGA Tour and Senior PGA Tour, Inglewood, California
The Foot/Shoe Interface

Paul J. Kiell, MD
Former Chief of Psychiatry, Muhlenberg Hospital, Plainfield, New Jersey
Running and Mood Disorders

Harvey S. Kohn, MD
Assistant Clinical Professor of Orthopaedics, Medical College of Wisconsin; Attending Physician at St. Francis Hospital, St. Michael's Hospital, and Mt. Sinai Hospital, Milwaukee, Wisconsin
Shin Pain and Compartment Syndromes in Running

Ronald M. Lawrence, MD, MS, PhD
Assistant Clinical Professor, Neuropsychiatric Institute, School of Medicine, University of California at Los Angeles; Director, Western Geriatric Research Institute, Los Angeles, California
Why Run?

Robert E. Leach, MD
Professor of Orthopaedic Surgery, Boston University Medical School, Boston, Massachusetts; Editor, American Journal of Sports Medicine, Waltham, Massachusetts
Stress Fractures

Brian P. H. Lee, MD
Adult Reconstruction Special Fellow in Orthopedics, Mayo Graduate School of Medicine, Rochester, Minnesota
Reconstructive Surgery of the Hip and Knee in Runners

Manfred Lehmann, MD
Professor and Director of Sport and Lifestyle Medicine, University Clinic, University of Ulm, Ulm, Germany
Overtraining Syndrome

Tom F. Novacheck, MD
Assistant Professor of Orthopaedics, University of Minnesota, Minneapolis, Minnesota; Director, Motion Analysis Laboratory, Gillette Children's Specialty Health Care, St. Paul, Minnesota
The Biomechanics of Running and Sprinting

John G. Paty, Jr., MD, FACP
Associate Clinical Professor of Medicine, University of Tennessee College of Medicine, Chattanooga, Tennessee
Arthritis and Running

Thomas A. Pietrocarlo, DPM
Clinical Instructor, Department of Family Practice, Medical College of Wisconsin; Podiatrist, St. Francis Hospital, Milwaukee, Wisconsin
Foot Pain in Runners

Marilyn M. Pink, PhD, PT
Director and Assistant Administrator, Biomechanics Laboratory, Centinela Hospital Medical Center, Inglewood, California
The Foot/Shoe Interface

Michael J. Shereff, MD
Associate Professor and Director, Foot and Ankle Division, Medical College of Wisconsin; Associate Staff, St. Francis Hospital and Columbia Hospital, Milwaukee, Wisconsin
Ankle Pain in Runners

Arthur J. Siegel, MD
Assistant Clinical Professor of Medicine, Harvard Medical School, Boston, Massachusetts; Chief of Internal Medicine, McLean Hospital, Belmont, Massachusetts
Medical Syndromes in Runners

Franklin H. Sim, MD
Consultant, Department of Orthopedics, Mayo Clinic and Mayo Foundation; Professor of Orthopedics, Mayo Medical School, Rochester, Minnesota
Reconstructive Surgery of the Hip and Knee in Runners

Guy G. Simoneau, PhD, PT, ATC
Assistant Professor, Program in Physical Therapy, Marquette University, Milwaukee, Wisconsin
Strengthening and Flexibility Concepts for Runners

Michael J. Stuart, MD
Consultant, Department of Orthopedics, Mayo Clinic and Mayo Foundation; Associate Professor of Orthopedics, Mayo Medical School, Rochester, Minnesota
Reconstructive Surgery of the Hip and Knee in Runners

Kevin E. Wilk, BS, PT

Adjunct Assistant Professor, Program in Physical Therapy, Marquette University, Milwaukee, Wisconsin; National Director, Research and Clinical Education, Healthsouth Rehabilitation Corporation; Director of Rehabilitation Research, American Sports Medicine Institute, Birmingham, Alabama
Strengthening and Flexibility Concepts for Runners

Annette M. Zaharoff, MD

Assistant Clinical Professor, Department of Physical Medicine and Rehabilitation, University of Texas Health Science Center, San Antonio, Texas
The Female Athlete Triad in Runners

Susan B. Zecher, MD

Resident, National Rehabilitation Hospital, Washington, DC
Stress Fractures

FOREWORD

Unlike the adults who will read this book, children are wonderfully self-limiting in their activities. When children undertake a physical activity, they continue until something internal tells them it is time to stop. Invariably, this stopping point is reached well before the activity has become too intense or chronically damaging. As they grow older, some people begin to set goals in their physical activities. Eventually, they encounter the physical and mental barriers beyond which lies the world of chronic injuries and fatigue.

I have been running for more than thirty years. The total number of miles I have run is more than one hundred thousand. During my time working out I have come to the conclusion that almost everyone possesses the mental ability to push his or her body beyond its physical and mental limits. When substantial long-term athletic goals are added to the training program, some sort of injury, either mental or physical, is the eventual but inevitable outcome.

I believe that everyone who exercises has what I term an "exercise quotient." This is the amount of exercise a person needs to do in a particular session before he or she feels satisfied. Why do I need to run eight miles on an easy training day rather than five? There is no real physiologic reason (yet discovered) in terms of the cardiovascular training effect. I just need to go that far. Over time, if my exercise quotient is greater than what I term my "orthopaedic limit," I break down. At this point in my life I have a 15-mile per day "exercise quotient" and an eight-mile per day body. I have resigned myself to cross-training, and, so, the information contained herein is of all the more interest to me.

I will readily admit that my knowledge in this area is the result of personal, anecdotal experience. Therefore, I am pleased to see that this book goes a long way toward bridging the gap between my kind of anecdotal experience and the much needed empirical research in this realm of sports injuries. It makes perfect sense to me, since the training habits of high-level athletes (in my case former athletes) have always provided the protocols for research in this area. For years, exercise physiologists have isolated the routines of successful athletes and, in essence, discovered the scientific reason for their successes.

As is often the case, answering many of the empirical questions in this area also results in the production of many more unanswered questions, but this is as it should be. I believe that being coached or coaching yourself is as much an art as it is a science. Basic training theory for endurance athletes is very simple to outline: develop a cardiovascular endurance base; add on some anaerobic training to produce as high an anaerobic threshold as possible; and then train as hard as possible without getting injured and/or mentally burned out. One combines art with science to tailor the theory to a particular athlete and to produce as much long-term, high-intensity training effect as possible.

Therefore, the information contained in this book will certainly educate health care professionals. However, it will also add verification (and justification) to what many athletes, elite and otherwise, have come to know through using their common sense as they strive to maintain these high levels of intensity. The best compliment that I can give is that it will be very easy for an athlete to read this book and nod his or her head in affirmation. There is tangible reinforcement in having one's long-time routine verified scientifically.

Just as this work will generate further research, it will also give coaches and athletes some new ideas on how to approach their training programs. The greater the knowledge, the greater the need and potential for adapting it to the particular, unique individual.

GARY N. GUTEN, M.D., EDITOR

PREFACE

Injuries in Running—A 25-Year Review

Do you remember where you were 25 years ago? I certainly do. Frank Shorter was winning the 1972 Olympic marathon as I sat watching the event on television—engrossed, excited, and amazed. That event sparked the "running revolution" in the United States and around the world. It caused me to vault my personal running program to new heights, along with millions of other runners. I then ran my first marathon in 1978.

The purpose and direction of this book are to pay tribute to the Frank Shorter victory and to review the changes in the sports medicine of running over the past 25 years. Running is not a static sport. It is evolving and revolving as the running revolution continues. Just as the runner is on the "go," the principles of sports medicine of running injuries are changing and evolving to enhance the benefits and reduce the injury rate.

The benefits of running are highlighted in an impressive 1995 study from the Cooper Aerobic Institute, which reviewed the mortality of 10,000 men. This study showed that there is a 44% reduction in mortality when a person changes from an "unfit" to a "fit" status.[1]

Along with the benefits of running come the risks and injuries. The focus of this book will be to review how to prevent and treat running injuries and how to rehabilitate the injured runner. The statistics on running injuries are alarming. Studies show that there are four injuries per 1000 hours of running. If a runner spends 5 to 10 hours a week at the sport, he or she runs for up to 500 hours a year. At this rate, the runner may have one or two injuries a year.[2]

Here is a list of general areas of change that I have seen in the last 25 years:

- Risks and rewards
- Training
- Biomechanics
- Alternative activities
- Shoes and orthotics
- Nutrition
- Surgery
- Rehabilitation
- New medical syndromes
- Bone and joint treatment

The focus and review of specific chapters are as follows:

CHAPTER 1: WHY RUN?

Ron Lawrence, MD, President and Founder of the American Medical Jogging Association, reviews the benefits of and reasons for running. He balances the 18 chapters on the injuries and risks of running with one chapter on the marvelous health benefits of aerobic exercise, jogging, and running.

CHAPTER 2: THE BIOMECHANICS OF RUNNING AND SPRINTING

Tom Novacheck, MD, Orthopedic Surgeon, reviews the past and latest techniques in kinematics and kinetics with three-dimensional studies of muscle and joint motion and function. This helps us understand normal running, mechanisms of injuries, and injury prevention.

CHAPTER 3: THE FOOT/SHOE INTERFACE

Marilyn Pink, PT, and Frank Jobe, MD, from the Biomechanics Laboratory, Centinela Hospital, show how the foot and shoe adapt to the forces that develop as the foot hits the ground. The research accomplished in the last

25 years is reviewed. We learn what happens to the body at foot impact and how shoes play a role in the prevention of injuries.

CHAPTER 4: STRESS FRACTURES

Robert Leach, MD, Orthopedic Surgeon, and Susan B. Zecher, MD, review the past and present ideas about the causes and treatment of stress fractures. Long-term results are reviewed for difficult stress fracture patterns. They address the question, "When and how can runners return to activity with a stress fracture?"

CHAPTER 5: THE ADOLESCENT RUNNER

Brian Black, MD, Children's Orthopedic Surgeon, answers the question, "Is it okay for children to run?" Our changing understanding over the past 25 years is reviewed. Growth plate injuries are reviewed with long-term case follow-up.

CHAPTER 6: BACK PAIN IN RUNNING

Charles Gatt, MD, Orthopedic Surgeon, presents the mechanics of spine and disc syndromes caused by running. Past and current treatment, rehabilitation concepts, and the question, "Can the runner with back surgery return to running?" are reviewed along with case presentations.

CHAPTER 7: OVERVIEW OF LEG INJURIES

Gary Guten, MD, Orthopedic Surgeon, reviews the office evaluation of the runner. Information is presented to the health care provider on how to recognize the specific syndromes and how to examine and treat the injured runner.

CHAPTER 8: ARTHROSCOPY OF THE KNEE IN RUNNERS

Gregg Foos, MD, and James Fox, MD, Orthopedic Surgeons, review the dramatic

changes that have occurred since 1972 in knee surgery with the introduction of the arthroscope in the late 1970s. The results of arthroscopy are reviewed with the results of meniscectomy, patella surgery, chondral debridement, and plica resection. "Can the runner return to running after arthroscopy?" This question is answered.

CHAPTER 9: RECONSTRUCTIVE SURGERY OF THE HIP AND KNEE IN RUNNERS

Brian Lee, MD, Adult Reconstruction Special Fellow in Orthopedics; Frank Sim, MD, Consultant, Department of Orthopedics; and Michael Stuart, MD, Consultant, Department of Orthopedics, review the changing concepts of the past 25 years in major knee and hip reconstruction. Results of long-term case follow-up are presented. The question, "Can the runner perform after major surgery?" is answered.

CHAPTER 10: SHIN PAIN AND COMPARTMENT SYNDROMES IN RUNNING

Harvey Kohn, MD, Orthopedic Surgeon, reviews the pain syndromes between the ankle and the knee—shin splints, stress syndromes, and compartment syndromes. Our changing concepts over the past 25 years are reviewed with case reports. The latest techniques for evaluation of compartment pressure are presented.

CHAPTER 11: ANKLE PAIN IN RUNNERS

Judy Baumhauer, MD, Michael Shereff, MD, and J. Gould, MD, Orthopedic Surgeons, present the syndromes of ankle pain, current and past. They review treatment and rehabilitation of specific cases with some long-term follow-up. The biomechanics of the ankle play an important role in our understanding of leg pain.

CHAPTER 12: FOOT PAIN IN RUNNERS

Tom Pietrocarlo, DPM, Podiatrist, reviews our past and current understanding of foot

syndromes. Office management with foot orthotics is presented. Conservative and surgical
long-term results are reviewed.

CHAPTER 13: OVERTRAINING SYNDROME

Carl Foster, PhD, Exercise Physiologist, and
Manfred Lehman, MD, review the new concepts in overtraining. They also discuss how
to recognize the syndrome and offer sugges-
tions for training and treatment.

CHAPTER 14: ARTHRITIS AND RUNNING

John Paty, Jr., MD, FACP, Rheumatologist,
reviews the question, "Does running cause
arthritis?" Long-term studies on the positive
and negative effects on joint function are discussed. Treatment plans for joint inflammation are reviewed.

CHAPTER 15: NUTRITION AND RUNNING

Ellen Coleman, RD, shows the evolution of
our concepts of nutrition and fluid replacement in the past 25 years. The current best
programs in nutrition, vitamins, supplements,
and fluid replacement are highlighted. "What
is the optimal nutrition program for a long
distance run?" This question is addressed.

CHAPTER 16: RUNNING AND MOOD DISORDERS

Paul Kiell, MD, Psychiatrist, reviews what
attracts certain mood disorder patients to running and how certain mood disorders develop
during the stresses of running injuries. What
brain chemicals are liberated by running and
how they affect the mood and motivation of
the athlete are discussed.

CHAPTER 17: THE FEMALE ATHLETE TRIAD IN RUNNERS

Annette Zaharoff, MD, presents our evolving concepts since 1972 of how we view and
treat the female athlete. New concepts regarding amenorrhea, osteoporosis, and stress
fractures are highlighted as they relate to running.

CHAPTER 18: STRENGTHENING AND FLEXIBILITY CONCEPTS FOR RUNNERS

Guy Simoneau, PhD, PT, Kevin Wilk, PT,
and William Clancy, MD, review the changes
in our understanding of exercise and rehabilitation of the injured runner. The current exercise programs of testing, strengthening, and
stretching are presented.

CHAPTER 19: MEDICAL SYNDROMES IN RUNNERS

Marvin Adner, MD, Hematologist, and Arthur Siegel, MD, Internist, review their experience in planning medical care during the
Boston Marathon. The 100th running of the
Boston Marathon occurred in April, 1996.
Changing medical syndromes and treatment
concepts are reviewed.

CHAPTER 20: CARDIOPULMONARY EFFECTS AND CONSEQUENCES OF RUNNING IN CHILDREN—GOOD OR BAD?

Stuart Berger, MD, reviews the cardiopulmonary information to date to make some
reasonable recommendations for training the
preadolescent and adolescent age group.

REFERENCES

1. Blair S: Changes in physical fitness and all-cause mortality. JAMA, 273(14), 1995.
2. Mechelen W: Prevention of running injuries by warm-
up, cool-down, and stretching exercises. Am J Sports
Med, 21(5), 1993.

ACKNOWLEDGMENTS

Running is both an individual sport and a team sport. The following is a list of those individuals who made this team effort possible:

Richard Lampert, Senior Medical Editor at the W.B. Saunders Company, for his insight and prompt communication with the production team.

Our contributors, whose expertise and thoroughness are on the leading edge of the running medical community.

The Audiovisual Department of the St. Francis Hospital, coordinated by Paul Ramsey, Photographer, and Carol Witkowski, Librarian, who helped develop the excellent photographic and scientific information.

The medical transcriptionists from our office, Marty Tans, Clare Bowe, Jane Frey, and Barbara Heffron, for their time, commitment, sense of humor, and patience for all of the "rewrites."

Our book coordinator, Judy Wichtoski, Medical Assistant, for her indispensable commitment to thoroughness, communication, running, and attention to fine detail.

CONTENTS

RONALD M. LAWRENCE

CHAPTER ONE

Why Run?

In 1971, I ran the Boston Marathon for the first time accompanied by about 25 other physicians who were part of the newly formed American Medical Joggers Association (established in 1969). The choice of running shoes was extremely limited. In fact, some of the doctors ran in their tennis shoes or sneakers. These sneakers were made of rubber and usually had a canvas top. Most of us used Japanese running shoes called Tigers, which consisted of a flat piece of rubber sole and a leather upper. No support was provided in the shoe base, and even the arch was unsupported. All of us, whatever our shoe choice, developed blisters over the plantar surfaces or the sides of our feet. Most of us lost our toenails because of subungual hematomas, and I actually lost all of my toenails. Each marathon run resulted in blisters and toenail injuries owing to the inadequate footwear. Distance runners expected those injuries and in fact considered them as "part of the game." Many running clubs had a Golden Toenail Award for the individual who lost the most toenails during the year.

All of this changed markedly with the development of the ethylene vinyl acetate (EVA) running footwear, which was developed during the mid and late 1970s by such pioneers as Bill Bowerman and Phil Knight.

The evolution of running shoes has probably been the most remarkable change we've seen during the past quarter century. In the 1980s, even more technologic advances by myriad manufacturers reduced foot and ankle injuries as well as knee, hip, and back problems. I have completed 200 marathons since 1970, and certainly the last 150 of them have been in comfortable shoes.

The other phenomenon that presents a glaring contrast between the 1960s and today is the larger number of people who are running not only the marathon but also the shorter events such as the 5- and 10-kilometer events. The actual number of those who complete a marathon has increased, but the number of major marathons has decreased. This is because of the high costs of marathon management due to requirements of insurance coverage (liability insurance mainly), police protection, and material cost increases. It is also true that the number of individuals who run the shorter races (i.e., 10-k) has increased much more than the number of those who run longer distances. The number of 5- and 10-k events has grown exponentially. All of this has resulted in an increased number of injuries. In fact, the field of sports medicine partially has evolved to its current level by virtue of the increasing number of injured runners who have sought care from health professionals since the 1970s.

The need to understand the basic physiology and science of running has markedly increased research in sports medicine. It is true that in recent years, cross-training (i.e., bicycling, swimming, and so forth), as required in the triathlon and biathlon competition, has somewhat reduced the potential for running injuries. Still, the greatest number of those starting leisure sports activities begin by running, and the number of injuries is always greatest in novices or beginners.

During the early years of the running movement, we physicians knew that running consistently enhanced our sense of well-being and our physical endurance and seemed to improve our health status. During the past 25 years, scientists have measured these effects carefully and have indeed shown that running enhances our cardiovascular and respiratory status as well as our psychologic profile. Indeed, the relevant books and articles number in the hundreds of thousands, and for the most part they extol the virtues to be gained from a long-term exercise program, particularly running.

As I have watched the more than 25,000 doctors who have been members of the American Medical Joggers Association (now the American Medical Athletic Association) during these past 25 years, I have an inherent sense that as a group they are healthier and more fit than a comparable group of their nonexercising peers. They seem to have fewer cardiac and respiratory diseases, and their active lifestyle has produced a more vigorous and engaging type of individual.

We now know that exercise, particularly running, not only improves the quality of our lives but actually increases the length of our lives, as shown in the classic studies by Paffenbarger and others. Steve Blair of the Cooper Institute has written about the reduction in cardiac disorders associated with moderate to high levels of fitness.[1] Cardiovascular disease is definitely retarded in runners and in many instances is prevented.

Jim Fixx's seminal work *The Complete Book of Running* was one of the first books for general readers to outline the widespread beneficial effects of running. Fixx's early demise due to a heart attack while running was used by the antiexercise establishment to attempt to discredit running for health. However, they failed to note that Jim survived longer than any male member of his family had in the past. Also, he came to running late in life, after most of his coronary vessel changes probably had developed. Running gave him many extra, quality-laden years of life.

The positive effects of running are numerous. They range from improved cardiovascular-respiratory status to enhanced mental health, evidenced by less depression, less anxiety, and a greater sense of tranquility. Years ago I was quoted in *Time* magazine as stating that "depression in the United States is more common than the common cold," and indeed a program of running is a simple, safe method of reducing mild to moderate depression. Regular running results in better sleep patterns, a better sex life, enhanced appetite, healthier weight, and a more stable (stronger) musculoskeletal structure.

Despite the fact that running injuries do affect large numbers of people, they are for the most part minor injuries. The cost-benefit ratio certainly encourages us to say to our patients, "Yes, get into a running program; the benefits far outweigh any risks involved." We should also, however, encourage them to obtain a careful, comprehensive prerunning physical examination, including a cardiovas-cular evaluation, especially for patients older than 40 years. They should start slowly and seek the advice of a coach, physician, or athletic trainer. This approach markedly reduces the number of running injuries.

Another opportunity that I have had is to observe a small group of children (ranging in age from 7 to 15 years) who began to run the marathon distance in the 1970s. At that time, the effect of long-distance running on juveniles was unknown. I am happy to say that 25 years or more after these youngsters started to run marathons, they are physically and psychologically in good shape. Our fears about the potential for problems developing, based only on this small group of 20 or so children, seems to be ill founded.

Dr. Terence Kavanagh brought a group of six runners, all of whom suffered from one or more prior heart attacks, to Boston in 1973. This was the first time that postcoronary runners participated in a major marathon. All of the original group of six finished the marathon, without a single problem. Since then, Kavanagh has brought other cardiac patients to run Boston and other marathons, and not a single fatality has occurred in the group. In fact, Kavanagh has for several years been working with a group of cardiac transplant recipients from England, and these people have finished not only a single marathon but multiple marathons without a mishap. This fact generally proves the reasonable safety of distance running.

It is hoped that during the next 25 years, research shall continue on the vital relationship between running and nutrition. We all now know that despite a good exercise or running program, one can develop cardiovascular disease, albeit at a slower rate. Jim Fixx's statement[2] that "the nutritional secret that lets runners eat foods absolutely forbidden to most dieters and lets them lose weight while doing it" no longer applies. Runners must obey the basic dietary rules, because running per se does not eradicate the need for a proper diet. Diet management not only helps runners prevent some injuries but also helps enhance performance as well. However, no amount of proper dieting produces a fit individual unless he or she exercises.

Except for walking, running is the easiest and least expensive means of enhancing exercise. Running, however, offers a more satisfactory physiologic approach to fitness as judged by today's standards, which require some exercise stress to produce more satisfactory cardiovascular conditioning. The triad of exercise (running), diet, and decreased mental stress (enhanced mental tranquility) all are necessary to produce a healthier individual. If one aspect is absent, the end result cannot be overcome by increasing the emphasis on the other two factors. During the next century, valid scientific inquiry will show the importance to health of the enrichment of the soul and spirit. I personally believe that the number of runners will not decrease and that by virtue of an expanding world population, the number of new runners will increase.

Increasing knowledge of the physiology of running as well as improvements in dietary control and biomechanics will result in not only fewer running injuries but also in slow, inexorable improvements in world record running times.

The future of running as it relates to health is a bright one. Certainly, orthopedists and sports medicine physicians shall continue to see numerous patients with injuries—that's a given! However, in my capacity as an adviser and officer of the American Running and Fitness Association, I believe that the general public is much more aware of injury prevention regimens. Therefore, the average runner is suffering less from the minor injuries that we sustained in the earlier days. The responsibility of the physician is to advise running patients about injury prevention. A book such as this one can offer health practitioners valuable information not only about treating injuries but also about preventing them.

REFERENCES

1. Blair SN, Kohl HW III, Barlow CE, et al: Changes in physical fitness and all-cause mortality. JAMA 273(14):1093, 1995.
2. Fixx J: The Complete Book of Running. New York, Random House, 1977, p xvi.

TOM F. NOVACHECK

CHAPTER TWO

The Biomechanics of Running and Sprinting

Walking, running, and sprinting all are forms of human bipedal locomotion. They range in speed from extremely slow walking at a steady velocity to sprinting at top speed with great acceleration. Discrete characteristics distinguish these three types of locomotion. This chapter describes the biomechanics of running and sprinting compared with normal walking. An explanation of the kinematics, kinetics, and muscle activity is included. Mechanisms for energy conservation and transfer within the body are also discussed. Understanding these concepts provides insight into injury mechanisms and training strategies. These concepts can be applied in an effort to avoid injury and enhance performance. The data presented in this chapter were gathered in the Motion Analysis Laboratory at Gillette Children's Specialty Healthcare (St. Paul, MN) and represent average information from 25 neurologically normal children.[8, 9] Because they were not highly trained athletes, their performance speeds are not world class. The movement patterns, however, are similar to those of higher levels of athleticism.

GAIT CYCLES

Normal human locomotion is a repetitive sequence of limb movements used to advance the body safely from place to place, at the desired speed, with a minimal expenditure of energy. The basic unit of locomotion is the gait cycle, or stride, which begins when one foot strikes the ground and ends when the same foot strikes the ground again. Just as you could not begin to understand what it means to run 100 miles if you had no concept of what a mile is, so it is with gait. The gait cycle is the basic unit of measurement of gait; understanding it is crucial. The gait cycle is commonly divided into two phases. Swing phase occurs when the foot is moving through space and is not contacting the ground. Stance phase, in contrast, occurs when the foot is in contact with the ground. The walking gait cycle comprises two periods of double support during which both feet are in stance phase and coincide with the subphases, loading response and preswing. It is during these periods that the two limbs are alternately loaded and unloaded as body weight is transferred from one leg to the other.

Running and sprinting, on the other hand, have no periods of double support. Instead, two periods of double float occur—one at the beginning and one at the end of swing phase. As a walker's speed increases, the movement strategy changes to a run abruptly in a single stride. The critical velocity at which walking changes to running for normal adults is approximately 5.6 miles per hour or 2.5 m/sec. It occurs at a slower velocity for children because of their shorter leg length. Walking and running generally differ in the time spent in swing and stance phase. Stance phase decreases from an average of 62% in normal walking to 22% for world-class sprinting. The transition from walking to running is made when less than 50% of the gait cycle is spent in stance and conversely more than 50% is spent in swing. As an athlete increases speed, the portion of the gait cycle spent in double float increases.

The differentiation between running and sprinting is based on which part of the foot initially contacts the ground. In running, initial contact is with the heel. The forefoot subsequently lowers to the ground. In sprinting, initial contact is with the forefoot. The heel then lowers to the ground (Fig. 2–1). However, elite sprinters may remain on their forefoot throughout stance phase. Other differences are also noted. Sprinting is typically a period of fast acceleration. An athlete's trunk is in a more forward, flexed position than in running. Runners accelerate more slowly and perform at slower speeds over longer distances. Examples include jogging, distance track events, and cross-country running.

Dividing the gait cycle into subphases makes it easier to understand. In walking, stance phase is divided into initial contact, loading response, midstance, terminal stance, and preswing (Fig. 2–2A). Swing phase is simply divided into initial, mid, and terminal swing. Unique events occur during each of these subdivisions. These events are quite different, however, in running and sprinting (Fig. 2–2B). Therefore, the divisions within both the stance and swing phases are different. Stance and swing phase are subdivided into two periods, absorption and generation. In stance, both the shock of contact with the ground and the energy of the moving body segments are initially absorbed by the stance phase limb while body weight is accepted. During this absorption period, the joints are flexing. Stance phase reversal marks the end of the absorption phase and coincides with the time when the center of gravity reaches its lowest point. Both kinetic and potential energy are at their lowest levels.

The muscles then begin to generate power, and the joints extend. The runner's body is propelled up and forward. This period is the

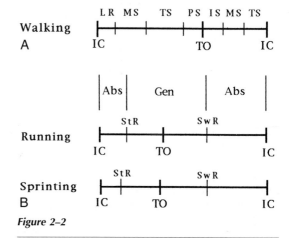

Figure 2–2

A: Walking gait cycle. (IC = Initial contact; TO = toe-off; LR = loading response; MS = midstance; TS = terminal stance; PS = preswing; IS = initial swing; MS = midswing; TS = terminal swing.) **B:** The running and sprinting gait cycles. (Abs = Absorption; Gen = generation; StR = stance phase reversal; SwR = swing phase reversal.)

generation phase. The muscles continue to generate power in swing phase as the leg is propelled forward. As in stance, there is a reversal point—swing phase reversal. Before swing phase reversal, energy is generated and the joints are generally flexing. At swing phase reversal, both kinetic and potential energy levels peak. After the swing phase reversal point, energy is generally being absorbed as the joints extend. The swinging leg decelerates in preparation for contact with the ground.

One can see why running and sprinting have been likened to a pogo stick with the musculotendinous units acting as the springs[7] and the center of mass rising to a peak and then falling to a low point. As just demonstrated, the running and sprinting gait cycles can be separated by four instantaneous events—initial contact, stance phase reversal, toe-off, and swing phase reversal. Abrupt changes in joint motion and the movements of the center of mass from high to low occur during these four phases.

KINEMATICS

Kinematics are a description of movement and do not consider the forces that cause that movement. Joint angles, displacements, velocities, and accelerations all are kinematic variables. We can graph kinematic variables as a function of the percentage of the total

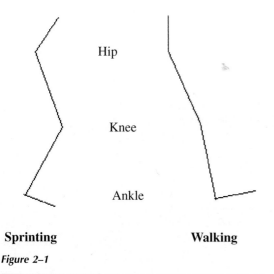

Sprinting   **Walking**

Figure 2–1

Diagrammatic stick figures walking versus sprinting.

gait cycle. For example, consider the plot of ankle plantar/dorsiflexion during walking, running, and sprinting (Fig. 2–3). The graph shows the changing position of the ankle for one complete gait cycle. The graph begins and ends at initial contact and therefore represents one gait cycle along the x-axis. The vertical lines represent toe-off for each situation. The portion of the graph to the left of the toe-off line depicts ankle motion during stance phase, and swing phase ankle motion is depicted to the right. The position of the ankle in degrees is represented along the y-axis. At initial contact during walking, the position of the ankle ranges from neutral to 5 degrees of plantar flexion. As the ankle moves through loading response, plantar flexion increases. During midstance and terminal stance, the ankle dorsiflexes, reaching on average a maximum of 10 degrees. In preswing, the foot begins to plantar flex in preparation for toe-off. Starting at initial swing, the ankle dorsiflexes. In terminal swing, the ankle begins to plantar flex slightly. Throughout this chapter, walking is represented by a lightly dashed line, running is a solid line, and sprinting is heavy-dashed. The corresponding toe-off line is plotted using the same line style. For all of the kinematic graphic data presented in the next section, the patterns of movement are important (e.g., At what point in the gait cycle is the joint in question flexing/extending?). The peak values in degrees of movement are not important because they depend on an athlete's level of training and speed. This is true in the subsequent kinetics section as well.

Motion in all three planes is considered. We must remember that the sagittal plane is a side view of the subject. In the transverse plane, the subject is viewed from above. The coronal plane is a frontal view of the subject.

SAGITTAL PLANE KINEMATICS

When observing sagittal plane motion, you can see the shift into flexion and the lowering of the center of mass as the motion changes from walking to running to sprinting. The pattern of movement in the tilt of the pelvis is similar at all speeds (Fig. 2–4). You might expect a greater amount of pelvic motion with faster velocities, but in fact motion increases very little. Pelvic motion is minimized to conserve energy and maintain efficiency in running and sprinting. As speed increases, however, the pelvis and trunk tilt farther forward. The center of mass is lowered, and the horizontal force produced in the propulsion phase is maximized.

The foot and ground exert an equal and opposite force on each other. This is called the *ground reaction force* (Fig. 2–5).[3] The position and acceleration of the runner's center of mass determine the direction and magnitude of the ground reaction force. Consider for example a sprinter accelerating from a standstill. During the initial phase of acceleration, the body is tilted forward and the center

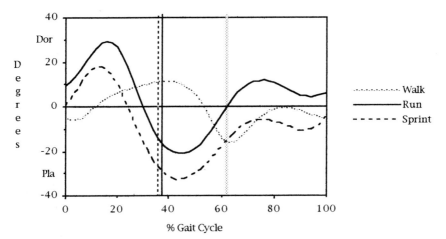

Figure 2–3

Sagittal plane ankle motion (kinematics).

PELVIC TILT

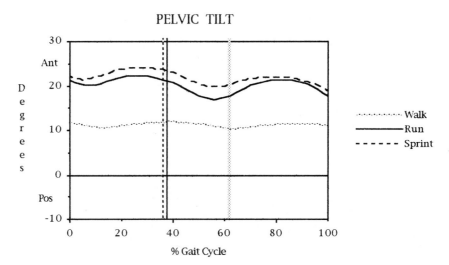

Figure 2–4

Pelvic tilt.

of gravity falls far ahead of the contact point. After several gait cycles, sprinters reach maximum velocity and their center of mass then moves backward. Athletes who tried to accelerate with their body upright would fall over backward because of the direction of the

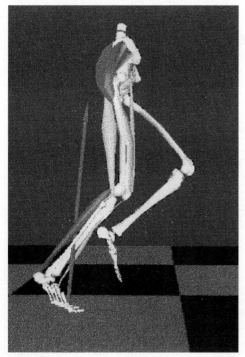

Figure 2–5

Ground reaction force.

ground reaction force. The forward trunk lean and pelvic tilt keep the ground reaction force in a position to allow forward acceleration.

Sagittal plane motion at the hip follows a sinusoidal pattern in walking (Fig. 2–6). Maximum hip extension occurs just before toe-off, and maximum flexion occurs in mid to terminal swing. In running and sprinting, maximum hip extension is similar to walking but occurs slightly later at the time of toe-off. As velocity increases, so does maximum hip flexion, leading to a longer step length.

Although the pattern of knee motion in walking, running, and sprinting is very similar, the extremes of motion are very different (Fig. 2–7). In running, during the absorption period of stance phase, the knee flexes to approximately 45 degrees. This is followed by knee extension to an average 25 degrees during the propulsion phase. In sprinting, the absorption period is shorter and the knee flexes less. Greater knee extension occurs during the propulsion period, peaking at 20 degrees. Swing phase also exhibits differences between walking, running, and sprinting. Maximum knee flexion during swing is about 60 degrees in normal walking. This is much less than the average of 90 degrees in running or the 105 degrees in sprinting. A highly trained athlete in a full sprint may exhibit up to 140 degrees of maximum knee flexion.

Initial contact during walking and running occurs with the heel. For walking, this occurs despite ankle plantar flexion because of the position of the tibia (see Fig. 2–3). In running,

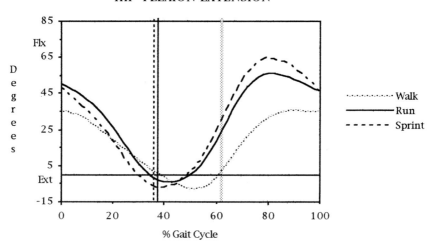

Figure 2–6

Hip kinematic (sagittal plane).

greater ankle dorsiflexion is required to achieve initial heel contact. In sprinting, initial contact occurs on the forefoot. Tibial position allows the ankle to be in a more neutral or slightly dorsiflexed position. In walking, the ankle initially plantarflexes as the forefoot is lowered to the ground. In contrast, during the absorption phase of running and sprinting, the ankle dorsiflexes as body weight is transferred to the stance leg. Maximum dorsiflexion during stance phase in sprinting is less than in running because of the relatively plantarflexed position at initial contact and the shorter duration of the absorption period.

During the generation phase of stance, maximum ankle plantarflexion is greater in sprinting than in running. Ankle dorsiflexion is less in sprinting than in both walking and running during swing phase. Dorsiflexion to a neutral position is not necessary for toe clearance during sprinting, given the increased amount of hip and knee flexion.

CORONAL PLANE KINEMATICS

Overall, coronal plane motion is more subtle than sagittal plane motion. It is, however,

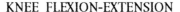

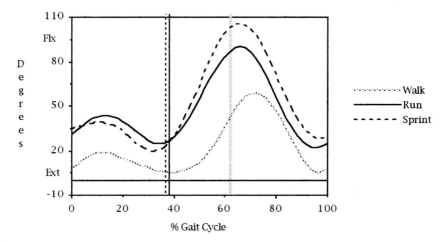

Figure 2–7

Knee kinematic (sagittal plane).

important in minimizing upper body movement. In this plane, motion of the knee and ankle is restricted by the collateral ligaments. In contrast, significant motion occurs at the hip. As the limb is loaded, the pelvis remains relatively stationary (Fig. 2–8A). The hip adducts relative to the pelvis (Fig. 2–8B). This is a shock-absorbing mechanism similar to that seen in the sagittal plane at the knee in running and the ankle in sprinting (as will be discussed later in the kinetics section). Throughout the rest of stance phase, the pelvis drops until the start of double float, where it is the most oblique. As the limb begins swing phase, this motion reverses. The pelvis now elevates to obtain foot clearance. Generally, in walking, running, and sprinting, the hip is adducted in stance phase and abducted during swing. Hip motion in this plane mirrors the movement of the pelvis. This nearly reciprocal motion combined with slight lumbopelvic motion minimizes shoulder and head movement. This is one of the most important mechanisms for decoupling the intense lower extremity motion from the trunk and head. The result is relatively minimal head and trunk motion, allowing balance and equilibrium to be maintained.

TRANSVERSE PLANE KINEMATICS

Motion in the transverse plane, as in the coronal plane, is small in magnitude com-

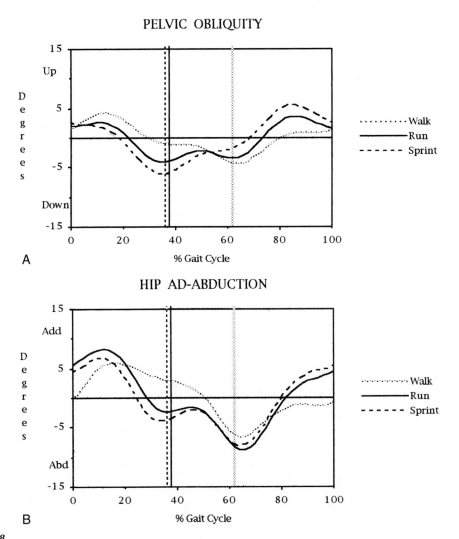

Figure 2–8

A: *Pelvic kinematic (coronal plane).* **B:** *Hip kinematic (coronal plane).*

pared with the sagittal plane. Joint rotations in this plane may be the most difficult to comprehend because they are difficult to see. The movement patterns in the transverse plane are important for energy efficiency, as discussed in greater detail later. The function and motion of the pelvis in the transverse plane while walking are very different from those in running and sprinting. In walking, pelvic rotation is an important method of lengthening the stride. The pelvis is maximally rotated forward at initial contact to achieve a longer step length (Fig. 2–9). The result is decreased horizontal velocity. During running and sprinting, maximum internal pelvic rotation occurs in midswing to lengthen the stride, but by the time of initial contact, the pelvis has rotated posteriorly. This maximizes horizontal propulsion force and avoids the potential loss of speed.

The pelvis in running and sprinting also functions as a pivot between the counter-rotating shoulders and legs. For example, when the right leg is maximally forward in midswing, the left shoulder is rotated forward and the pelvis is neutral.

Another important motion, pronation/supination, occurs in an oblique plane in the foot. Pronation occurs during the absorption phase while the limb is loaded. The foot then supinates during the generation phase, providing a stable lever for push-off. In addition to the bony and ligamentous structures of the foot, the posterior tibialis helps to control this motion. This complex motion is difficult to

quantify biomechanically because the motions are small in magnitude, and the body segments about which they occur are small and defy accurate localization.

KINETICS

Unlike kinematics, kinetics involves the study of forces responsible for joint movements. This type of analysis includes ground reaction forces, musculotendinous and ligament forces, joint moments, and joint powers. The study of kinetics begins to answer the how and why of the movement we observe. Force plates embedded in the floor can measure the ground reaction force. By combining kinematics with the measured ground reaction force, joint moments and powers can be calculated. The mathematic method used for this calculation is inverse dynamics.

To understand these concepts better, several terms require definition. The moment due to a force acting at some distance from the axis of rotation can cause a body to rotate. The moment of force (M) is the product of the force (F) times the distance (d) and can be expressed in Newton-meters.

$$M = F \times d$$

The distance (d) is called the lever arm. Unbalanced moments result in movement. For example, consider two children on a teeter-totter (Fig. 2–10).[4] The weight of each child

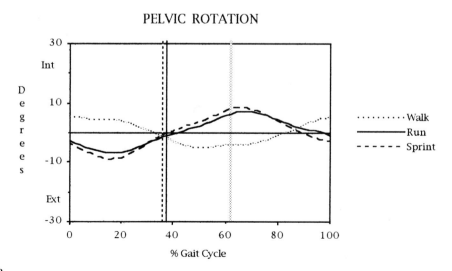

PELVIC ROTATION

Figure 2–9

Pelvic kinematic (transverse plane).

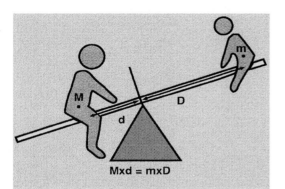

$$Mxd = mxD$$

Figure 2–10

Moment of force.

creates a moment around the axle to which the teeter-totter is attached. If one child is lighter and both sit an equal distance from the axle, the lighter child rises. The rotation of the teeter-totter about its axis is caused by the difference in the magnitude of the moments created about the axle by each child. The lighter child can balance the heavier child if the lighter child sits farther from the axis, thereby lengthening the lever arm and increasing the moment created about the axle. Both internal and external forces affect how our bodies move. For a person to remain upright without falling, the external forces must be balanced by the internal forces. External forces include ground reaction forces and inertial forces caused by moving body segments. Internal forces are created by muscle, tendon, ligament, or joint capsules. These forces act on the bones that provide the lever arms. The axis of rotation passes through the joint centers.

Movement requires power. Muscles and other soft tissues both generate and absorb power. The net power contributed by all of the structures crossing a particular joint is calculated by multiplying the net internal joint moment (F × d) by the joint angular velocity (ω). This is expressed in watts per kilogram of body weight and represented mathematically as

$$P = F \times d \times \omega$$

When the joint moment and the joint angular velocity are in the same direction, an increase in either indicates increased power generation by the muscles crossing the joint and represents a concentric contraction. In contrast, when the moment and velocity are in opposite directions, an increase in the joint moment, or the joint angular velocity, indicates increased power absorption (an eccentric contraction). The calculated net joint moments and powers can be graphed for the gait cycle. As with the kinematic graphs, the x-axis depicts the percentage of the gait cycle. On the moment graph, the y-axis represents the net joint moment, which is standardized for body weight and is named for the dominant muscle group (Fig. 2–11A). The power graph is similar to the moment graph. Power output is displayed on the y-axis and is also standardized for body weight (Fig. 2–11B). Power absorption (eccentric muscle contraction) is below the zero line, and power generation (concentric contraction) is above. Remember that understanding the patterns and timing of the moments and powers is important. The absolute values of the peaks and valleys on the y-axis are not important because they depend heavily on the speed of movement and level of training.

SAGITTAL PLANE

The most interesting kinetics occur in the sagittal plane. During running, the ankle moment pattern is similar to that in walking (see Fig. 2–11A). Initial contact is with the heel. The forefoot is lowered to the ground under the control of eccentric contraction of the anterior tibial muscles. The onset of the ankle plantar flexion moment occurs at 5% to 10% of the running gait cycle. In contrast, during sprinting there is no initial dorsiflexor moment because initial contact is on the forefoot, followed by immediate dorsiflexion. The total energy absorbed at the ankle is greater in sprinting than in running (see Fig. 2–11B). In walking, running, and sprinting, the period of absorption is followed by a period of power generation. The power generated provides energy for forward propulsion. The magnitude of the ankle power generation is directly related to the athlete's speed.

The knee moment pattern is very similar in sprinting and running (Fig. 2–12A). To prepare for initial contact, the hamstrings become dominant, producing a knee flexor moment. This moment controls rapid knee extension in the second half of swing phase. Shortly after initial contact, the quadriceps become dominant, producing a knee extensor moment. The magnitude of the peak knee extensor moment tends to be greater in run-

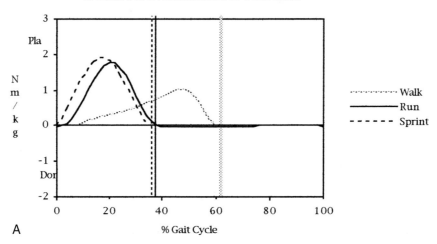

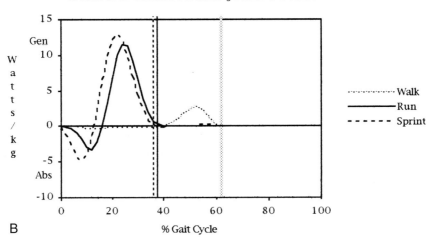

Figure 2–11

A: *Ankle moment (sagittal plane).* **B:** *Ankle power (sagittal plane).*

KNEE FLEX-EXT MOMENT

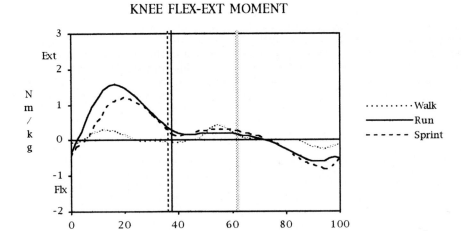

A

SAGITTAL PLANE KNEE JOINT POWER

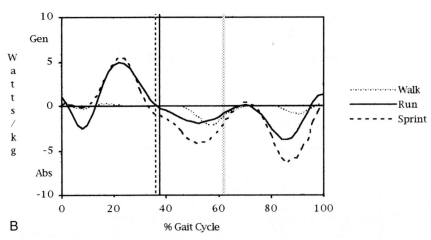

B

Figure 2–12

A: *Knee moment (sagittal plane).* **B:** *Knee power (sagittal plane).*

ning than in sprinting. This is related to the runner's greater degree of knee flexion as the limb is loaded. In running, as the knee flexes after initial contact, the quadriceps contract eccentrically. This is seen as power absorption and reflects their essential role as shock absorbers (Fig. 2–12B). In sprinting, however, the ankle absorbs much of the shock of contact with the ground (see Fig. 2–11B). Therefore, little power is absorbed at the knee. In both running and sprinting, the knee extends in the second half of stance phase. The quadriceps contract concentrically, and power is generated. In swing phase, very little power is generated by the muscles crossing the knee. Instead, the muscles absorb power to control the movement of the swinging leg. The rectus

femoris contracts eccentrically in early swing to prevent excessive knee flexion. During late swing phase, the hamstrings contract eccentrically to control the momentum of the tibia and prevent knee hyperextension as the knee is rapidly extending.

The hip moment pattern is similar in all conditions of forward locomotion (Fig. 2–13A). Just before and just after initial contact, the hip extensors are dominant. In contrast, the hip flexors are dominant in the second half of stance through the first half of swing. Both the hip flexors and extensors are responsible for increased power generation in running and sprinting (Fig. 2–13B). Peak hip flexion occurs in the second half of swing in both running and sprinting. After peak flexion,

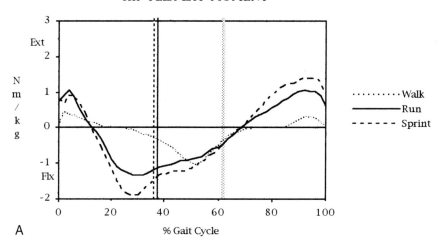

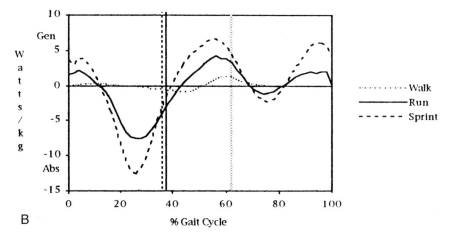

Figure 2–13

A: Hip moment (sagittal plane). *B:* Hip power (sagittal plane).

the hip extensors contract concentrically to extend the hip in preparation for initial contact. The power graph depicts power generation for running and sprinting before initial contact. The hip extensors continue to generate power through the first half of stance phase. The hip continues to extend rapidly. After this, the hip flexors become dominant and decelerate the hip in preparation for swing. During this time, the psoas tendon is stretched. The energy absorbed in stretching the tendon is returned at toe-off.

CORONAL PLANE

Although the magnitudes of coronal plane moments are substantial, the muscles and lig-aments that create them function primarily as stabilizers. Motion is minimal; therefore, power generated and absorbed is much less than in the sagittal plane. During stance phase, a continuous hip abductor moment is produced primarily by the gluteus medius (Fig. 2–14A). The hip adducts in the absorption phase because the ground reaction force falls medial to the hip. The gluteus medius contracts eccentrically to control this motion (Fig. 2–14B). During the propulsion phase, the gluteus medius contracts concentrically, abducting the hip. At the knee and ankle, moments are generated but little motion occurs. Therefore, ligaments, bone-on-bone contact forces, and tendons neither generate nor absorb significant power.

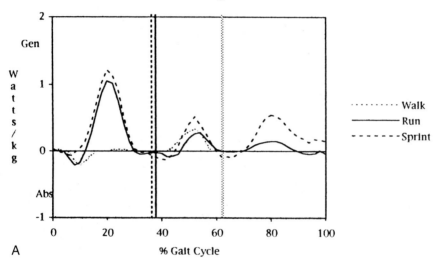

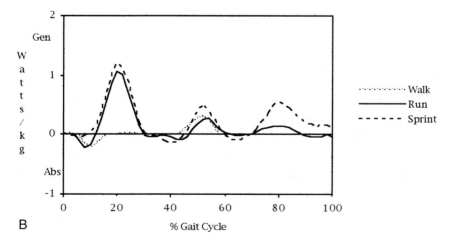

Figure 2–14

A: Hip moment (coronal plane). *B:* Hip power (coronal plane).

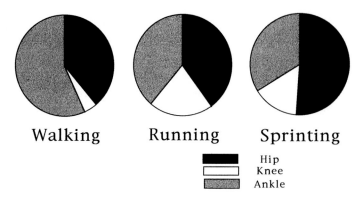

Walking   Running   Sprinting

■ Hip
□ Knee
▨ Ankle

Figure 2–15

Sources of energy.

KINETICS OVERVIEW

The movement strategy changes as one increases speed. This is apparent by considering the sources of power generation for forward propulsion. By examining the power curves (Figs. 2–11B, 2–12B, 2–13B, and 2–14B), one can see that the main sources of power generation are from the hip extensors during the first half of stance, the hip flexors at the time of toe-off, the knee extensors during the second half of stance, the ankle plantar flexors just before toe-off, and the hip abductors. Some researchers also believe that the arms generate some of the power for lift.[5]

Essentially, the hamstrings and gluteus maximus pull us forward by actively extending the hip after initial contact when our foot is ahead of our body. Then during the second half of stance phase, the quadriceps and gastrocnemius-soleus contract to push us forward by extending the knee and plantar flexing the foot. Almost simultaneously, the hip abductors contract to provide lift. Finally, the psoas propels the limb into swing by flexing the hip. The total amount of power generated increases as speed increases, and the relative contribution from each of these muscle groups changes such that relatively more power is generated proximally as speed increases (Fig. 2–15). The muscle mass of a horse (an animal that is able to run much faster than a human) is concentrated proximally, reflecting this change in movement strategy. Horses have long tendons connecting their muscles to distal structures. This anatomy concentrates weight proximally, thereby minimizing the inertia of the rapidly moving distal segments.

One should also note that each of these essential power generators stretches eccentrically just before generating its burst of power.

It has been shown that tendons stretch and then efficiently return most of that energy when they recoil (Fig. 2–16). The small amount of energy that is not returned is dissipated as heat. In addition, muscles that are pretensioned and then contract generate more power per unit of activation than those that are not.[2] In essence, the tendons can be thought of as springs and the muscles as the tensioners of the springs.

ENERGY CONSERVATION

Walking is generally an efficient way to move from one place to another. Each one of us naturally adjusts our step length and cadence to assume a walking speed with the lowest energy expenditure. Walking at a faster than normal pace decreases energy efficiency. Also as speed increases, a point is reached at which running is more efficient than walking.[2] We have explained that muscles absorb as well as generate mechanical energy. During walking, running, and sprinting, various mechanisms allow the energy supplied by the muscles to be used effectively. These mechanisms include

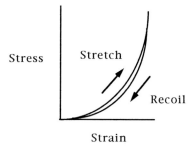

Figure 2–16

Tendon stretch/recoil.

1. Storage and later return of elastic potential energy by stretch of the ligaments, tendons, and other elastic structures
2. Transfer of energy from one body segment to another by two-joint muscles such as the rectus femoris and the hamstrings
3. Reduction of accelerations not contributing to forward progression
4. Effective interchange between kinetic energy and gravitational potential energy

The action of the Achilles tendon is an example of the first mechanism for improving energy efficiency—*storage and later return of elastic potential energy.* During running or sprinting, the Achilles tendon may stretch as much as 15 mm.[1] However, more than 90% of the energy required to stretch the tendon is returned at toe-off when the foot leaves the ground. The arch of the foot also stores elastic potential energy. As the foot is loaded, the arch flattens and the muscles, tendons, and ligaments are stretched. Approximately 80% of the energy absorbed to flatten the arch is returned when the foot is unloaded.[9]

The second mechanism, *transfer of energy between body segments by two-joint muscles,* also contributes to energy efficiency. For example, in the later part of swing phase, both the hip and knee extend while the hamstrings contract. An extensor moment is produced by the hamstrings at the hip when the hip is extending. At the same time in the cycle, the knee is also extending and the hamstrings generate a flexor moment. The moment produced at the knee is opposite the knee motion. In effect, the hamstrings absorb energy at the knee and generate energy at the hip. However, because the overall change in length of the hamstrings is minimal, the muscles as a whole neither absorb nor generate energy. In this instance, the hamstrings can be thought to function as an energy strap, transferring energy from the moving tibia to the pelvis to aid in hip extension. As the knee extends, energy from the tibia is supplied to the pelvis to augment hip extension.

The third mechanism, *reduction of accelerations not contributing to forward progression,* is best exemplified by pelvic motion in the transverse plane. The motion of the pelvis assists in both maximizing acceleration of the center of mass in the direction of progression and minimizing acceleration in all other directions. In walking, the pelvis is in a position of maximum forward rotation at initial contact. The ground reaction force is directed posteriorly. The posterior component of the ground reaction force creates a braking effect on horizontal motion (walking speed). Horizontal velocity decreases until the direction of the ground reaction force shifts forward during terminal stance, at which time the velocity of the center of mass again increases. In contrast, during running and sprinting, the athlete prepares for contact with the ground by rotating the pelvis posteriorly, or away from the direction of progression. At the same time, the hamstrings contract concentrically to extend the hip. This pulls the forward leg back just before initial contact, helps to decrease the posterior component of the ground reaction force, and thereby minimizes the horizontal braking force. In this way, efficiency improves.

The motion of the pelvis also helps to decrease acceleration in directions other than in the line of progression. The pelvis acts as a pivot. It balances rotational acceleration in the transverse plane. For example, rotations of the lower extremities are balanced by the shoulders and arms. As the shoulders rotate forward, the legs rotate posteriorly, and vice versa. The power generated by the swinging arms does not directly contribute to increased speed but balances the rotational energy of the swinging legs.[5] If this were not the case, the rotational accelerations of the body would be significant and energy would be needlessly wasted.

The final mechanism to enhance energy conservation is the effective interchange between kinetic energy and gravitational potential energy. This relationship in running and sprinting differs from that in walking. In each case, however, the interchange facilitates the effective use of the mechanical energy supplied by the muscles. Specifically, in running and sprinting, the kinetic and potential energy are in phase (Fig. 2–17A). This means that when kinetic energy is high, potential energy is also high, and vice versa. In walking, they are out of phase, with kinetic energy being high when potential energy is low (Fig. 2–17B). Because of these differences, the sum of kinetic and potential energy fluctuates more in one gait cycle of running or sprinting than in one gait cycle of walking. If these large fluctuations of energy in running and sprinting were not modulated by the storage and transfer of energy, inefficiency would be great. For example, in midswing, potential and kinetic energy peak. As the center of mass falls toward the ground, potential en-

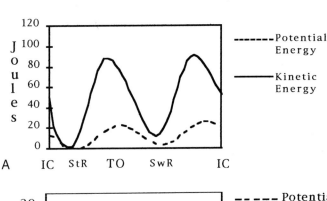

A   IC   StR   TO   SwR   IC

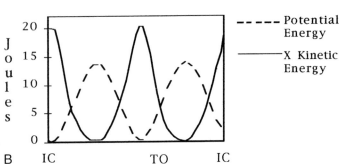

B   IC   TO   IC

Figure 2–17

*A: Kinetic/potential energy in running. **B:** Kinetic/potential energy in walking.*

ergy is lost. As the foot contacts the ground, kinetic energy is lost. Much of the lost potential and kinetic energy is converted into elastic potential energy and stored in the muscles, tendons, and ligaments. During the generation phase, the center of mass accelerates upward and both potential and kinetic energy increase. Energy for this movement is supplied by active contraction of the muscles and release of the elastic potential energy stored in the ligaments and tendons. Storage of energy in the elastic structures of the lower extremities thus has a more important role in running and sprinting than in walking.

The goal of an athlete is to maintain energy efficiency. This is accomplished through these four mechanisms. These represent some of the ways that an athlete conserves energy, increases speed, and maximizes endurance.

CONCLUSION

The descriptions of running and sprinting in comparison with normal walking in this chapter provide basic information in the study of human locomotion. This information offers further insight into injury mechanisms and therefore training strategies for injury prevention and performance enhancement. As more knowledge and experience are gained, this type of analysis will be used to better understand forward human bipedal locomotion.

Acknowledgments

The author acknowledges Lisa Schutte, PhD and Joyce Phelps Trost, RPT, for their assistance in the preparation of this manuscript, and the staff of the Motion Analysis Laboratory at Gillette Children's Specialty Healthcare (St. Paul, MN) for gathering and processing the data presented in this chapter. This information is also available in a video or CD-ROM through Gillette Children's Specialty Healthcare Foundation, 200 East University Avenue, St. Paul, MN 55101.

REFERENCES

1. Alexander RM: Running. The Human Machine. London, National History Museum Publications, 1992, pp 74–87.
2. Alexander RM: Walking. The Human Machine. London, National History Museum Publications, 1992, pp 59–73.
3. Delp SL, Loan JP, Hoy MG, et al: An interactive, graphics-based model of the lower extremity to study orthopaedic surgical procedures. IEEE Trans Biomed Eng 37:757–767, 1990.
4. Gage JR: Gait Analysis in Cerebral Palsy. London, MacKeith Press, 1991, p 80.

5. Hinrichs RN: Upper extremity function in distance running. In Cavanagh PR (ed): Biomechanics of Distance Running. Champaign, IL, Human Kinetics Publishers, 1990, pp 107–133.
6. Ker RF, Bennett MB, Bibby SR, et al: The spring in the arch of the human foot. Nature 325:147–149, 1987.
7. McMahon TA: Spring-like properties of muscles and reflexes in running. Multiple Muscle Systems: Biomechanics and Movement Organization. New York, Springer-Verlag, 1990, pp 578–590.
8. Novacheck TF: Walking, running, and sprinting: A three-dimensional analysis of kinematics and kinetics. Instr Course Lect 44:497–506, 1995.
9. Novacheck TF, Trost JP, Schutte L: Running and Sprinting: A Dynamic Analysis (Video/CD-ROM). St. Paul, MN, Gillette Children's Hospital, 1996.

MARILYN M. PINK ■ *FRANK W. JOBE*

══════ *CHAPTER THREE*

The Foot/Shoe Interface

Running is a natural extension of walking. Babies learn to walk, and later, as children, they speed up and teach themselves to run. Both walking and running are very natural, yet technically different, developmental events. Those differences include an airborne phase in running that is not present in walking. The lower extremity ranges of motion are much larger in running.[38] The muscle firing amplitudes are much greater in running.[29, 39] The forces on the foot have different locations in walking and running.[37] The total forces encountered when running are 2 to 3.6 times higher than in walking.[40, 43] The time during which the forces are accumulated is much shorter in running.[41] All of these differences have been deduced to cause at least a fourfold increase in strain on the supportive structures,[35] which can cause injury not only to the foot but also to other body segments.[3, 10, 15]

It is important for clinicians to know what and where the loads are on the foot during running and to understand the role that shoes have in mediating these forces. Thus, the purpose of this chapter is to describe the pressures on the foot during running and to discuss the components of running shoes that are relevant to clinicians.

PRESSURES ON THE FOOT DURING RUNNING

DISTRIBUTION OF PRESSURE

When discussing the phases of walking, one typically begins with heel strike.[36] This is an appropriate description of how the foot comes in contact with the ground when ambulating. The heel carries most of the load when walking, and the first and second metatarsal heads carry about the same load.[18]

In running, between 75% and 90% of runners make initial contact with the ground at the heel.[14, 22, 43] The literature extrapolates from this and the walking data and discusses the heel as a major point of concern during an assumed impact-type landing during running.[11, 20, 21, 28]

Until recently, the actual distribution of forces on the foot during running was not known. With the development of technology that uses multiple sensors within an insole that can be placed between the foot and shoe, the relative pressures on the foot can be measured. In a study of 25 men and 25 women, the second metatarsal head was found to bear the most pressure, closely followed by the first and third metatarsal heads and extending up to the great toe (Fig. 3–1).[37] These same areas were found not only to bear the peak instantaneous pressure but also to bear the pressure over a relatively longer time than the other parts of the foot. The heel bore much less pressure for a shorter period. It appears that even though the heel may typically be the first part of the foot to come in contact with the ground, relatively little force is encountered at that time.

This may at first appear confusing in light of the observation that the posterolateral outsole of a running shoe commonly demonstrates signs of wear. This wear quite likely is the result of an anterior-posterior shearing force that occurs as the foot contacts the ground.[30] The peak vertical force does not, however, occur until later in the stance phase. Many researchers have demonstrated that the peak vertical force during running occurs about halfway through the stance phase.[5, 7, 30] At this point, the heel is typically off the ground. This observation supports the research results that revealed the highest pressures in the forefoot rather than in the heel.

The calcaneus is obviously a much larger sur-

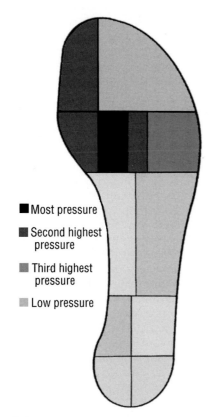

■ Most pressure

■ Second highest pressure

■ Third highest pressure

■ Low pressure

Figure 3–1

Distribution of forces on the foot.

face area over which to distribute forces than are the metatarsal heads. The fat pad under the calcaneus is relatively thick. Steinback and Russell[42] found the heel thickness of Caucasians to be approximately 17.8 mm and of African-Americans to be approximately 20.1 mm. These fat pads may decrease the magnitude of peak forces by 20% to 28%.[33] Although the fat pads at the metatarsal heads have not yet been measured, they are notably qualitatively less than at the heel. The body appears to be better designed to accommodate to pressures on the heel, which is satisfactory during walking. Perhaps this is an evolutionary practicality. Because humans spend more time walking than running, our bodies may have evolved to be best suited for walking. During running, however, the heel does not appear to be the area at risk; the first three metatarsal heads and the great toe may be more at risk. The surface area is smaller at the metatarsal heads, which have less biologic cushioning, and less attention has historically been focused on the role of pressure on the metatarsal heads.

It is not surprising then that injury might occur on the forefoot during running—and indeed, that is the case. Lysholm and Wiklander[25] have shown that the foot is the most common area of injury in marathon runners. Also, Eisele and Sammarco[13] have reported that the most common fatigue fractures in the forefoot are of the shaft or neck of the second or third metatarsal. The first ray may be spared because it is larger and the muscles attached to it are stronger.[18] Because the first ray has been projected to be about four times stronger than the second ray, it may be better equipped to endure the loads. However, the sesamoids under the head are subject to fatigue fractures.[13]

With this in mind, clinicians may want to examine the inside of the running shoe at the level of the medial metatarsals and great toe when a runner presents with an injury. Rather than focusing on the heel area, it may be more appropriate to make certain that the pressure-absorbing characteristics of the shoe are intact on the medial forefoot.

EFFECT OF SPEED ON PRESSURE

The effect of running pace has been suggested to have a role in how the forces are distributed on the foot. Hoshikawa and colleagues[17] found that as the speed of running increased, the stance time decreased. This has lead to a widely accepted extrapolation that average (i.e., slower) runners are characteristically rearfoot strikers and that elite (pace of 5.36 m/sec, i.e., faster) runners generally make initial contact much farther forward on the shoe.[34, 44]

Contrary to this thought, it now appears that recreational and competitive runners tend to select one pattern of running, which they maintain even when changing paces between a training pace (7.8 miles per hour) and a running pace (9.6 miles per hour).[37] Some subtle differences in the distribution of pressure within the foot are noted when running at different paces, however.

At faster paces, less pressure appears to be placed on the medial midfoot and more pressure on the lateral four toes. This may indicate that the foot was in less pronation or more supination at the faster pace,[37] although this was found only in women runners. Male runners had no differences in their pressure distribution. This may be because the men's feet were more rigid and thus did not have as much pronation into which to move at the faster pace. In women runners, as the stance time decreased (a faster pace), the runners may not have had the time to pronate as much. Thus, the fear that at faster paces the pronation increased or the rate of pronation increased may not be valid.

This leads us directly into a discussion of gender differences related to pressure distribution.

GENDER DIFFERENCES IN PRESSURE DISTRIBUTION

Men tend to place slightly more pressure on the lateral aspect of the midfoot and forefoot than do women.[37] Clinical inference drawn from this may be limited, however, in that the areas of differences were areas of relatively low pressure. Thus, the discussion of differences may be a bit academic, but let's proceed with the subtleties.

In that men placed more pressure laterally, they may have a more rigid foot than do women. They appear to have a smaller surface area over which to distribute the pressures, as well as a higher concentration of pressure. If this were due to foot rigidity, loss of shock-attenuating ability might be noted in the lower extremity.[16] The combination of small surface area and loss of shock-attenuating ability could potentially lead to injury.

Overall, women are thought to have more joint flexibility than men, and their foot may be no exception. During lower extremity weight-bearing, women have been noted to pronate more than men. If excessive, prolonged, or rapid pronation occurs, clinical problems could be found not only in the foot but also at the knee because the tibiofemoral relationship could be skewed.[19] Chondromalacia patellae or patellofemoral pain (which may be caused in part by a skewed tibiofemoral relationship) has been suggested to be almost twice as common in the general female population than in the male population.[1]

This study of pressure distribution in the foot was not designed to show that one gender has too much rigidity or that the other gender has too much pronation, because the actual degree of supination/pronation was not measured. The findings from this study simply point out the subtle differences in the pressure distribution between the two groups. These subtleties will be considered valid

only if they are supported by injury incidence differences in the two genders, and at this point, the jury is still out. Some studies suggest that overall, the injury rates are similar in the two groups. During a cohort study of 252 men and 48 women who were observed for a year, 52% of the men and 49% of the women reported at least one running injury. Of these injuries, 37% of those incurred by men and 38% of those incurred by women were severe enough to require a decrease in weekly mileage.[26] In a separate study,[24] the new injuries per person-year of running were basically the same for women and men at 10 different body sites. These studies, however, may not be specific enough to sort out the differences in injury that could be suggested by the different pressure distributions. As with much of science, this new information may generate additional thoughts and research to either support or reject the subtleties of different pressure distributions in men and women.

With this as a background, let's now discuss the most common strategy for accommodating/adapting/absorbing the loads on the foot during running. That strategy is, quite simply, shoes.

RUNNING SHOES

HISTORICAL PERSPECTIVE: TO BE (SHOD) OR NOT TO BE (SHOD)

Sandals thought to be about 10,000 years old were found by archaeologist Luther Cressman in 1932 in an Oregon cave under a 5-ton rock. They were made of sagebrush bark that had been knotted together to form a tight material. Ridges had been added on the outsole to improve traction. The sandals had a covering where the forefoot would be and had straps that probably went around the back of the heel. A secondary source projected that these sandals may have been used for running, because one of the main preoccupations at that time was hunting for food[4]—or else avoiding becoming someone else's food. To hunt successfully without being hunted, one must have had to be an accomplished runner.

In the first Olympics, when running was a form of recreation and sport rather than a necessity, shoes were not worn. This was in the eighth century B.C. The starting line for the longest race of the Olympics (the dolichos, which was 3846 meters) was made of two narrow grooves in stone. The athletes ran barefoot and probably put their toes into the grooves, which served as a type of starting block. Etchings in vases from this time also depict runners without footwear.

As the Roman Empire emerged and later dominated, running footwear came into being (and by 393 A.D., the Olympics had been outlawed by a Roman decree). The Roman armies appear to have used runners to send messages, and at least one emperor issued an edict that specified single-soled shoes, or *gallicas*, for the runners. Although gallicas were a far cry from today's shoes, this appears to be one of the earlier acknowledgments of specific requirements for runners.

Fast forward to 1839: A man by the name of Charles Goodyear was heating up some crude rubber from trees and mixing it with sulfur. He created a pliable substance that is rubber as we know it. One of the ultimate applications of this product was in running shoes. This undoubtedly made the sport much more comfortable than with hard-soled shoes.

By 1865, specialized running shoes were being made. Spalding catalogs and later Sears catalogs began showing running shoes that could be ordered at prices of $3.00 to $6.00, which amounted to approximately a quarter to half of an average weekly salary.

Adi Dassler advanced the development of running shoes when he formed Adidas in 1948 and began manufacturing running shoes in Germany. His brother, Rudi, formed a rival company called the Puma Company. The brothers' heated competition most surely furthered the innovation of running shoes.

Tiger Marathon shoes came into existence in 1951 as the Japanese entered the marketplace. Their first running shoes separated the big toe from the four lateral toes (Fig. 3–2). They were modeled after traditional Japanese shoes, the Geta.

New Balance had been making orthopedic shoes in the Boston area since 1906, and in the early 1960s, the owners began to transfer their knowledge to running shoes to make use of their spare production capacity.

Nike came into existence a decade later (1972) as the founders decided to cease distributing Tiger shoes and to develop their own company.

The year 1972 was also the year that Frank Shorter won the Olympic marathon. The shoes he wore were made from a pair of track spikes. The bottoms had been removed, and

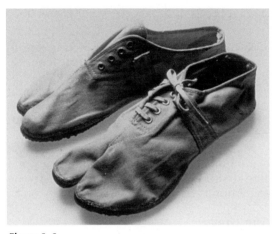

Figure 3–2

Tiger Marathon shoes, 1951. (Courtesy of ASICS Tabby Toe.)

a layer of midsole material had been glued onto the shoes. The outsole was then glued to the midsole.

As running for sport increased in the United States, so did competition for the percent of market share for running shoes. Shoe testing and biomechanical testing of shoes became popular. Companies attempted to distinguish themselves by demonstrating sound knowledge of the mechanics of running and running shoes.

In the 1990s, most of us wouldn't think of going for a run without donning some high-tech running shoes; however, let's think for a moment about running in other cultures. In a recent Olympic marathon, we saw Abebe Bikila from Ethiopia run barefoot. Having not trained in shoes as we know them, he chose not to compete in them for his first Olympic marathon. (He did, however, wear them in his second Olympic appearance.) Think also of the Tarahumara Indians, who live in Copper Canyon, Mexico. They run their rarjíparo, which continues for several days and covers 100 to 200 miles of rocky mule track. These Indians also hunt deer by running them down until they (the deer) collapse from exhaustion. They accomplish these amazing feats while wearing truck tire sandals.

As we now continue with a description of the components of running shoes as we know them, let us remember that humans from the end of the ice age may already have had functional running shoes, just as do the Indians currently living in Copper Canyon.

ANATOMY OF RUNNING SHOES

The purpose of a running shoe is to absorb the loads and control/stabilize the foot. No perfect shoes have yet been devised to do this. The majority of running injuries and resultant treatments are related to these two functions of the shoe.[2] It is therefore important for clinicians to have an understanding of the shoe.

A shoe has two basic parts, the upper and the bottom. The upper covers the sides and top of the foot, and the bottom is between the ground and the foot (Fig. 3–3).

The Upper

The vamp is the portion of the shoe covering the forefoot. The toe box is at the front of the vamp and may have a leather overlay that extends toward the laces. This overlay is called a *wingtip*. If the leather does not cover near the laces, it is called a *mudguard tip* or a *moccasin toe box*. The throat is the area of the shoe around the laces, and the collar is the padded material around the upper that makes contact with the foot. At the back of the shoe is the heel counter and the pull-tab or Achilles tendon protector. The heel counter should be firm, because its intent is to stabilize the rearfoot. By squeezing the sides of the heel counter with the fingers, one can get an idea of the heel counter durability.

The Bottom

The outermost surface of a running shoe is called the *outsole*. The outsole is built mainly for traction and durability.

The wedge is on top of the outsole and is designed to lift the heel and to absorb shock. The heel is ideally elevated approximately ½ inch to relieve stress on the gastrocnemius and soleus.[12]

The midsole is the next layer. The purpose

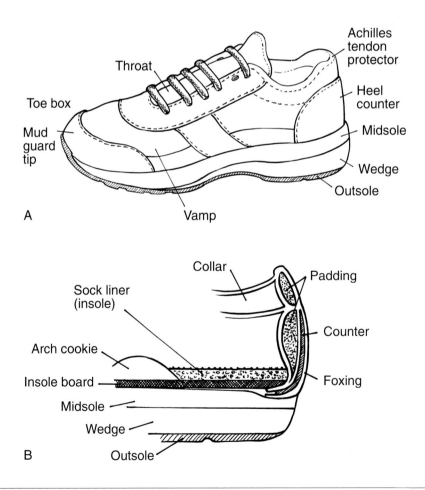

Figure 3–3

Anatomy of the running shoe.

of the midsole is for absorption of load. Development of the midsole and wedge has been the major change in shoe design in the past 25 to 30 years. In the 1970s, the polymeric foams such as ethylene vinyl acetate (EVA) were refined to the point of application in shoe design.

In shoes that are cement lasted, the insole board is the next layer of the shoe. The board must balance stability and flexibility because it provides a rigid base for the shoe without excessively restricting the foot. One of the areas where flexibility is notably important is under the metatarsophalangeal joints. At toe-off, the metatarsophalangeal joints dorsiflex 25 to 30 degrees. If the shoe offers insufficient flexibility, the gastrocnemius and soleus endure the imposed additional stress.[12]

The sock liner or insole is the portion of the shoe that touches the foot. It must absorb perspiration and loads while allowing a slight shearing motion to occur without chafing the undersurface of the foot.

Some shoes also place an "arch cookie" at the longitudinal arch of the foot. This is made of foam rubber and is intended to minimize overpronation. Some runners like this feature, but many pull it out of the shoe because it is difficult to obtain a comfortable fit with the cookie.

The heel of the shoe may flare outward. As styles of shoes have changed, so has the width of the flare. If the flare is too wide, some think it may cause the foot to pronate too rapidly.[12]

CONSTRUCTION

The shoe-manufacturing process is labor intensive. Before a shoe leaves the assembly line, some 25 people have probably helped to construct it. One of the steps in making a shoe entails putting it on a last. A last is a metal or wooden foot-shaped form around which a shoe is constructed. Lasts are tightly guarded secrets in the shoe industry. A last holds the basic shoe design and affects both the fit and support of the shoe. There are four basic lasts, and the type of last used is easiest to determine by looking at the bottom of the shoe.

The curvature of the last is an important component of the shoe design. The degree of curvature extends on a continuum from straight to curved (Fig. 3–4). (Categoric names such as semicurved or slightly curved are

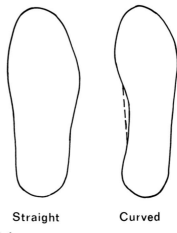

Straight   **Curved**

Figure 3–4

The continuum of curvature in a shoe.

sometimes given to the degree of curvature.) A shoe that is straight-lasted has no forefoot adduction. It tends to offer the most medial support for a foot and is typically the preferred last for overpronators, but it may feel awkward to some runners. At the opposite end of the spectrum is a curve-lasted shoe, which offers the greatest inward flare and the least medial support. Curve-lasted shoes tend to be more flexible than straighter-lasted shoes.

A shoe is pulled together on the bottom of the last in one of three basic ways. To determine the type of construction, simply remove the sock liner and look. A board-lasted, or cement-lasted, shoe has the uppers pulled over a last and cemented to the innersole board. A board can be seen when looking under the sock liner. Board-lasted shoes are supposed to provide stability and a solid platform for orthotic devices. However, the stability (and the longevity of that stability) is debatable because the board is made of cardboard or cardboard-like material and quite likely breaks down very quickly. A slip-lasted shoe looks like a moccasin underneath the sock liner. In a slip-lasted shoe, the upper is stitched together on the undersurface and slipped onto the last. This type of construction is said to provide flexibility. A shoe that is combination-lasted is board-lasted in the rearfoot for stability and slip-lasted in the forefoot for flexibility.

EFFECT OF THE SHOE ON THE FOOT

Many researchers have investigated the effect of the shoe on the foot. When studying heel deformation, De Clercq and colleagues[11] found that barefoot running deformed the heel approximately 61% but running in shoes deformed it only 36%. The rationale for this may be that the shoe absorbed some of the forces and may have also dispersed the forces over a larger surface area.

As mentioned earlier, the midsole's function is to absorb the loads during running. If the material is soft, it is said to be *point elastic,* with impact affecting mostly the material under the point of impact. Harder materials are called *surface elastic* because the impact forces are supposedly distributed over a larger surface area.[14] The actual effect of the midsole hardness is not established, however.

Komi and associates[23] found that ground reaction forces were not as dependent on the shoe material as they were on the velocity. Nigg and coworkers[31] reported that midsole hardness did not influence the magnitude or loading rate of external vertical impact forces. They also found that viscoelastic shoe insoles did not change the forces.[32] Clarke and colleagues[7] substantiated that the magnitude of the peak vertical impact force was unchanged with different hardness/softness of shoes. They did find, however, that the softer shoe had a significantly longer rise time to the peak force. Cook and his research team[9] studied shock absorption of approximately 40 models of shoes tested after 0 to 500 miles of use. They found very little difference in energy absorbed at heel strike between models. Additionally, they noted significant reduction in shock absorption at the heel with increased mileage when bench testing the shoes. This, however, was not borne out when the shoes were field tested (i.e., people ran in them). Clarke and associates[6] likewise found no correlation between bench testing and force plate testing. In regard to Clarke's and others' work, it may be that bench testing measured the forces between the foot and the shoe whereas the force plate measured it between the shoe and the force plate. An error may well be associated with applying the results of the latter to the actual interface of the foot and shoe. Also, because we now know that very little pressure is borne at the heel during running, the difference in findings between the bench testing (heel compression) and field testing (minimal heel compression) may simply mean that the bench tested the heel whereas the field was more of a test for the forefoot and did not challenge the heel.

It is also interesting to note the apparent inverse relationship between shock absorption and stability/motion control.[2, 14] Given that much of the motion is thought to be controlled through the rearfoot but the absorption of forces is needed at the forefoot, it will be interesting to see if shoes in the future will be designed to be firmer under and around the heel (thus affording rearfoot control) with more cushion in the forefoot (to absorb the forces). This would conflict with the idea that shoes need to emphasize protection of the foot from impact forces at 0% to 60% of the shoe heel[5] but would be supported by concentrating design attention under the forefoot, where the forces and pressures are the largest.[5, 37]

Another idea that has been suggested is to design different shoes for rearfoot and midfoot strikers.[5] Because we now know that maximal pressure is on the forefoot regardless of the type of initial contact and regardless of the speed of the runner, this concept may not be applicable.

In their study of design of running shoes, Bates and colleagues[2] searched for one shoe type that was best for all runners. They identified multiple important concepts in shoe design and tested them. They determined there was no single best shoe type. Thus, to summarize their findings, they averaged the rankings on the different variables that were measured. As clinicians, we must be aware, however, that an average of rankings may not meet the needs of any runner. Thus, we must look at each person's individual needs—which brings up the next topic, evaluation of an injured runner's shoes.

SHOE EVALUATION

Shoes are designed for the "universal foot" which most of us normal humans do not possess. Shoes must "toe" a fine line between shock absorption and control/stabilization of the foot because one has been thought to contradict the other. The current clinical thought is that people with too much pronation need a shoe that has more rearfoot control but can have a bit less shock absorption, whereas those with a more rigid foot need additional shock absorption but less rearfoot control. The pattern of foot pronation/supination is summarized next to aid in our understanding of this idea. (A more thorough description of foot mechanics is found elsewhere in this book.)

When a foot makes contact with the ground, it is in a supinated position and quickly begins to move into pronation. About halfway through the stance cycle, the foot reaches maximum pronation and begins to supinate again.[8] When a foot is pronated, it is better able to absorb the forces incurred during running as the joints are unlocked. When a foot is supinated, it is more rigid and functions as a solid lever over which the body weight is propelled. There is a time and place for each of these functions. Obviously, it is advantageous if a foot can have some flexibility and absorb forces, yet become a rigid lever at toe-off.

One of the problems that can evolve occurs when a foot is too flexible. Excessive subtalar joint pronation has been associated with injuries on the medial aspect of the lower extremity. These injuries include patellofemoral pain syndrome, tibial stress syndrome, and posterior tibial tendinitis. Other problems can develop when a foot is too rigid. Injuries due to foot rigidity tend to be on the lateral aspect of the lower extremity and include iliotibial band friction syndrome, peroneus tendinitis, stress fractures, trochanteric bursitis, and plantar fasciitis.[27]

Thus, when a patient presents with a running injury, the clinician wants to check the flexibility of the foot and examine the shoes for signs of overpronation or foot rigidity. If the patient can run with the injury, a clinical assessment of the foot in action is advantageous. It has been suggested that runners with excessive pronation may benefit from running shoes that are board-lasted and straight-lasted with a stable heel counter and extra medial support. A person with a more rigid foot may want to try slip-lasted, curve-lasted shoes with more cushioning.[27] Many times, however, the solution is not as simple as selecting shoes with more shock-absorbing or control/stabilization characteristics. Custom-made orthotics are sometimes necessary to minimize the problem.

In *The Running Shoe Book*, Cavanagh[4] describes an interesting project in which he advertised in the Penn State student newspaper to "Give your old running shoes to science and get $3.00." He described the response as both overwhelming and worrisome. Some of the shoes had been worn "until they were falling apart, until they had no outsoles, holes in the uppers, midsoles that were rock hard and counters that were completely shredded." Perhaps the main lesson to be learned from this is that no shoes should be worn to this level of destruction. A closer look at the various components of shoe wear can lead to recommendations for preventing further injury.

If the heel counters and medial aspect of the heel fall over the medial sole, the patient probably has excessive pronation. A varus heel wedge could help this problem, as could shoes with good rearfoot control (i.e., firm heel counters and board-lasted). If the lateral aspect of the heel counter is leaning off the lateral sole, a rigid foot is suggested. In this case, the shoes should not have a varus wedge. Flimsy heel counters reduce manufacturing costs but can affect both the life of the shoes and the health of the lower extremity. Thus, heel counters should be examined for firmness.

If wear is noted on the uppers at the area of the big toe, the runner may have a rigid hallux. Thus, she or he could have problems with shock absorption and with rigid forefoot flexibility for dorsiflexion at toe-off. These individuals need to make sure their shoes have a high toe box. An orthotic device may also be required. Likewise, if a person has black toenails, a higher toe box or wider shoe may be necessary.

The midsole and wedge should be palpated from the inside to be certain they are not too hard (i.e., loss of shock-absorbing capabilities). As mentioned earlier, particular attention should be paid to the medial forefoot. Overall, the shoes should be flexed to ensure that the materials have not become brittle.

If wear patterns are readily apparent on the outsole, the shock-absorbing characteristics are probably depleted. The material of the outsole is quite durable (especially in light of the fact that wear on the outsole is largely reflective of shearing forces rather than impact forces), thus wearing away of the material may represent excessive mileage for the shoes.

SUMMARY

The foot/shoe interface is important for clinicians to understand in order to minimize injury in runners. Some of the key points from this chapter follow:

1. The medial forefoot bears the majority of forces during the running cycle.
2. The running pace does not appear to dictate the distribution of force on the foot.

3. Some subtle differences in force distribution between males and females could be reflective of foot rigidity or flexibility.

4. An evaluation of worn running shoes may give clues to the pathology of running injuries.

REFERENCES

1. Atwater AE: Gender differences in distance running. In Cavanagh PR (ed): Biomechanics of Distance Running. Champaign, IL, Human Kinetics Publishers, 1990, pp 321–354.
2. Bates BT, Osternig LR, Sawhill JA, et al: Design of running shoes. Presented at the International Conference on Medical Devices and Sports Equipment, ASME Centennial Program Century II, Emerging Technology Conference, San Francisco, CA, August 1980.
3. Burdett RG: Forces predicted at the ankle during running. Med Sci Sports Exerc 14:308–316, 1982.
4. Cavanagh PR: The Running Shoe Book. Mountain View, CA, World Publications, 1980.
5. Cavanagh PR, LaFortune MA: Ground reaction forces in distance running. J Biomech 13:397–406, 1980.
6. Clarke TE, Frederick EC, Cooper LB: Biomechanical measurement of running shoe cushioning properties. In Nigg BM, Kerr BA (eds): Biomechanical Aspects of Sport Shoes and Playing Surface. University of Calgary, Alberta, Canada, 1983, pp 25–33.
7. Clarke TE, Frederick DC, Cooper LB: Effects of shoe cushioning upon ground reaction forces in running. Int J Sports Med 1:247–251, 1983.
8. Clarke TE, Frederick EC, Hamill C: The study of rearfoot movement in running. In Frederick EC (ed): Sport Shoes and Playing Surfaces. Champaign, IL, Human Kinetics Publishers, 1984, pp 166–169.
9. Cook SD, Marcus AK, Brunet ME: Shock absorption characteristics of running shoe. Am J Sports Med 13:248–253, 1985.
10. Copozzo A: Force actions in the human trunk during running. J Sports Med 23:14–22, 1983.
11. De Clercq D, Aerts P, Kunnen M: The mechanical characteristics of the human heel pad during foot strike in running: An in vivo cineradiographic study. J Biomech 27:1213–1222, 1994.
12. Drez D: Running footwear. Am J Sports Med 8:140–141, 1980.
13. Eisele SA, Sammarco GJ: Fatigue fractures of the foot and ankle in the athlete. J Bone Joint Surg Am 75:290–298, 1983.
14. Frederick EC, Clarke TE, Hamill CL: The effect of running shoe design on shock attenuation. In Frederick EC (ed): Sport Shoes and Playing Surfaces. Champaign, IL, Human Kinetics Publishers, 1984, pp 190–198.
15. Garbutt G, Boocock MG, Reilly T, et al: Running speed and spinal shrinkage in runners with and without low back pain. Med Sci Sports Exerc 22:769–772, 1990.
16. Hamill J: Understanding rear foot motion. J Biomech March:87–90, 1995.
17. Hoshikawa T, Matsui H, Miyashita M: Analysis of running pattern in relation to speed. Biomechanics III 8:342–348, 1973.
18. Hutton WC, Dhanendran M: A study of the distribution of load under the normal foot during walking. Int Orthop 3:153–157, 1979.
19. James SL, Bates BT, Osternig LR: Injuries to runners. Am J Sports Med 6:40–50, 1978.
20. Jørgensen U, Bojsen-Møller F: Shock absorbency of factors in the shoe/heel interaction, with special focus on the role of the heel pad. Foot Ankle 9:294–299, 1989.
21. Jørgensen U, Ekstrand J: Significance of heel pad confinement for the shock absorption at heel strike. Int J Sports Med 9:468–473, 1988.
22. Kerr BA, Beauchamp L, Fisher V, et al: Footstrike patterns in distance running. In Nigg BM, Kerr BA (eds): Biomechanical Aspects of Sport Shoes and Playing Surfaces. Calgary, Alberta, Canada, University Press, 1983, pp 135–142.
23. Komi PV, Gollhofer A, Schmidtbleicher D: Interaction between man and shoe in running: Considerations for a more comprehensive measurement approach. Int J Sports Med 8:196–202, 1987.
24. Koplan JP, Powell KE, Sikes RK, et al: An epidemiologic study of the benefits and risks of running. JAMA 248:3118–3121, 1982.
25. Lysholm J, Wiklander J: Injuries in runners. Am J Sports Med 15:168–171, 1987.
26. Macera CA, Pate PR, Powell KE, et al: Predicting lower extremity injuries among habitual runners. Arch Intern Med 149:2565–2568, 1989.
27. McKenzie DC, Clement DB, Taunton JE: Running shoes, orthotics, and injuries. Sports Med 2:334–347, 1985.
28. Misevich KW, Cavanagh PR: Material aspects of modeling shoe/foot interaction. In Frederick EC (ed): Sport Shoes and Playing Surfaces. Champaign, IL, Human Kinetics Publishers, 1984, pp 47–75.
29. Montgomery WH, Pink M, Perry J: Electromyographic analysis of hip and knee musculature during running. Am J Sports Med 22:272–278, 1994.
30. Munro CF, Miller DI, Fuglevand AJ: Ground reaction forces in running: A reexamination. J Biomech 20:147–155, 1987.
31. Nigg BM, Bahlsen HA, Luethi SM, et al: The influence of running velocity and midsole hardness on external impact forces in heel-toe running. Biomechanics 20:951–959, 1987.
32. Nigg BM, Herzog W, Read LJ: Effect of viscoelastic shoe insoles on vertical impact forces in heel-toe running. Am J Sports Med 16:70–76, 1988.
33. Paul IL, Munro MB: Musculo-skeletal shock absorption: Relative contribution of bone and soft tissues at various frequencies. J Biomech 11:237–239, 1978.
34. Payne AH: Foot to ground contact forces of elite runners. In Matsui H, Kobayashi K (eds): Biomechanics III-B, Champaign IL, Human Kinetics Publishers, 1983, pp 746–753.
35. Perry J: Anatomy and biomechanics of the hindfoot. Clin Orthop 177:9–15, 1983.
36. Perry J: Phases of gait. In Perry J (ed): Gait Analysis: Normal and Pathological Function. Thorofare, NJ, Slack, 1992, p 11.
37. Pink M, Huynh T, Perry J, et al: Pressures on the foot during running. Am J Sports Med (in press).
38. Pink M, Perry J, Houglum P, et al: Lower extremity range of motion in the recreational sport runner. Am J Sports Med 22:541–549, 1994.
39. Reber L, Perry J, Pink M: Muscular control of the ankle in running. Am J Sports Med 21:805–810, 1993.

40. Rodgers MM: Dynamic foot biomechanics. J Orthop Sports Phys Ther 21:306–316, 1985.

41. Scranton PE, Rutkoski R, Brown TD: Support phase kinematics of the foot. In Bateman JE, Trott A (eds): The Foot and Ankle. New York, Thieme-Stratton, 1980, pp 195–205.

42. Steinback HL, Russell W: Measurement of the heel-pad as an aid to diagnosis of acromegaly. Radiology 82:418–423, 1964.

43. Voloshin AS: Shock absorption during running and walking. J Am Podiatr Med Assoc 78:295–299, 1988.

44. Williams KR, Cavanagh PR, Ziff JL: Biomechanical studies of elite female distance runners. Int J Sports Med 8:107–118, 1987.

ROBERT E. LEACH ■ SUSAN B. ZECHER

CHAPTER FOUR

Stress Fractures

Stress fractures are among the more common injuries that occur in runners.[3, 26, 35, 38] They are a source of disability, but that disability is usually brief. With early diagnosis, treatment usually becomes simple and the period of disability is lessened. Thus, it is important that those people caring for runners be aware of the typical history, physical findings, and any laboratory tests that help to make the diagnosis of a stress fracture. The magnitude of the problem is considerable, because it has been estimated that between 4.7% and 15.6% of all injuries to runners are stress fractures.[33]

The first medical description of what we now call stress fractures was reported in 1855 and concerned military recruits.[6] During the next 110 years, many reports in the literature described "march" or "fatigue" fractures in military recruits. Only with the increased awareness of fitness and particularly with the running boom, beginning in the 1960s, did these same types of fractures in runners begin to be recognized. At that point, the term *stress fracture* came into general use.[13]

A simple definition of a stress fracture is any bone fracture that does not occur as a result of a single traumatic episode sufficient to cause a fracture of the involved bone. Stress fractures may occur when abnormal stress is applied to normal bone or when normal stress is applied to weakened bone. In either instance, this could result in what we clinically identify as a stress fracture, which fits into the category of the overuse injuries that are so commonly encountered in many athletes but particularly in runners.

Stress fractures occur in all sports that require repetitive running and jumping but are far more common in long-distance runners than in any other athletes. A distinct difference is observed in the bony sites where stress fractures occur in military recruits versus the sites in which they occur in runners (Figs.

4–1 and 4–2). A question thus arises about the cause of stress fractures in the two groups or at least about the various factors affecting the production of the fractures.

Military recruits are frequently people in relatively poor physical condition who, when they start training, are rapidly made to undertake significant physical fitness activities including running and marching. Both the skeletal and muscular systems are rapidly loaded under the military training system. Giladi and colleagues reported that changing the military footwear and the training surfaces and using orthotic devices dramatically decrease the incidence of stress fractures in a military population.[19] The calcaneus and the metatarsals are the most common sites of stress fractures in military personnel. Metatarsal stress fractures are also noted in runners but far less commonly than those in the tibia, whereas calcaneal stress fractures are uncommon in runners.

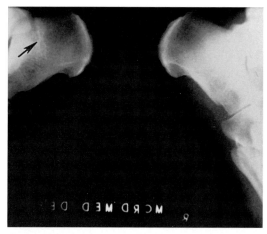

Figure 4–1

The arrow points to an area of sclerosis in the os calcis denoting a stress fracture.

Figure 4–2

The typical area for stress fracture in military recruits is encircled.

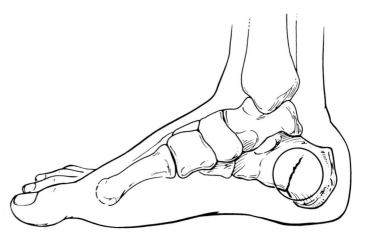

Runners have the highest incidence of stress fractures for all athletes—more than in all other sports combined—as shown by one large series. Of the 320 stress fractures reported by Matheson and associates, 221 were due to running and the other 90 were due to various other sports, most of which entailed running.[33] In that particular series, the tibia was the most commonly affected bone, being involved 49% of the time, and the weekly running mileage of the afflicted patients ranged from 25 to 44 miles per week.

CAUSE OF STRESS FRACTURES

It is interesting that despite all of the clinical material about stress fractures that has been collected during the past 25 years and the voluminous reports in the literature,[45, 47] we do not know the precise cause of stress fractures.[41] A great deal of information shows that frequent running causes an overload to the bony skeleton that in some way subverts the usual dynamic reparative process that we associate with normal bone repair. The amount of running and the time in which this stress is delivered seem to be important.[35] In Sullivan and colleagues' 1983 study of stress fractures in 51 runners, only 5 would have been classified as joggers (i.e., running less than 20 miles per week).[50] Personal experience and reading the literature indicate that 20 miles per week is a reasonable cutoff, in the sense that the vast majority of stress fractures occur in people who are running more than 20 miles per week. It appears that the inability of bone to withstand certain stresses is dose related.

Under the usual circumstance, normal bone reacts to both direct and muscular stress by an adaptation response called Wolff's law. We know that bone can respond by remodeling, and either too much or too little stress can cause changes in the normal biologic response of bone. The early literature refers only to the direct effect of weight-bearing stress on the bones as being a primary cause of stress fractures. Later reports refer to the effect of muscle forces acting on the bone, particularly in certain areas. In either case, the forces exceed the stress-bearing capacity of the affected bone.

Guoping and coworkers[21] and Johnson[25] have investigated the histology of stress fractures, and their findings have been well summarized by McBryde.[34] Continued repetitive stress on the bone leads to a normal remodeling response that is gradually overcome, and trabecular microfractures occur. Osteoclastic resorption results from accelerated cortical bone remodeling, which should lead to increased periosteal new bone formation and reinforcement. At this point, if the newly formed bone is not strong enough to accept the stress being exerted, the osteoclastic activity continues. At some point, the structural integrity is broached and a stress fracture occurs.

Marymont and colleagues,[32] McBryde,[34] and others believe that certain other conditions occurring in runners such as the ubiquitous shin splints, medial tibial stress syndrome, and tibial periostitis are preroentgenographic stress fractures. They believe that these clinical syndromes represent a continuum that, if runners continue to run, would eventuate in the production of a clinical and roentgenographic stress fracture. Although this is an attractive hypothesis in some ways, in actuality, many patients do run despite certain of these syndromes and regardless of pain and never develop an actual stress fracture. Also, bone scans taken of patients with a medial tibial syndrome usually show a longer hot area of involvement along the posterior tibia and not the focal point seen in stress fractures. This may indicate a related but not necessarily a continuing pathologic entity.

EVALUATION OF RISK FACTORS

Various studies have evaluated the risk factors for stress fractures in both runners and military recruits. One factor that seems destined to receive more attention with regard to stress fractures is the amount of muscle mass present in the lower extremities of those suffering these fractures. Garrett and colleagues have shown that one of the major roles of muscles is energy absorption.[18] When muscles become fatigued, they act differently from unfatigued muscles. They have difficulty absorbing the same amount of energy, and they thus probably have a role in the production of stress fractures as muscle fatigue does become intensified with long periods of running. The relatively lesser muscle mass of the lower leg, particularly around the tibia, may explain the abundance of tibial stress fractures. This structural difference could also be a factor in the higher incidence of stress fractures in women than in men.

Other physical variables have been studied with reference to risk factors. Giladi and associates, studying 300 military recruits, found only two independent variables that they considered major risk factors.[19] These were a narrow tibia and increased external rotation of the hip. These factors were independent of each other, and the study concerned military recruits, not running athletes. However, the concept of a narrow tibia being susceptible to stress fractures conforms to certain biomechanical concepts. Stress fractures are caused by numerous repetitive loads. In a tubular structure such as the tibia, the compression strength is proportional to the square of its radius. This means that an increase in the tibial bone width of 4 mm from 24 mm to 28 mm would increase the bone's compression strength by 36%. In the same bone, torsional and bending strength are proportional to the fourth power of the radius, which means that the same increase of 4 mm would increase bending and torsional strength by 86%. Thus,

small differences in a tubular bone such as the tibia could cause major differences in the susceptibility to stress fracture.

In this same study by Giladi and coworkers, aerobic physical fitness, body type, and leg strength, which could be an index of muscle mass, were not found to be related to the incidence of stress fracture.[19] This study was of military recruits, and we have reason to believe that the pathogenesis of stress fractures in military recruits and runners may be somewhat different given the different bones primarily affected.

Pronation of the feet has commonly been linked to stress fractures, particularly fractures of the tibial or tarsal bones. Although this association has been cited frequently, we do not know how much pronation might be indicative of a problem. Feet have to pronate to absorb energy; thus, many runners have pronated feet. Rigid cavus feet have been found in association with certain stress fractures such as that of the tarsal navicular. Most people with rigid cavus feet do not do much running, so we may not have a true incidence of stress fractures in relation to this entity. Varus alignment of the lower extremity, including genu varum, tibia vara, or forefoot varus has been commonly seen, but no strong correlation has been drawn. We simply do not have a good biomechanical explanation about why an increased incidence of stress fractures might be related to certain structural conditions.

Most studies of stress fractures cite training factors, particularly increases in the amount of running over a relatively short period, as being the most significant factor in the production of stress fractures.[26] In Matheson and colleagues' study, 22.4% of all stress fractures were thought to be due to training errors.[33] The problem is defining a training error. This usually means that a person has increased his or her mileage or increased his or her speed or changed to a different surface. However, other runners have often done much the same thing and not suffered a stress fracture. Therefore, training errors appear to be an independent variable—that is, one individual can run a certain mileage and increase it without ill effects, but others cannot. What we as physicians say is that a stress fracture represents a training error, but we have not developed parameters that forecast a stress fracture under certain conditions. In Matheson and associates' study, the lowest amount of mileage producing stress fractures was around 25 miles per week.[33] Clinically, most runners who develop stress fractures do so within 2 to 12 weeks of a training modification, indicating that the body reacts relatively quickly to these training errors. Other physical causes of stress fractures include the running surface, particularly when one changes from a running surface that is more resilient to a stiffer, harder surface. Indoor running tracks with their relatively tight turns are another training modification often cited as increasing the incidence of stress fractures.

RISK FACTORS IN WOMEN RUNNERS

It has been well recognized that women runners have a particular problem with stress fractures (Fig. 4–3). Major menstrual irregularity has also been a well-recognized consequence of distance running.[10, 30] In 1988, Barrow and Saha reported that stress fractures occurred in 49% of those women runners with a very irregular menstrual history, in 39% of the runners with an irregular menstrual history, but in only 29% of runners with a regular menstrual history.[2] They also found that 47% of amenorrheal runners had an eating behavior disorder, compared with 7% of the regular group having an eating behavior disorder.

Amenorrhea is associated with a hypoestrogenic state that could well lead to early osteoporosis in these runners.[15] Along with amenorrhea, other significant risk factors in women include lower bone density and decreased muscle mass in the lower limbs. If women athletes with these risk factors maintain minimal body weight but increase their running mileage, their chances of a stress fracture are markedly increased.

DIAGNOSIS

It is probable that both the real incidence and the reported incidence of stress fractures have increased dramatically in the past few decades. This is because of the increased number of people running and because those people are running for longer distances. In addition, physicians and other medical personnel are much more aware of the possibility of a stress fracture, and fewer cases are undiagnosed.

In the majority of patients, the diagnosis of a stress fracture should be made on the basis of the clinical history. Any runner who complains of pain localized to a bone in the lower extremity should be considered to have a stress fracture until this diagnosis is disproved. If the history is accompanied by local tenderness over the bone, further workup should include radiographs or bone scans. The usual history consists of the onset of aching pain with no major precipitating factor other than running. The pain gradually increases during activity. At this point, a carefully taken history often reveals a change in the training regimen sometime during the past 2 to 6 weeks.

The most striking aspect of the physical examination is local tenderness over the involved bone. In instances in which the bone is subcutaneous, some edema and even a thickening of the periosteum may be noted, most frequently over the tibia.

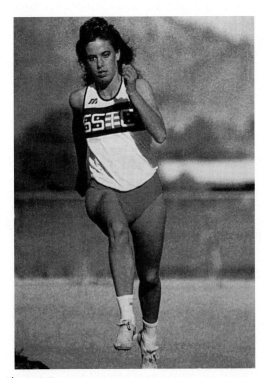

Figure 4–3

Women runners have an increased incidence of stress fractures.

RADIOGRAPHS

Early in the clinical history of a stress fracture, plain radiographs may not be revealing.

Despite this, we believe that radiographs should be taken because they may disclose the fracture and they may show the rare case of some displacement of a fracture such as in the tarsal navicular or femoral neck. If the radiograph is nondiagnostic but a stress fracture is suspected, a bone scan must be performed.[31]

The most important test for diagnosing a stress fracture is a bone scan performed with technetium 99m methylene diphosphonate (Fig. 4–4).[38] This bone scan has a sensitivity of virtually 100% for the diagnosis of stress fractures. Results can be positive within less than 72 hours of the apparent clinical appearance of symptoms, and the scan results may remain positive for 6 to 24 months. The accuracy of the bone scan depends on the vascular supply that delivers the technetium 99m to the area of increased metabolic activity.[36, 55] Anything interfering with the vascular supply such as infection could yield a false-negative result. Although the sensitivity is excellent, the specificity is less so; therefore, a triple-phase bone scan consisting of an angiogram phase, a blood pool phase, and a delayed image phase is used. With a stress fracture, all three phases would be positive, but results would be helpful in differentiating a stress

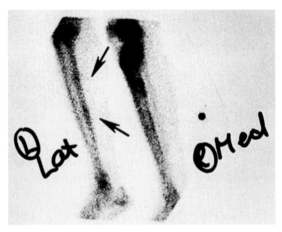

Figure 4–5

Positive bone scan with a diffused hot area more consistent with medial tibial syndrome.

fracture from a medial tibial stress syndrome because this latter yields positive findings in the delayed image phase only.

The medial tibial stress syndrome is one example of a possible diagnostic dilemma with runners because it also causes bone tenderness when running.[40] A triple-phase bone scan should show uptake during the delayed image phase and a linear, more longitudinal uptake involving the tibia than would a stress fracture (Fig. 4–5). Stress fractures tend to show small fusiform lesions, although at their earliest, they may show bone lesions that are more diffuse. As the lesion matures, the margins become sharper.

Magnetic resonance imaging (MRI) is expensive but could be used in rare instances when the lesion on bone scan is indistinct. Hemorrhage and edema around the fracture should be seen as a low signal intensity on the T_1W images and high signal intensity on the T_2W. The problem is that these findings are not pathognomonic of a stress fracture, but MRI could be helpful in distinguishing a stress fracture from an infection or a suspected bone tumor.[29]

Computed tomography (CT) scans are generally not as useful as bone scans but may be helpful for certain stress fractures such as that of the tarsal navicular or the lateral process of the talus. In this instance, they may show early separation of the fragments, which might need early internal fixation.

GENERAL TREATMENT PLAN

It is possible to make a general treatment plan for most stress fractures. The concepts

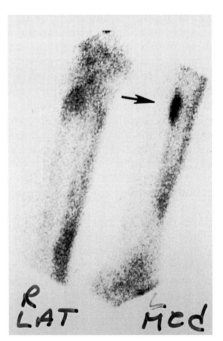

Figure 4–4

Positive bone scan with a focal hot area typical of a stress fracture.

are simple. The individual must stop running and by so doing decrease the excess stress that is causing the stress fracture. This should lead to bone healing. Pain can usually be controlled by the use of nonsteroidal antiinflammatory drugs (NSAIDs) and in rare instances by immobilization with a cast or splint. Displacement of stress fractures is uncommon except in particular instances such as a tarsal navicular fracture or the tension type of femoral neck fracture.

During the nonrunning phase, alternate forms of exercise are needed to maintain aerobic conditioning. Swimming, biking, and use of a stair-climber all are possibilities. This hiatus also offers an excellent chance to increase muscle mass and muscle strength in the upper extremities and particularly the lower extremities. Inadequate muscle mass may be one of the factors related to insufficient energy absorption and thus to stress fractures. During the nonrunning phase, it is reasonable to take this opportunity to increase muscle mass and improve general flexibility.

We believe that follow-up can generally be directed by the degree of local tenderness. When that has disappeared, a final radiograph can be evaluated, and the runner is then gradually reintroduced to a schedule. At this point, one has to know the previous history and be sure that return is gradual.

PELVIS AND SACRUM

Stress fractures of either the pelvis or the sacrum are relatively rare in runners.[28, 46] Because of the rarity, the diagnosis may be missed. Various muscle or tendon maladies may initially be suspected. In the pelvis, the most common site is the ischiopubic ramus. This location, with local pain, may lead a physician to consider adductor strain or even osteitis pubis (Fig. 4–6).

Only in recent years have the first cases of stress fractures of the sacral wing been reported.[1, 23] These probably were previously misdiagnosed because the symptoms could easily represent lumbosacral strain. The diagnosis would be very difficult to make on traditional roentgenograms.

For both the pelvis and the sacrum, the diagnosis is likely to be made on the basis of a bone scan. In the sacrum, it is conceivable that an osteoid osteoma could be confused with a stress fracture, but the clinical history is completely different. Osteoid osteoma usu-

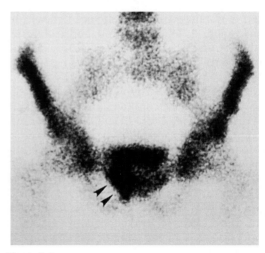

Figure 4–6

Positive bone scan of the pelvis typical of a stress fracture.

ally causes pain at night, whereas stress fractures cause pain with activity and are not painful when the runner is resting.

Treatment of a stress fracture in either the pelvis or the sacrum requires rest. Once local tenderness has disappeared, one could reasonably expect to send the athlete back to his or her routine with a slow buildup. Monitoring such a patient with serial scans is unnecessary provided the pain gradually disappears.

Stress fractures of the anterior iliac apophysis may occur in adolescent runners.[9] Pain and tenderness are localized over the anterior iliac crest. Radiographs may show a separation of the anterior iliac crest. If separation has not occurred, we assume that this is apophysitis. Separation represents a stress fracture. Rest for 4 to 6 weeks usually suffices to decrease symptoms and allow the runner to begin training gradually.

FEMORAL NECK

Stress fractures of the femoral neck are much less common in runners than they are in military recruits.[17] They do, however, have a high possibility of complications including displacement of the fracture and avascular necrosis. An affected runner usually complains of pain in the groin area or, in some instances, some anterior thigh pain. An antalgic gait and some loss of range of motion or pain with motion are common. In some instances, routine radiographs show sclerosis in the femoral neck. However, if the routine film is nondiagnostic, a bone scan should be performed. A report by Shin and colleagues suggests that MRI may be as sensitive as and more specific than a bone scan in detecting stress fractures of the hip.[49]

If a stress fracture involves the inferior cortex, as a result of compression, it is unlikely to displace (Fig. 4–7). Cessation of running, range-of-motion exercises, and some type of cross-training should be used while waiting for healing. As a general rule, 2 to 3 months is required for complete healing of stress fractures of this type. Fractures involving the superior cortex, thought to result from tension, are more likely to displace. These less common fractures in the athletic population are well treated by surgical fixation.

FEMORAL SHAFT FRACTURES

Johnson and colleagues' 1994 report stated that stress fractures of the femoral shaft are much more common than previously documented.[24] In a 2-year study of college athletes at the Division I AA level, during a 2-year period, 34 stress fractures were found in 914 athletes. Seven (21%) of these stress fractures were in the femoral shaft, a much higher number of femoral stress fractures than found in previous studies.[33]

One way that Johnson and coworkers were

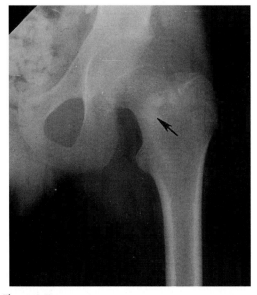

Figure 4–7

Plain radiograph shows bony sclerosis of the femoral neck with a compression stress fracture.

able to identify so many fractures of the femoral shaft was by using a clinical test they called the *fulcrum test.*[24] In this test, with the patient seated, the examiner's arm is placed under the distal thigh of the affected extremity and gentle pressure is applied distally to the dorsum of the femur near the knee. A patient with a stress fracture feels pain deep within the femur in the area where the examiner's arm is providing a fulcrum. The examiner's arm is moved from distal to proximal along the thigh as pressure is applied to the dorsum of the knee with the opposite hand. The researchers found this to be a very effective clinical test for diagnosing stress fractures of the femur. All suspected stress fractures were then evaluated with technetium 99m bone scans. The positive findings on the bone scan determined the final diagnosis of stress fracture. They found that initial radiographs were often nondiagnostic, although after 3 weeks, several of these routine radiographs did show bony sclerosis.

In this study and in a previous study by Hershman and associates, the majority of these stress fractures were found in the midmedial, posterior medial cortex of the proximal femoral shaft.[22] This location is in contrast to the stress fractures of the femoral shaft in military personnel, in whom approximately half are found in the distal third of the femur. Although only two of the seven stress fractures of the femoral shaft in the Johnson series occurred primarily as a result of running, this is an injury that must be sought in runners with thigh pain.

A runner with a stress fracture of the femur usually reports a history of a vague deep thigh or groin pain. The occurrence of groin or thigh pain may lead the physician to think of a muscle strain, because hamstrings, adductors, and quadriceps all can be involved in runners. A careful physical examination should distinguish between a stress fracture of the shaft and a muscle strain. An antalgic gait is noted in many instances, and running always increases the pain. Another clinical test for a stress fracture is the hopping test, in which the patient simply hops on the affected side, causing pain in the involved bone. (This test, however, is not specific to the femur.) Once the index of clinical suspicion has been raised, a bone scan is necessary to establish the final diagnosis.

Treatment in virtually all instances simply is rest, but 6 to 14 weeks may be required to decrease symptoms. The fulcrum test can be used as a clinical indicator of how healing is progressing, and when results are negative, the athlete should gradually return to full activity. Only in the event of displacement of a stress fracture would other treatment be necessary, and this is exceedingly rare in runners.

TIBIA

Tibial stress fractures are the most common stress fractures in athletes in general and in runners in particular.[12] In Matheson and colleagues' study, 49% of the stress fractures occurred in the tibia (Fig. 4–8).[33] In Barrow and Saha's study of women runners, 63% of the stress fractures occurred in the tibia, with approximately half of these in the distal portion of the tibia, one quarter in the proximal, and the remainder in the midportion.[2] In the proximal tibia, a common site is just below the medial tibia plateau. Although this may be difficult to see on routine radiographs, a bone scan quickly establishes the diagnosis (Fig. 4–9).[53] Most of these fractures heal once

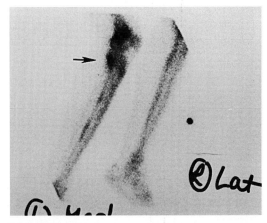

Figure 4–9

Bone scan shows a focal hot spot typical of a proximal medial tibial stress fracture.

a patient stops running, and complications such as an intraarticular extension are unusual.[48]

A more troublesome tibial stress fracture is that of the anterior cortex of the tibia in the midshaft region.[42, 43] These occur in runners but are even more likely in certain other athletes, particularly basketball players. They are characterized by marked local tenderness. Routine roentgenograms show a radiolucent cortical defect surrounded by sclerosis. This has been characterized as the "dreaded black line" stress fracture, which has a disturbing tendency not to heal even with decreased activity (Fig. 4–10). This fracture also has a tendency to be bilateral, and we have seen several patients who have had similar successive stress fractures during different calendar years.

If simply stopping physical activity does not cause healing, electric stimulation has been tried with some success. Those that do not respond to this may need operative excision and bone grafting. Simple cortical drilling through the fracture site has not been successful in our experience.

Runners and other athletes frequently ask if they can play through the pain of a stress fracture, particularly in the tibia or fibula. We have in some instances gone against our usual advice of not playing until the bone is completely nontender, by using some type of splint or an Aircast stirrup device.[14] If the athlete is able to be active with the device in place and pain does not increase, we are willing to continue with that regimen (Fig. 4–11). Whitelaw's group found this to be effective in

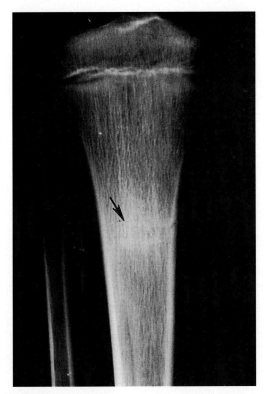

Figure 4–8

Plain film shows reactive sclerosis of a tibial stress fracture in an adolescent runner.

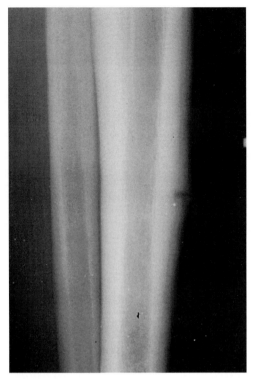

Figure 4–10

Anterior sclerosis of the midtibia with a radiolucent black line.

allowing some athletes to resume sports earlier than usual.[54]

Tibial stress fractures in runners may occasionally be confused with the medial tibial syndrome or more rarely with an anterior exertional compartment syndrome.[8, 37] In the latter instance, the pain always occurs during exercise and ceases once the exercise is stopped. There is no bone tenderness. The medial tibial syndrome does produce pain along the posteromedial border of the tibia. The pain is not as localized as it is with a stress fracture and in many instances is acute with even normal walking. A bone scan does show not the usual focal uptake of a stress fracture but a more diffuse and longer uptake along the posteromedial border of the tibia. Stress fractures of the medial malleolus are rare but important as healing is often delayed.[44, 48]

FIBULA

Fibula stress fractures are not common in runners, but in one study they did affect 6.5% of 320 athletes. The majority occurred in the distal third of the bone and were more rarely noted in the proximal third.[5] Runners complain of pain with running, and that pain is well localized. In some instances, with distal fibula stress fractures near the ankle joint, the pain might be thought to be intraarticular (Fig. 4–12). The subcutaneous location of the fibula makes it easy to make the diagnosis because pain is felt with palpation directly over the area of the stress fracture. Early in the course, radiographs are unlikely to be diagnostic, although at 3 weeks or later they may show an area of sclerosis extending across the bone. A bone scan would be diagnostic.

Differential diagnosis might possibly include an anterior exertional compartment syndrome or peroneal nerve entrapment. With tenderness over the bone and a diagnostic bone scan, however, the fracture is obvious. Avoidance of running and passage of time are the two essentials in the treatment of this stress fracture. When local tenderness abates, training can be resumed. By about

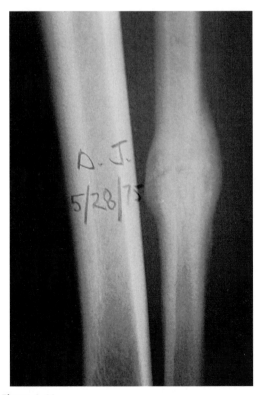

Figure 4–11

Healed fibula stress fracture in a runner who continued to run despite pain.

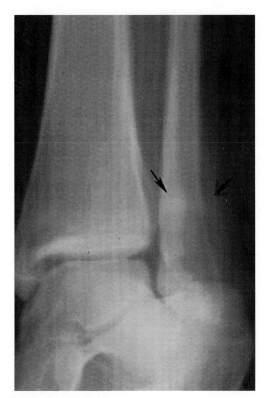

Figure 4–12

The mild area of sclerosis in the distal fibula could be easily overlooked.

6 weeks after the diagnosis, tenderness has usually subsided.

TARSAL BONES

Tarsal bones are frequently involved by stress fractures, as shown in the study by Matheson and coworkers.[33] Twenty-five percent of their 320 patients had stress fractures of the tarsal bones. Various tarsal bones have been noted to have stress fractures, including the calcaneus, the navicular, the medial cuneiform, and the lateral process of the talus.[4, 27, 39]

In military recruits, calcaneal stress fractures were one of the most common reported, but they are less common in runners.[20] Stress fractures involving the tarsal navicular are difficult to diagnose because affected athletes confuse the symptoms with an arch strain or possibly inflammation of the posterior tibial tendon.[51] The frequent history of some trauma accompanying the tarsal bone stress fractures may also interfere with the diagnosis. In the calcaneus and the navicular, local tenderness on palpation is usually striking. Routine radiographs are infrequently diagnostic. Technetium bone scans are the most useful diagnostic test, although in some instances a CT scan shows a fracture (Fig. 4–13). Pronated feet are often noted to be associated with stress fractures of the tarsus, but whether or not they are causative is still undetermined. Interestingly, in some basketball players, cavus feet have been found to be associated with tarsal and metatarsal stress fractures in one study.

Diagnosis of tarsal navicular stress fractures is exceedingly important because they have a disturbing tendency to displace if an athlete continues to be active.[16, 50] Athletes often feel the pain but continue to run despite it, and this may lead to displacement. If this occurs, the fracture must be treated with internal fixation. Even after the cessation of running, the fracture may not heal for 8 to 12 weeks, and local tenderness and pain with activity are the best way to judge how the fracture is healing.

In the calcaneus, the diagnosis is less anxiety provoking. The pain, being localized over the bone, usually in the body of the calcaneus posterior to the talus, should make it relatively easy to differentiate from Achilles tendinitis and other conditions in that area. In some of these patients, the radiographs are diagnostic at 3 weeks, making the diagnosis easier. With calcaneus stress fractures, resumption of running may be possible at 4 to 5 weeks.

METATARSALS

Metatarsal stress fractures were initially the most commonly diagnosed stress fractures when these fractures were thought to occur only in military recruits. Although these fractures remain relatively common in military recruits, they involve a lower but significant number of runners. In Matheson and associates' study, metatarsal stress fractures accounted for 9% of all stress fractures.[33] In my experience (REL), metatarsal stress fractures have been more common than that, particularly in women distance runners.

Pain is brought on by running but in many instances is not intense when walking. The fracture usually occurs in the neck area or in the distal shaft, with the second and third metatarsals much more commonly involved

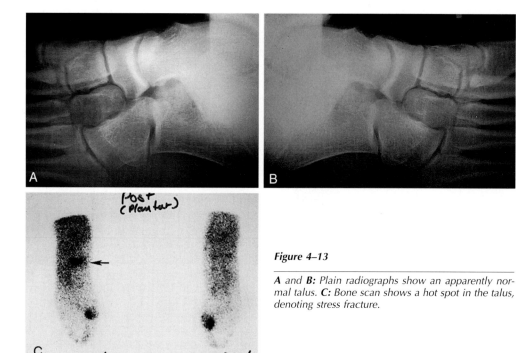

Figure 4–13

A and B: Plain radiographs show an apparently normal talus. C: Bone scan shows a hot spot in the talus, denoting stress fracture.

than others. Some local swelling or point tenderness is present over the bone. This is one of two stress fractures, the other being that of the distal fibula shaft, that we have seen patients literally run through the pain without a splint. However, most people do not run through the pain. Radiographs, if taken after several weeks of involvement, may show sclerosis, a radiolucent line across the bone, or callus. A bone scan is diagnostic. In most instances, it is not necessary to perform a bone scan to establish the diagnosis.

It is rare that these fractures need any immobilization. Four to 6 weeks without running usually suffices to permit healing. The pain disappears quickly after the cessation of running, and runners tend to want to return as soon as they no longer feel pain. Our rule has always been that they should not return to running until they have no tenderness on manual palpation. We have encountered some stress fractures in metatarsals of patients who have worn down a pair of running shoes, thus causing a change of the foot strike. Some runners may benefit from having a metatarsal pad placed behind the area of the fracture to help distribute stress more evenly.

DeLee and colleagues have described the stress fracture of the fifth metatarsal that occurs 1.5 cm distal to the fifth metatarsal tuberosity.[11] This particular fracture is more common in basketball players than in runners. The usual history is a prodromal period of pain with a sudden onset of more acute pain after a misstep, jump, and so on. Radiographs may show a radiolucent line or sclerosis of the medullary canal or, in some instances, an apparent developing nonunion. DeLee and associates recommended internal fixation of this fracture using an intramedullary screw. If this does not secure healing, a bone graft may be needed, but that is unlikely with early fixation. Although this is obviously an important fracture in athletes, it is less common in runners than in certain other athletes.

SESAMOID

A stress fracture of the sesamoid bone of the foot is particularly disabling for a distance runner.[7, 52] The pain usually develops gradually but is exacerbated with faster running. However, because of the exposed position of the sesamoid bone, this stress fracture may cause pain with certain other normal activities such as going up and down stairs. In our experience, the medial sesamoid is involved more frequently than the lateral, but either is a possibility. Localized swelling and pain with

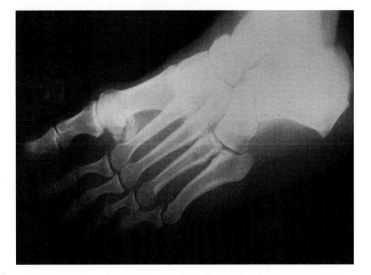

Figure 4–14

Routine films show a fragmented sesamoid as a result of a stress fracture.

direct pressure over the injured bone lead to the correct diagnosis.

This is one instance in which a standard radiograph may be very helpful. Runners with a sesamoid fracture frequently have had symptoms for a while before they seek medical treatment (Fig. 4–14). Standard anteroposterior, lateral, and oblique radiographs should be performed, and they may show the fracture. However, an axial radiograph of the sesamoid is likely to be of even more help. Radiographs must be taken of the contralateral foot because of the possibility of a bipartite sesamoid mimicking a fracture. Bipartite sesamoids are more likely to be bilateral than are stress fractures. The differentiation is important because pain with a bipartite sesamoid may be related to sesamoiditis rather than to a stress fracture. Separation of the sesamoid fragments and irregular edges suggest a stress fracture rather than a bipartite sesamoid. Bone scans may be helpful, but many runners normally have an increased uptake over the first metatarsal head, hindering differentiation between that and the adjacent sesamoid.

Treatment is rest in an orthotic to decrease stress on the sesamoid while transferring weight along the first metatarsal, which may be very helpful. We have found this even more effective than simply making a donut to take pressure off the sesamoid. In some instances, the pain continues and, particularly where the fragments have separated, avascular necrosis of the sesamoid may occur. In these instances, surgical excision may be necessary and curative. One has to be very care-

ful in shelling out the sesamoid not to cut the flexor hallucis brevis tendon, which envelops the sesamoid. Runners can return to competitive long-distance running after a sesamoid excision.

REFERENCES

1. Atwell EA, Jackson DW: Stress fractures of the sacrum in runners: Two case reports. Am J Sports Med 19:531–533, 1991.
2. Barrow GW, Saha S: Menstrual irregularity and stress fractures in collegiate female distance runners. Am J Sports Med 16:209–216, 1988.
3. Belkin SC: Stress fractures in athletes. Orthop Clin North Am 11:735–742, 1980.
4. Black KP, Ehlert KJ: Stress fracture of the lateral process of the talus in a runner. J Bone Joint Surg Am 3:441–443, 1994.
5. Blair WF, Hanley SR: Stress fracture of the proximal fibula. Am J Sports Med 8:212, 1980.
6. Breithaupt MD: Zur Pathologie des Mensch Lichen Fussess. Medizin Zeitung 24:169–177, 1855.
7. Chillag K, Grana WA: Medial sesamoid stress fracture. Orthopedics 8:819–821, 1985.
8. Chisin R, Milgrom C, Giladi M, et al: Clinical significance of nonfocal scintographic findings in suspected tibial stress fractures. Clin Orthop 220:200–205, 1987.
9. Clancy WG Jr, Foltz AS: Iliac apophysitis and stress fractures in adolescent runners. Am J Sports Med 4:214–218, 1976.
10. Cook SD, Harding AF, Thomas KA, et al: Trabecular bone density and menstrual function in women runners. Am J Sports Med 15:503–507, 1987.
11. DeLee JC, Evans JP, Julian J: Stress fracture of the fifth metatarsal. Am J Sports Med 11:349–353, 1983.
12. Devas MB: Stress fractures of the tibia or "shin soreness." J Bone Joint Surg Br 40:227–239, 1958.
13. Devas MB: Stress Fractures. New York, Churchill Livingstone, 1975.
14. Dickson TB, Kichline PD: Functional management of

stress fractures in female athletes using a pneumatic leg brace. Am J Sports Med 15:86, 1987.

15. Drinkwater BL, Nilson K, Chesnut CH III, et al: Bone mineral content of amenorrheic and eumenorrheic athletes. N Engl J Med 311:277–281, 1984.

16. Eisele SA, Sammarco GJ: Fatigue fractures of the foot and ankle in the athlete. J Bone Joint Surg Am 75:290–298, 1993.

17. Fullerton LR: Femoral neck stress fractures. J Sports Med 9:192–197, 1990.

18. Garrett WE Jr, Safran MR, Seaber AV, et al: Biomechanical comparison of stimulated and nonstimulated skeletal muscle pulled to failure. Am J Sports Med 15:448–454, 1987.

19. Giladi M, Milgrom C, Simkin A, Danon Y: Stress fractures: Identifiable risk factors. Am J Sports Med 19:647–652, 1991.

20. Gilbert RS, Johnson HA: Stress fractures in military recruits—a review of twelve years' experience. Milit Med 131:716–721, 1966.

21. Guoping L, Shudong Z, Chen G, et al: Radiologic and histologic analysis of stress fracture in rabbit tibias. Am J Sports Med 13:285–294, 1985.

22. Hershman EB, Lombardo J, Bergfeld JA: Femoral shaft stress fractures in athletes. Clin Sports Med 9:11–19, 1990.

23. Holtzhausen LM, Noakes TD: Stress fracture of the sacrum in two distance runners. Clin Sports Med 2:139–142, 1992.

24. Johnson AW, Weiss CB, Wheeler DL: Stress fractures of the femoral shaft in athletes—more common than expected. Am J Sports Med 22:248–256, 1994.

25. Johnson LK: The kinetics of skeletal remodeling symposia, In Bergsma, Milch (eds): Structural Organization of the Skeleton. Birth Defects. Original Article Series, Rochester, MN, National Foundation 11:66–142, 1966.

26. Jones BH, Harris J, Vinh TN, et al: Exercise-induced stress fractures and reactions of bone: Epidemiology, etiology and classification. Exerc Sport Sci Rev 17:379–472, 1989.

27. Khan KM, Brukner, PD, Bradshaw C: Stress fracture of the medial cuneiform bone in a runner. Clin Sports Med 3:262–264, 1993.

28. Latshaw RF, Kantner TR, Kalenak A, et al: A pelvic stress fracture in a female jogger. Am J Sports Med 9:54, 1981.

29. Lee JK, Yao L: Stress fractures: MR imaging. Radiology 169:217–220, 1988.

30. Lloyd T, Triantafyllou SJ, Baker ER, et al: Women athletes with menstrual irregularity have increased musculoskeletal injuries. Med Sci Sports Exerc 18:374–379, 1986.

31. Martire JR: The role of nuclear medicine bone scans in evaluating pain in athletic injuries. Clin Sports Med 6:713–737, 1987.

32. Marymont JV, Lynch MA, Henning CE: Exercise-related stress of the sacroiliac joint, an unusual cause of low back pain in athletes. Am J Sports Med 14:320–323, 1986.

33. Matheson GO, Clement DB, McKenzie DC, et al: Stress fractures in athletes: A study of 320 cases. Am J Sports Med 15:46–58, 1987.

34. McBryde AM Jr: Stress fractures in runners. In D'Ambrosia R, Drez D Jr (eds): Prevention and Treatment of Running Injuries, 2nd ed. Thorofare, NJ, Slack, 1989, pp 43–82.

35. McMaster JH, Scranton PE, Stanitski CL: On the nature of stress fractures. Am J Sports Med 6:391–396, 1978.

36. Mettler FA, Guiberteau MJ: Essentials of Nuclear Medicine, 2nd ed. Philadelphia, WB Saunders, 1985, pp 269–272.

37. Milgrom C, Chisin R, Giladi M, et al: Negative bone scans and impending tibial stress fractures: A report of three cases. Am J Sports Med 12:488–491, 1984.

38. Monteleone GP Jr: Stress fractures in the athlete. Orthop Clin North Am 26:423–433, 1995.

39. Motto SG: Stress fracture of the lateral process of the talus. J Sports Med Br 27:275–276, 1993.

40. Mubarak SJ, Gould RN, Lee YF, et al: The medial tibial stress syndrome: A cause of shin splints. Am J Sports Med 10:201–205, 1982.

41. Orava S: Stress fractures. Br J Sports Med 14:40–44, 1980.

42. Orava S, Hulko A: Stress fractures of the mid tibial shaft. Acta Orthop Scand 55:35–37, 1984.

43. Orava S, Hulko A: Delayed unions and nonunions of stress fractures in athletes. Am J Sports Med 16:378–382, 1988.

44. Orava S, Karpakka G, Taimela S, et al: J Bone Joint Surg Am 77-A:362–365, 1995.

45. Paul IL, Munro MB, Abernethy PJ, et al: Musculoskeletal shock absorption: Relative contribution of bone and soft tissues at various frequencies. J Biomech 11:237–239, 1978.

46. Schils J, Hauzeur J: Stress fracture of the sacrum. Am J Sports Med 20:769–770, 1992.

47. Scott SH, Winter DA: Internal forces at chronic running injury sites. Med Sci Sports Exerc 22:357–369, 1990.

48. Shelbourne KD, Fisher DA, Rettig AC, McCarroll JR: Stress fractures of the medial malleolus. Am J Sports Med 16:60–63, 1988.

49. Shin AY, Morin WD, Gorman JD, et al: The superiority of magnetic resonance imaging in differentiating the cause of hip pain in endurance athletes. Am J Sports Med 24:168–176, 1996.

50. Sullivan D, Warren RF, Pavlov H, Kelman G: Stress fractures in 51 runners. Clinical Orthop Rel Res 187:188–192, 1984.

51. Torg JS, Pavlov H, Cooley LH, et al: Stress fractures of the tarsal navicular. A retrospective review of twenty-one cases. J Bone Joint Surg Am 64:700–712, 1982.

52. Van Hal ME, Keene JS, Lange TA, Clancy WG Jr: Stress fractures of the great toe sesamoids. Am J Sports Med 10:122–128, 1982.

53. Walter NE, Wolf MD: Stress fractures in young athletes. Am J Sports Med 5:165–170, 1977.

54. Whitelaw GP, Wetzler MJ, Levy AS, et al: A pneumatic leg brace for the treatment of tibial stress fractures. Clin Orthop Rel Res 270:301–305, 1991.

55. Wilcox JR Jr, Monoit AL, Green JP: Bone scarring in the evaluation of exercise-related stress injuries. Radiology 123:699–703, 1977.

CHAPTER FIVE

The Adolescent Runner

In the past several years, running as a sport has become increasingly popular among children and adolescents of both sexes. Consequently, running injuries in children and adolescents have become more common.

The majority of pediatric running injuries are due to overuse and involve the apophyses. The apophyses are growth plates under tension from a musculotendinous insertion. Patellofemoral pain is another common problem among adolescent runners. Some of these injuries result from parents' and coaches' pressure to excel, as well as lack of knowledge about injury prevention.

It is safe for children to run. Children have been running in sports such as basketball and soccer for decades without too many problems. Guidelines for children's sports participation in running as a sport should be proper footwear, gradual progressive increase in distance and speed, and realistic and reasonable goals for children such as local competitions and shorter distances. Children should not run in marathons, for instance.

Some of the general treatment guidelines for children's running injuries are to modify the activity level, change to alternative exercises temporarily, and obtain better support for the legs and feet. Thermal treatments such as ice or heat and medications such as vitamins and nonsteroidal antiinflammatory drugs (NSAIDs) or acetaminophen may be tried. In addition, a good surface and proper equipment help child runners return more readily to running as a sport. Healthful nutrition and appropriate adequate fluids are also necessary for these young athletes.[2]

The following sections describe specific running injuries in adolescents and children and highlight their treatment.

OSGOOD-SCHLATTER DISEASE

Osgood-Schlatter disease[5–9] should not be called a disease. It is a traction apophysitis of the tibial tubercle caused by repetitive traction trauma to the apophysis with a resulting tender prominence of the tibial tubercle. A lateral radiograph of the knee reveals this prominence, and a separate ossicle formation is often noted (Fig. 5–1). Treatment consisting of temporary activity moderation, icing after running, and optional use of a Chopat knee strap is usually adequate. Severe recalcitrant cases can occasionally be treated in a knee immobilizer or cylinder cast. Very painful lesions persisting into adulthood sometimes re-

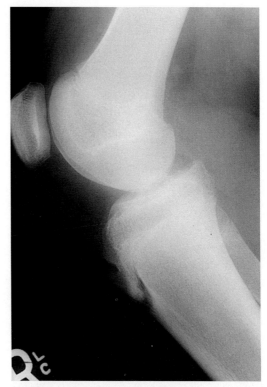

Figure 5–1

Separate ossicle formation and prominence of the tibial tubercle in a 16-year-old patient with Osgood-Schlatter disease.

quire surgical removal of the ossicle through a patellar tendon-splitting approach. In the majority of cases, all pain is resolved by skeletal maturity.

SINDING-LARSEN-JOHANSSON SYNDROME

Sinding-Larsen-Johansson syndrome[5-9] is a traction apophysitis of the inferior patellar pole. Radiographically, slight separation and elongation of the inferior patellar pole is seen on the lateral view of the knee (Fig. 5-2). Nonsurgical treatment is essentially the same as that of Osgood-Schlatter disease. All of these lesions adequately resolve by skeletal maturity without any need for surgery.

ADOLESCENT HIP POINTER

Adolescent hip pointer[10] is an avulsion injury of a musculotendinous origin from its pelvic apophysis (Fig. 5-3). It may be either

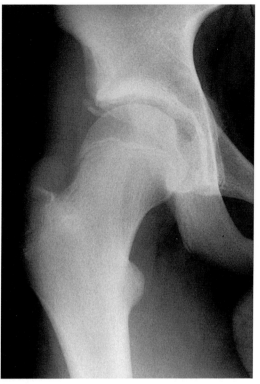

Figure 5-3

Acute avulsion fracture at anterior inferior iliac spine (adolescent hip pointer).

an acute or chronic injury. Treatment consists of rest, NSAIDs, and physical therapy modalities. These lesions heal at varying rates without the need for surgery. They are at times painful enough to require crutches temporarily.

PATELLOFEMORAL PAIN SYNDROME

Patellofemoral pain syndrome[1] presents as generalized complaints of anterior knee pain without any history of trauma. This condition is particularly prevalent in female cross-country runners. Malalignment of the lower extremity is related to the development of patellofemoral pain syndrome. The malalignment findings typically are a constellation of foot pronation, external tibial torsion, genu valgum, and increased internal rotation at the hips. This malalignment causes the patella to track abnormally laterally.

Runners with patellofemoral pain syndrome typically complain of anterior knee

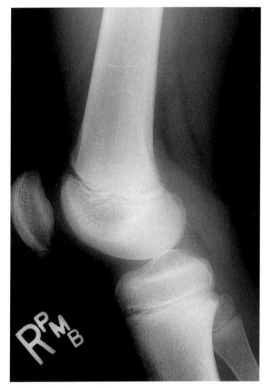

Figure 5-2

Elongation of the inferior patellar pole in an adolescent with Sinding-Larsen-Johansson syndrome.

pain, patellar instability, painful cracking from the patella, and the knee giving way. Their pain is increased by climbing stairs and hills.

Physical examination should evaluate patellar tracking with active knee flexion and extension. When the patella is passively pushed laterally, patients usually have apprehension from a sensation that the patella will subluxate or dislocate. The previously mentioned malalignment findings are usually present. The Q angle is greater than 20 degrees. Patellofemoral compression elicits pain.

Radiographic examination may reveal lateral tilting or subluxation on the patellar views (Fig. 5–4). A lateral radiograph may demonstrate patella alta. The normal ratio of patellar length to patellar tendon length is no greater than 1:1.2. Increased patellar tendon length indicates patella alta, and a decrease indicates patella baja.

An appropriate physical therapy program should be faithfully pursued for at least 3 months before surgery is considered. Temporary use of a patellar stabilizing brace may allow patients to remain more asymptomatic during conservative treatment. Patients with pronated feet may find benefit from orthotics.

For the occasional patient who fails to respond to conservative management, surgical intervention is considered. Arthroscopic lateral release is usually the primary procedure of choice for a runner. The rehabilitation time is much shorter than with more extensive procedures. However, the surgeon and patient must be aware that lateral release has a high rate of failure (20%) and complications. Contraindications to lateral release are patella alta and excessive passive medial glide on examination.

For those runners for whom lateral release surgery fails or for whom it is contraindicated, proximal realignment procedures may be considered even for skeletally immature patients. Distal realignment procedures are contraindicated in skeletally immature patients but may be required for mature patients. Rehabilitation and a return to running are much more difficult for patients who undergo realignment procedures.

Adolescent and child runners also may be candidates for an additional procedure that is different from that in adults because of a child's open growth plates. Several of my patients with the malalignment syndrome and genu valgum have been successfully treated for their patellofemoral pain by distal medial femoral physeal stapling. Obviously, this technique cannot be useful in skeletally mature patients.

Three staples are placed, bridging the distal medial physis extraperiosteally without damage to the perichondral ring or growth plate or to the joint surface. The staples are removed after adequate correction or slight overcorrection is obtained. Some rebound genu valgum may occasionally occur after staple removal.

SEVER'S APOPHYSITIS

Sever's apophysitis[5, 6, 9] is a painful inflammatory condition of the apophysis of the calcaneal tuberosity. The pain may also extend into the plantar fascia or tendo Achillis. Sever's apophysitis may be unilateral but most often occurs bilaterally. Heel pain occurs with weight-bearing activities. Tenderness on palpation of the calcaneal apophysis is noted on examination. An element of Achilles tendon contracture is often observed. Radiographs are essentially nondiagnostic and are taken to rule out other pathologic conditions. Treatment consists of rest or activity modifi-

Figure 5–4

Laterally tilted, mildly subluxated patellae in an adolescent girl with malalignment and patellofemoral pain syndrome.

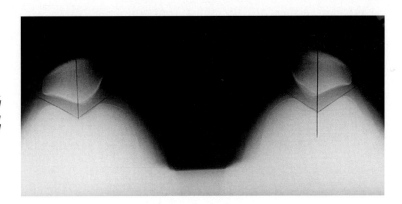

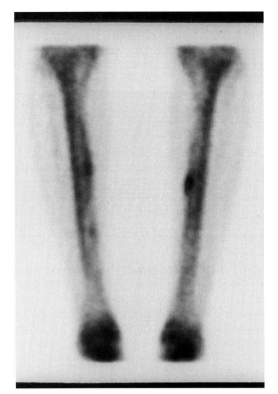

Figure 5–5

Bilateral tibial stress fractures, seen as areas of increased uptake on bone scintigraphy, in an adolescent girl.

cation, the use of viscoelastic heel cups or pedorthotics, NSAIDs, icing, tendo Achillis stretching, and in severe recalcitrant cases walking casts. Sever's apophysitis invariably resolves with closure of the calcaneal apophysis at skeletal maturity.

STRESS FRACTURES

Stress fractures are rare in young runners and not uncommon in adolescents.[3, 4, 9] Tibial or metatarsal sites are the most common. Runners often report a history of a recent increase in miles. Bone scan is the best early diagnostic tool because radiographs are often nondiagnostic (Fig. 5–5). Rest is required until the symptoms resolve. This typically takes 4 to 6 weeks. Orthotics and proper shoes, both for better shock absorption, help prevent recurrence, particularly in runners with flat feet.

CONCLUSION

As running continues to grow in popularity for young patients, overuse injuries will continue to become more prevalent. In general, all of the conditions described in this chapter are alleviated by modification of activity and other conservative measures. In many cases, as Frank Shorter has noted, "children are wonderfully self limiting." However, as running for sport becomes more important to young athletes and to their parents and coaches, orthopedists will continue to see increasing numbers of young runners with injuries and musculoskeletal problems.

REFERENCES

 1. Brody D: Running Injuries. Ciba Clin Symp 32:2–34, 1980.
 2. Burrington JD: Exercise and children. Compr Ther 6:60–67, 1980.
 3. D'Ambrosia R: Prevention and treatment of running injuries. Clin Symp 39:1–7, 1987.
 4. Maffulli N: Intense training in young athletes. Sports Med 9:229–243, 1990.
 5. Micheli L: Sports injuries in children. Curr Probl Pediatr 12:1–54, 1982.
 6. Micheli L: The traction apophysites. Clin Sports Med 6:389–405, 1987.
 7. Micheli L: Overuse injuries in children's sports; the growth factor. Orthop Clin North Am 14:337–360, 1993.
 8. Micheli L, Fehlandt A: Overuse injuries to tendons and apophysis in children. Clin Sports Med 11:713–726, 1992.
 9. Micheli L, Ireland L: Prevention and management of calcaneal apophysites in children: An overuse syndrome. J Pediatr Orthop 7:34–38, 1987.
10. Paty J, Swafford D: Adolescent running injuries. J Adolesc Health Care 5:87–90, 1984.

CHARLES J. GATT, JR.

CHAPTER SIX

Back Pain in Running

Within the general population, as many as 70% of people will complain of back pain at some time in their lives. In general, these are self-limiting episodes and require no formal medical treatment. For the running population, back pain is not as common as injuries of the lower extremities. In a survey of 10,754 runners, back pain was last on the list of the 12 most common running injuries, accounting for 1.8% and 2.0% of the injuries in men and women, respectively.[11] The typical patient with back pain has traditionally been thought of as a middle-aged, overweight individual leading a sedentary lifestyle. Because typical runners are neither sedentary nor overweight, few are affected by back pain.

Through the years, *Runner's World* has educated the running population about injuries. The articles related to knee, ankle, and foot pain have been plentiful. On the other hand, little attention has been paid to low back pain in runners. In fact, only about three articles in the past 15 years have addressed the topic of low back pain. Although the earliest of the articles discussed the controversy about the positive and negative effects of running on the low back,[9] the other two more recent articles described how running can help prevent or treat low back pain.[24, 34]

ANATOMY OF THE SPINE

The spine is an articulation of bony segments called *vertebrae*. These vertebrae protect the spinal cord, located in the vertebral foramen, from injury. The transverse processes and the spinous processes provide sites for ligament and muscle attachments (Fig. 6–1). To allow motion, the vertebral bodies are connected by interposed intervertebral discs as well as by the intervertebral ligaments and muscles. The two synovial joints in the poste-

rior aspect of the vertebral body are referred to as the *facet joints* and are composed of superior and inferior articular processes (Fig. 6–2).

The spine is composed of a total of 33 vertebral bodies, which are thought of as divided into five sections. The cervical spine, comprising seven vertebrae, is in the neck area. The thoracic spine, composed of 12 vertebrae, articulates with the ribs. The lumbar spine, which has five vertebral bodies and is in the lower part of the back, is of most interest to the running population. It also is the lowest area that allows movement between the vertebral motion segments or between one vertebral body and another. The remaining vertebral bodies of the sacral and the coccygeal spine are fused.

Superior View

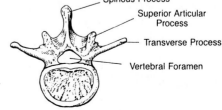

Lateral View

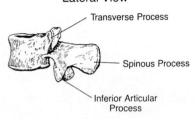

Figure 6–1

Anatomy of the vertebral body. (From Stover CN, McCarroll JR, Mallon WJ [eds]: Feeling up to Par: Medicine from Tee to Green. Philadelphia, FA Davis, 1994, p 101.)

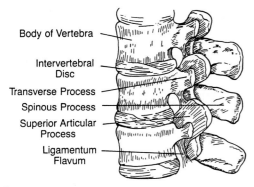

Figure 6–2

Anatomy of the spinal motion segment. (From Stover CN, McCarroll JR, Mallon WJ [eds]: Feeling up to Par: Medicine from Tee to Green. Philadelphia, FA Davis, 1994, p 101.)

The ligaments and intervertebral discs allow motion in the cervical, thoracic, and lumbar regions of the spine. Intervertebral discs act as thick-walled, deformable shock absorbers that contain fluid under pressure. When subjected to stress, a disc responds by developing a corresponding increase in intradiscal pressure or by remodeling.[1] The other load-sharing structures of the lumbar motion segment are the facet joints. Facet joints help in the distribution of stress applied to the lower back by working in tandem with the intervertebral discs. Studies have shown that the facets carry as much as 20% of the spinal compression load in the upright, standing position and more than 50% of the anterior shear load affecting the lumbar spine in the forward flexed position.[29]

BIOMECHANICS OF THE SPINE

A general overview of spine mechanics helps put into perspective the forces generated in the low back during running. As a mechanical model, each spinal motion seg-

ment has six degrees of freedom. That is to say, each motion segment is affected by a combination of three forces and three moments (Fig. 6–3). Linear forces acting on the spine are (1) compressive, in a craniocaudal direction; (2) shear, in an anteroposterior direction; and (3) lateral shear, in a laterolateral direction. Rotational moments act about each of the three coordinate axes. Flexion-extension moments cause rotation about the transverse (laterolateral) axis. Lateral bending moments lead to rotation about the midsagittal (anteroposterior) axis. Rotation about the longitudinal (craniocaudal) axis is due to axial rotation moments.

Compressive forces have been by far the most extensively studied. This is mostly because of the interest in herniated nucleus pulposus and the effect that compressive loads have on the intervertebral discs. Adams and Hutton demonstrated that an average compression load of 5448 N produced prolapse of the intervertebral disc in a cadaver spine.[1] Although normal discs are well suited to withstand these compression loads, with aging, discs degenerate and lose their viscoelastic properties, increasing susceptibility to injury and increasing the amount of load resisted by the facet joints and posterior vertebral structures. This increased loading of the facet joints may also lead to development of low back pain and disability. Although the lumbar facet joints are well oriented to resist shear loading, when shear loading is combined with compression forces, the facets resist approximately one half to one third of the shear force while the intervertebral disc between the vertebral bodies resists the remaining force.

Some of the most clinically useful studies of forces on the intervertebral discs were performed by Nachemson.[31] In his studies, a needle pressure transducer was inserted into the lumbar intervertebral discs of subjects to measure pressures as they performed various ac-

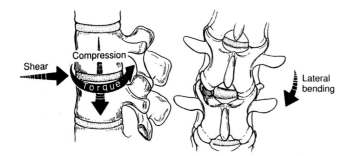

Figure 6–3

Spinal motion in three planes. (From Stover CN, McCarroll JR, Mallon WJ [eds]: Feeling up to Par: Medicine from Tee to Green, Philadelphia, FA Davis, 1994, p 102.)

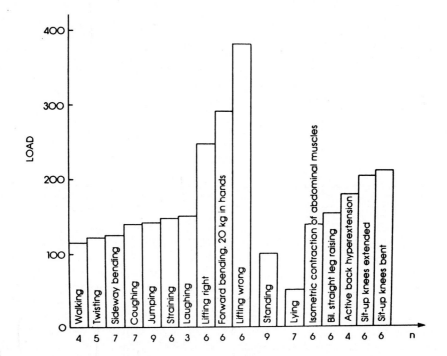

Figure 6–4

Intradiscal pressure generated during various activities. (From Nachemson A, Elfstrom C: Scand J Rehabil Med Suppl 1:31, 1970.)

tivities. Lying in the supine position generated a force of approximately 250 N; standing upright, a force of 1000 N; unsupported sitting, a force of 1500 N; and standing with a 20-degree forward lean, holding a 20-kg weight, a force of approximately 2200 N (Fig. 6–4).

Mathematic modeling and motion analysis have been used to estimate forces on the lumbar spine in weightlifting,[17] rowing,[20] golf,[21] and football blocking.[15] In all of these activities, the compression forces on the lumbar spine have been shown to exceed five times body weight. Participants in all of these activities have a higher incidence of low back pain than the general population.[2]

BIOMECHANICS OF WALKING AND RUNNING

During walking and running, the musculoskeletal system generates forces to propel the body forward. Because the net movement of the body is forward and posture is basically upright, shear and lateral shear forces are not of great magnitude. The same is true of axial rotation and lateral bending moments. However, in order to move forward, the musculo-

skeletal system must generate enough force to raise the body's center of gravity and then absorb the force of heel strike. As a result, the compressive forces and flexion-extension bending moments generated during running are of significant magnitude.

Lumbar spine forces during level walking have been predicted by gait analysis studies.[6, 8] A combination of video data and electromyographic (EMG) data provided the information necessary for mathematic modeling to predict the lumbar spine forces. According to Cappozzo, the most significant trunk muscular activation occurs in the trunk extensor muscles (erector spinae).[6] This occurs at the time of heel strike to decelerate the trunk and stabilize it over the pelvis. The trunk lateral benders (one-sided erector spinae and abdominal obliques) also contract at the time of contralateral heel strike to prevent excessive lateral trunk movement as the center of gravity of the trunk is shifted over the supporting limb.[8] Because little side-to-side motion occurs during walking, studies have focused on the compression forces in the spine. During level walking, the estimated compression force on the lower lumbar spine is approximately 1.2 times body weight (or approximately 840 N).[6, 8]

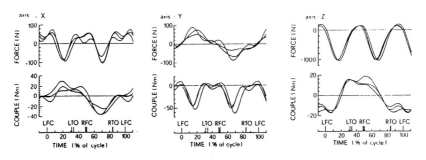

Figure 6–5

Intersegmental force and couple components. (From Cappozzo A: Force actions in the human trunk during running. J Sports Med 23:14–22, 1983.)

Cappozzo used the same modeling techniques to estimate the forces on the lumbar spine during running.[7] He found that the patterns of muscular activation did not differ from those of level walking (Fig. 6–5). As in walking, the compressive forces were of far greater magnitude than the horizontal components. The peak compressive forces were approximately 3.1 times the weight of the portion of the body above L4. The force along the anteroposterior axis was 0.4 times the upper body weight, and the force along the laterolateral axis was also 0.4 times body weight. The rotational couple of greatest magnitude, ranging from 50 to 110 Nm, was about the laterolateral (flexion-extension) axis. This was a flexion couple that was resisted by the erector spinae muscles. The lateral bending couple about the anteroposterior axis was between 60 and 100 Nm. EMG tracings demonstrated that erector spinae muscles were activated to control lateral bending (Fig.

6–6). Based on his observations, Cappozzo concluded that muscular engagement of trunk muscles should not be significantly different between running and walking. However, he did note that running posture did affect muscle activity. Two runners in the study who ran with excessive forward lean generated substantially greater flexion-extension couples than the rest of the study group.

In general, the forces and moments generated in the spine during running are of magnitudes that do not place the spine at risk for injury. However, biomechanical abnormalities may increase the force and lead to aggravation or exacerbation of existing low back problems. The example of excessive forward leaning has already been mentioned. Another biomechanical deviation not uncommon to runners is excessive pronation of the feet. Pronation leads to increased internal tibial rotation, which places increased stress on the lower back, probably because of increased

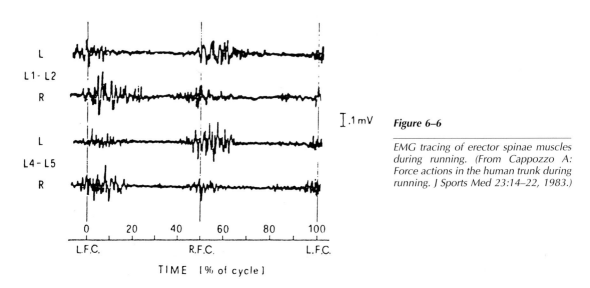

$\text{I}.1\,\text{mV}$

Figure 6–6

EMG tracing of erector spinae muscles during running. (From Cappozzo A: Force actions in the human trunk during running. J Sports Med 23:14–22, 1983.)

transverse plane motion in the lower extremities.[27] Hill training is another example of a biomechanical deviation from running on a level surface. Many runners are told to lean into the hill when faced with a hill. As a result, they assume a more forward flexed posture, moving the upper body center of gravity more anterior to the lumbar spine, resulting in increased lumbar extensor muscle activity and therefore increased compression forces on the spine.

MUSCULAR LOW BACK PAIN

The vast majority of patients evaluated for acute low back pain are eventually found to have some type of muscular or ligamentous strain. The vague nature of the diagnosis stems from the fact that in most cases, the symptoms resolve with minimal if any treatment and diagnostic studies usually do not lead to a specific diagnosis. In general, runners usually do not seek treatment for acute low back pain for fear of being told they must take a few days off from their training schedule. The attitude is one of expectancy. They wait for the symptoms to persist before seeking medical advice.

Because most low back pain is short lived and most affected individuals do not seek treatment, it is difficult to report on the natural history of acute low back pain. It has been reported that the natural history of low back pain is that 50% of patients recover by 2 weeks and 90% by 3 months.[14] Although many different forms of treatment have been tried during the past 25 years, studies have failed to demonstrate the efficacy of corsets, bed rest, transcutaneous nerve stimulation, or conventional traction. In fact, 2 days of bed rest has proved as effective as 7 days for patients with acute low back pain. Furthermore, patients who received 2 days of bed rest missed 45% fewer days of work than those who received 7 days of bed rest.[10]

The history of acute low back pain is highly variable. Patients' presenting complaint is pain in the low back. The onset can be insidious, such as waking up in the morning with a stiff low back. Some patients report a day of heavy work around the house that led to nighttime soreness in the lower back. Others associate their symptoms with a minor incident such as bending over to pick up a light object. In any case, the pain in the low back may be anywhere from the midline to one side or radiating to the top of the buttocks. The quality of the pain is also highly variable, ranging from a burning pain to a deep, dull ache. It is helpful to ask if similar episodes have occurred in the past, how long they lasted, and how they were treated.

Physical examination is also of little help in arriving at a specific diagnosis. However, it is important to pay attention to detail during the examination to avoid missing the diagnosis of a herniated disc, spinal stenosis, or other anatomic pathologic cause of the symptoms. Palpation of the lumbar spine and paraspinal muscles may reveal areas of tenderness or spasm. Flexion, extension, and side bending may be restricted owing to pain. It may be helpful to perform resistive muscle testing in flexion, extension, and side bending in an attempt to identify a muscle group that may have sustained a strain injury. Next, a detailed neurologic examination is conducted to rule out compression of the spinal cord or nerve roots. These are discussed in more detail in the following sections. The straight-leg raise may cause pain in the low back but should not result in radiating pain in the posterior aspect of the leg, especially distal to the knee.

Radiologic studies add very little to the workup. Plain radiographs of the lumbar spine are initially obtained. Anteroposterior and lateral views of the lumbar spine are usually adequate for patients presenting with acute low back pain and no physical examination findings consistent with neurologic involvement. These films almost always show normal findings (Fig. 6–7). They may occasionally show a loss of lumbar lordosis. This may be a result of the patient's posture, the radiographic technique, or extensive muscle spasm. The plain films are most helpful in precluding a pathologic source of the pain, such as a neoplastic process. Magnetic resonance imaging (MRI) is frequently ordered to rule out a herniated disc. It is surprising how many patients present to the office with an MRI scan in hand and no plain radiographs. MRI is very expensive compared with plain radiographs, and recent studies have cited the high rate of false-positive interpretations of MRI findings. In a study of asymptomatic individuals with no history of back pain, 20% of subjects younger than 60 years had MRI findings consistent with a herniated lumbar disc. Fifty-five percent of those older than 60 had positive findings on MRI scan.[4]

It is obvious from this discussion that providing patients with a specific diagnosis such

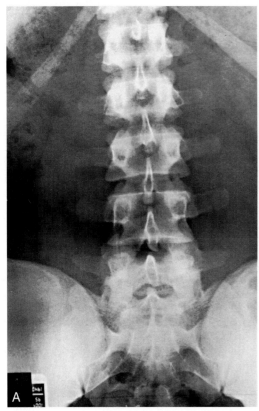
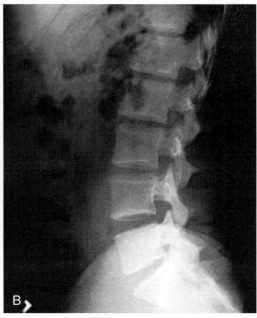

Figure 6–7

A and *B:* *Radiographs of the lumbar spine.*

as a strain of the right musculus iliocostalis lumborum is unlikely. Most patients leave the office with a diagnosis of an acute musculo-ligamentous injury of the lower back. This lack of specificity does not alter or diminish the attention paid to treatment of the injury. As with any acute muscular or ligamentous injury, rest and ice are helpful in alleviating the acute symptoms. For runners, 2 days of bed rest may be intolerable. It is more practical to ask them to cut back on distance and pace for a few days until the symptoms have resolved. Stretching and a longer warm-up than normal usually allow runners to complete a workout with minimal discomfort. Avoidance of hilly terrain is also a wise recommendation. Ice applied to the lower back after a run may lessen the next day's soreness and reduce any inflammation that may occur as a result of the run. Aspirin or nonsteroidal antiinflammatory drugs (NSAIDs) also help to diminish the inflammatory response to the acute injury. Patients in general, but especially runners, need to be reassured that the symptoms should resolve within a few weeks and that return to work or workouts should be guided by their symptoms. An acute epi-

sode of low back pain that is not completely resolved within 2 months may warrant a more extensive workup.

LUMBAR DISC DISEASE

The vast majority of patients who are evaluated for low back problems have isolated low back pain and are diagnosed with lumbar strains. When patients present complaining of low back pain with associated symptoms in one or both legs, a herniated lumbar disc must be considered in the diagnosis. Compared with the 70% lifetime incidence of low back pain, the incidence of back pain with radiating leg pain ranges from 13% to 40%.[2]

Running has not been implicated as one of the risk factors for herniated lumbar disc. Frymoyer[13] reviewed the epidemiology of lumbar disc disease. Studies analyzing the risk factors have found that men have a slightly higher incidence of lumbar disc disease than women. In both groups, the peak incidence is in the fifth decade of life, rarely occurs before age 20 years, and declines after the fifth decade. Patients in the highest quintile for height and weight may have a minimally increased risk for disc disease, but runners rarely fall into this category. Smoking, vibration, and occupation are three associations that have been thoroughly evaluated as risk factors. The vibration associated with disc problems occurs at a frequency similar to that of vehicular driving. Occupations that require heavy lifting present a greater risk for lumbar disc herniations.

Although the affected intervertebral disc probably has preexisting disease, most patients report a history of a specific incident that led to the onset of their symptoms. If they are questioned carefully, a prior history of mild low back pain with radicular symptoms can often be elicited. Patients usually complain of pain on one side of the lower back, radiating down the back of one leg. After prolonged periods of activity, they complain of tingling in the same distribution. It is not common for patients to complain of weakness. However, they do notice decreased sensation and usually describe a dermatomal distribution of the numbness. Use of a pain drawing can be helpful in documenting the presenting complaints (Fig. 6–8).

On physical examination, mild to severe paraspinal spasm may be noted. Extension of the spine does not increase symptoms, but patients are quite reluctant to flex at the spine. Results of straight-leg raise test and sometimes a contralateral straight-leg raise test are positive. Sensory examination demonstrates decreased perception to light touch in a dermatomal distribution. Motor examination may reveal decreased strength. Again, the deficit should correlate with involvement of a single nerve root. For instance, a problem at the L4–L5 level is manifested as extensor hallucis longus weakness, because this muscle has essentially isolated L5 innervation. Examination of unilateral diminished reflexes should include both the patellar tendon reflex for L4–L5 disc involvement and the Achilles tendon reflex for L5–S1 involvement.

Radiographic evaluation should begin with plain radiographs of the lumbar spine. Disc space narrowing may be apparent and may occur in conjunction with degenerative changes at the suspected level of involvement. In the past, computed tomography (CT) scans with or without a myelogram have demonstrated a disc bulge impinging on the dural sac and nerve roots. MRI has become the radiographic study of choice for most clinicians because it does not involve exposure to x-rays and the anatomy is clearly demon-

Please fill out the pain drawing. This will tell us where your pain is now and something about it.

Mark the areas on your body where you feel pain. Use the following patterns:
NUMBNESS━━ PINS and NEEDLES OOO BURNING XXX
STABBING / / / ACHING +++ OTHER ∗∗∗

Figure 6–8

Pain drawing by a patient with a herniated lumbar disc. (From Brown MD: The pathophysiology and diagnosis of low back pain and sciatica. Instr Course Lect 41:217–224, 1992.)

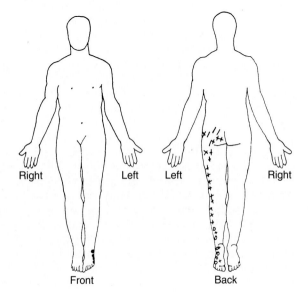

Right   Left   Left   Right

Front   Back

strated without the need for contrast dye in the spinal canal. The herniated portion of the disc can usually be visualized, as well as compression of the dural sac and nerve roots.

If running exacerbates a patient's symptoms, it may prove helpful to watch him or her run. Some runners maintain an exaggerated forward lean while running, resulting in loss of lumbar lordosis and increased activity of the lumbar paraspinal extensor muscles. This leads to increased compression forces in the lumbar spine and may aggravate a preexisting diseased disc level.

For patients presenting with a relatively acute onset of radicular symptoms, rest is the first line of treatment. Breaking the spasm with narcotic pain medications, NSAIDs, and muscle relaxants may help patients shorten the early phase of the injury. In the past, prolonged rest and pelvic traction were often prescribed as definitive treatment. Obviously, this form of treatment was not well accepted by the running population. Through the years, the period of rest has shortened, and mobility, strengthening, and activity have been emphasized as soon as symptoms permit. Williams or McKenzie exercises under the supervision of a physical therapist trained in these techniques can speed recovery and, more importantly, avoid a rehabilitation routine that may exacerbate symptoms rather than alleviate them.[30]

If a course of rest and physical therapy is unsuccessful in alleviating symptoms, some minimally invasive procedures may help. Chymopapain injections were popular several years ago but have fallen out of favor because of anaphylactic reactions. Epidural steroid injections provide a mechanism for delivery of a strong antiinflammatory directly to the site of involvement. For patients who have not had a favorable response to physical therapy and who wish to avoid surgery, this is an option. The literature on epidural steroid injections for acute herniated lumbar discs is equivocal.[12]

The only absolute indication for immediate lumbar disc excision is cauda equina syndrome.[5] This is a massive prolapse of a lumbar disc that results in severe back pain, bilateral leg pain, inability to stand or void, and neurologic deficits in both lower extremities. Patients may also have decreased rectal tone and perianal anesthesia. Functionally significant muscle weakness is a strong relative indication for surgical treatment. However, most patients undergo surgery for pain. In the past,

lumbar disc excision included bilateral laminectomies at the involved level, and recovery time was long. Now, more attention is paid to removing the disc with minimal surgical trauma. In many cases, an open diskectomy requires minimal muscle stripping from the posterior aspect of the spine, excision of the ligamentum flavum at the involved level, a small foraminotomy, and finally excision of the herniated disc. Percutaneous lumbar diskectomies are being performed at several centers around the country, with good results in properly selected patients.[16]

CASE REPORT

A 37-year-old man presented complaining of a 6-week history of low back pain with radiation to his right lower extremity. At the onset, the patient had mild low back pain that he attributed to a busy work schedule. He was a salesman who spent a lot of time in the car and had to carry heavy boxes to his meetings. In addition, the patient was a 40- to 50-mile-a-week runner with no recent increase in training or mileage. At the onset, the patient was able to maintain his usual mileage without difficulty. Approximately 2 weeks later, he bent over to pick up a box and on arising had excruciating pain in the back of his right leg.

Physical examination revealed signs consistent with a herniated L5–S1 disc. He had moderate paraspinal spasm. Ipsilateral straight-leg raise caused pain down the back of his leg and into his foot. Contralateral straight-leg raise also caused pain radiating down the back of his right leg. He had 5/5 strength on manual muscle testing of the quadriceps, hamstrings, ankle dorsiflexors, ankle plantar flexors, ankle evertors, hallux dorsiflexors, and hallux plantar flexors. Sensory examination demonstrated decreased sensation on the lateral aspect of the right foot. Patellar tendon reflexes and Achilles tendon reflexes were equal and symmetric.

Results of radiographs of the lumbar spine were normal. An MRI verified a herniated lumbar disc at the L5–S1 level, with impingement of the right S1 nerve root (Fig. 6–9).

The initial treatment consisted of rest, NSAIDs, and a narcotic pain medication. After 3 days, the severity of the pain was significantly decreased and the patient was started

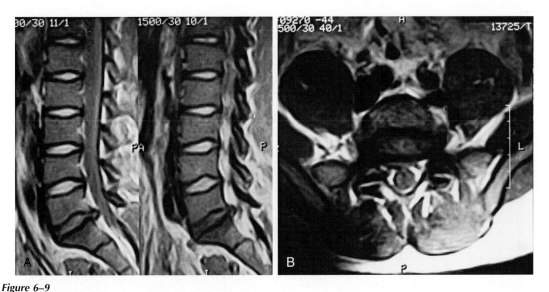

Figure 6–9

A and B: MRI scans showing L5–S1 disc herniation.

on physical therapy. This consisted of local modalities such as ultrasound and hot and cold massage. In addition, a program was begun to improve lumbar flexibility and strength. After 2 weeks, with further improvement of his condition, the patient felt ready to resume running. He started running on flat, soft surfaces every other day. By 6 weeks from his first evaluation, he had returned to his usual weekly mileage, was working, and had incorporated some of his low back exercises into his daily routine.

This case was presented to demonstrate that even in the presence of true radicular symptoms and an MRI scan that clearly established a herniated disc, nonoperative treatment is the first line of treatment. Had this patient had a progression of his symptoms despite the physical therapy, surgery would have been indicated.

SPINAL STENOSIS

More a condition of the elderly, spinal stenosis accounts for a significant percentage of patients evaluated for back pain. Spinal stenosis has been defined as an abnormal narrowing of the osteoligamentous vertebral canal or the intervertebral foramina. It is responsible for compression of the dural sac or the caudal nerve roots.[32] Note that this definition appropriately excludes disc hernia-

tion, because the two conditions have different prognoses.

The average age of onset is between the fifth and sixth decades of life. Men reportedly are more commonly affected than women, but this has been disputed.[18] Running has not been implicated as a risk factor for spinal stenosis. However, several studies have cited occupations that involve heavy manual labor as a risk factor.[25] Although many syndromes and disease states have been associated with the development of spinal stenosis, the vast majority of cases are due to degenerative changes in the lumbar spine.

Patients present complaining of low back pain that is mechanical in nature. Activity exacerbates the pain, and rest relieves it. The pain usually radiates bilaterally to the buttocks and produces a burning sensation in the back of the thighs. Bending forward does not produce significant discomfort, but extension of the spine worsens the symptoms. Patients occasionally complain of radicular symptoms. A more common complaint is neurogenic claudication. Patients complain of pain, numbness, or cramping in both lower extremities. The distribution does not follow a dermatomal pattern. Walking or standing usually leads to the onset of these symptoms, and they are alleviated by sitting or leaning forward.

Peripheral vascular disease is not a common condition in the running population. However, this condition can be confused with neurogenic claudication. Patients with vascu-

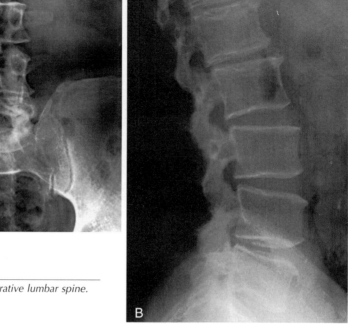

Figure 6–10

A and B: Radiographs of degenerative lumbar spine.

lar claudication complain of pain and cramping in the calf muscles associated with activity. With continued activity, such as walking or running, the pain migrates proximally. Cessation of the activity alleviates the symptoms because muscle demand for blood supply is decreased. In neurogenic claudication secondary to spinal stenosis, a position change such as sitting or leaning forward controls the symptoms. It is believed that bending forward stretches the thickened ligamentum flavum, thereby decreasing its thickness and increasing the volume of the spinal canal.

Paraspinal muscle spasm is not a usual finding in the physical examination of patients with spinal stenosis. Patients can usually bend forward, but extension of the lumbar spine is limited and painful. Straight-leg testing usually does not elicit pain. Manual muscle testing and sensory testing are also inconsistently affected in patients with spinal stenosis. Reflex testing usually reveals symmetric findings.

Radiographs usually show evidence of degenerative changes (Fig. 6–10). Anteriorly, osteophytes may be present on the superior and inferior aspects of the vertebral bodies. Posteriorly, sclerosis and hypertrophy of the facet joints usually are present. Imaging studies that display the spinal canal in cross section such as CT scan, CT myelogram, or MRI demonstrate the decreased area of the canal and the encroachment of the degenerative processes on the exiting nerve roots (Fig. 6–11).

Running involves repeated hyperextension of the spine; therefore, symptoms of spinal

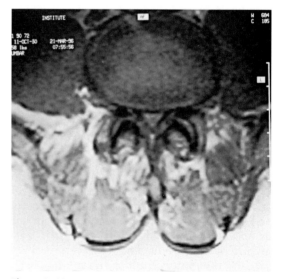

Figure 6–11

MRI scan showing lumbar spinal stenosis.

stenosis are usually exacerbated by prolonged running. Because stenosis is more a problem of the elderly and is associated with advanced degenerative changes, most patients with this condition have curtailed their running long before presenting for evaluation. If a runner does present with symptoms of spinal stenosis, however, rest is the first line of treatment. NSAIDs may help patients in the early phase of treatment as well as long term. As in disc disease, exercise under the supervision of a physical therapist may help alleviate symptoms to the point where running is again comfortable. The therapy should concentrate on improving lumbar flexibility and developing strength and endurance of the muscles supporting the lumbar spine.

If a course of rest and physical therapy is unsuccessful in alleviating symptoms, some minimally invasive procedures may help. Injection of facet joints with corticosteroids is a common practice and has reportedly mixed results. For patients who have not had a good response to physical therapy and wish to avoid surgery, this is an option.

If nonoperative treatment fails, surgical decompression has reported success rates of 75% to 90%. A spine fusion at the time of decompression remains controversial. The indications for a fusion remain unclear. The dilemma lies in the determination of instability associated with spinal stenosis. In general, fusion is indicated if evidence suggests segmental instability, such as degenerative spondylolisthesis.[19] An associated fusion significantly delays a return to running because

most surgeons want fusion to be well established before such an activity is resumed.

SPONDYLOLYSIS AND SPONDYLOLISTHESIS

Spondylolysis and spondylolisthesis are common causes of back pain in the athletic population. Participants in gymnastics, diving, football, and weightlifting have a greater incidence than the 5% incidence cited for the general population.[33] Spondylitic defects are not a result of running but may become symptomatic owing to stresses on the spine generated during running.[22]

Spondylolisthesis is a result of a defect of the pars interarticularis that allows anterior "slippage" of a superior vertebral body on an inferior vertebral body. In spondylolysis, no forward displacement occurs (Fig. 6–12). Five types of spondylytic defects have been described—dysplastic, isthmic, degenerative, traumatic, and pathologic. Of these, the isthmic type generally affects the athletic population. The L5–S1 segment is most commonly involved, followed by the L4–L5 segment.

Most people affected by spondylolysis or spondylolisthesis are asymptomatic and become aware of a defect only as a result of radiographs of the lumbar spine. In the early stages, symptomatic patients complain of a dull midline low back pain with activity. In running, the backache may begin after a certain amount of time into the run and resolve shortly after the run is completed. As symp-

Figure 6–12

Spondylolysis and spondylolisthesis. (From Stinson JT: Spondylolysis and spondylolisthesis in the athlete. Clin Sports Med 12:517–528, 1993.)

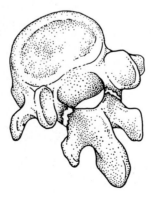
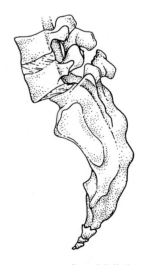

Spondylolysis   **Spondylolisthesis**

toms progress, the pain becomes more constant. Athletes occasionally complain of pain radiating into the buttocks.

Hamstring tightness or spasm is the classic physical examination finding. This is a result of the hamstrings attempting to extend the pelvis and stabilize the affected segment.[23] Paraspinal spasm may also be evident in acutely symptomatic patients. Radicular symptoms are uncommon but may present as irritation of the L5 or S1 nerve root.

When diagnosed with symptomatic spondylolysis or spondylolisthesis, patients are usually concerned about the risk of progression to a slip if one has not occurred or progression of an existing slip. As long as the patient is past skeletal maturity, the risk is minimal.[33] For a skeletally immature runner who is asymptomatic, periodic follow-up is recommended and radiographic evaluation is performed if the patient does become symptomatic.

If a patient presents with symptoms of hamstring tightness or spasm, conservative treatment is usually successful in resolving symptoms. A period of rest, followed by lumbar and abdominal strengthening and hamstring stretching, allows the patient to return to running when the symptoms resolve. In resistant cases, medication or brace immobilization may be indicated.[28]

The indications for surgical treatment, which is uncommon, are refractory pain, slip progression, persistent abnormal gait, persistent neurologic deficit, or a high slip angle. Most cases are managed by in situ fusion. In cases with neurologic deficit, a decompression may be performed at the time of fusion.

STRESS FRACTURES

Most runners have heard of stress fractures and fear that a serious case of shin splints might progress to a stress fracture of the tibial shaft. Not many runners have considered that back pain that has not responded to conventional measures may signal a stress fracture of the lumbar spine.

Although uncommon, stress fractures of the lumbar spine have been reported in runners.[26] As previously discussed, spondylolysis is a form of a stress fracture of the pars interarticularis. In addition, stress fractures of the sacrum have been described in runners.[3]

Stress fractures are believed to occur secondary to the pull of muscles on the bone. They most commonly occur after a sudden change in training frequency or intensity, possibly because muscles adapt more rapidly to activity changes than does bone.[3] Early after the fracture, patients complain of low back pain after the run is well under way. In some cases, pain begins after a fixed distance or time into the run. As symptoms progress, the onset of pain is earlier in the run. The pain usually subsides shortly after the activity is stopped. In patients who have ignored the symptoms for long periods, the pain may become almost constant.

Physical examination may reveal paraspinal muscle spasm or hamstring tightness. It may be possible to palpate an area of point tenderness. Results of neurologic examination are usually normal. Radiographs of the lumbar spine are usually not helpful. Overlying bowel gas patterns make it difficult to detect the areas of sclerosis associated with stress fractures. If suspicion is high, a bone scan may show an isolated area of increased uptake (Fig. 6–13). CT scan or single-photon emission CT scan shows the vertebrae in cross section and further delineates the site of involvement. MRI has proved useful in the detection of stress fractures, demonstrating marrow changes and occasionally cortical hypertrophy.[3]

If a spinal stress fracture is diagnosed, cessation of running is indicated. During this time, therapy is pointed toward improving lumbar

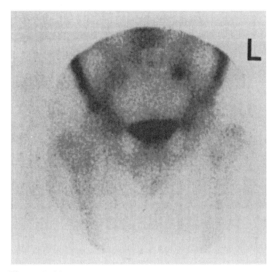

Figure 6–13

Bone scan showing a sacral stress fracture. (From Atwell EA, Jackson DW: Stress fractures of the sacrum in runners: Two case reports. Am J Sports Med 19:531–533, 1991.)

flexibility and maintaining anaerobic endurance with non–weight-bearing activities. As soon as symptoms have resolved, usually in 3 to 6 weeks, running may be resumed. Of course, as with any overuse injury, the return should be gradual, and recurrence of symptoms usually reflects premature resumption of running.

SUMMARY

Low back pain is not one of the common complaints of the running population. Most runners are not overweight and do not lead a sedentary lifestyle—both risk factors for low back problems. In addition, evidence suggests that running may actually decrease the chances of an individual's having problems with the lumbar spine.

Most cases of low back pain are musculo-ligamentous in character and have a relatively short, self-limiting course. Through the years, prolonged rest and avoidance of strenuous activity as treatment for low back ailments have been replaced by early mobilization of the lumbar spine and strengthening of the supporting musculature. As a result, affected patients are returning to work and workouts much earlier.

In general, running does not cause lower back problems but may exacerbate existing conditions. Attention should be paid to the presence of neurologic involvement in conjunction with low back pain. Most cases of mechanical low back pain, herniated disc, spinal stenosis, spondylolysis, and stress fractures can be managed nonoperatively. By incorporating lumbar and abdominal flexibility and strengthening routines into their workout routine, those affected by lower back problems can keep the frequency of exacerbations to a minimum and avoid interruptions in their running schedule.

REFERENCES

1. Adams MA, Hutton WC: Mechanics of the intervertebral disc. In Ghosh P (ed): The Biology of the Intervertebral Disc, vol 2. Boca Raton, FL, CRC Press, 1988.
2. Andersson GBJ, Pope MH, Frymoyer JW, et al: Epidemiology and cost. In Pope MH, Andersson GBJ, Frymoyer JW, et al (eds): Occupational Low Back Pain: Assessment, Treatment and Prevention. Chicago, Mosby-Year Book, 1991, pp 95–113.
3. Atwell EA, Jackson DW: Stress fractures of the sacrum in runners: Two case reports. Am J Sports Med 19:531–533, 1991.
4. Boden SD, Davis DO, Dina TS, et al: Abnormal magnetic resonance scans of the lumbar spine in asymptomatic subjects. J Bone Joint Surg Am 72:403–408, 1990.
5. Brown MD: The pathophysiology and diagnosis of low back pain and sciatica. Instr Course Lect 61:217–224, 1992.
6. Cappozzo A: The forces and couples in the human trunk during level walking. J Biomech 16:265–277, 1983.
7. Cappozzo A: Force actions in the human trunk during running. J Sports Med 23:14–22, 1983.
8. Cromwell R, Schultz AB, Beck R, Warwick D: Loads on the lumbar trunk during level walking. J Orthop Res 7:371–377, 1989.
9. Crossen D: Getting back to running. Runner's World Oct:72–75, 1980.
10. Deyo RA, Diehl AK, Rosenthal M: How many days of bed rest for acute low back pain? A randomized clinical trial. N Engl J Med 315:1064–1070, 1986.
11. Ellis J: Running Injury Free: How to Prevent, Treat and Recover from Dozens of Painful Problems. Emmaus, PA, Rodale Press, 1994.
12. Fadale PD, Wiggins ME: Corticosteroid injections: Their use and abuse. J Am Acad Orthop Surg 2:133–140, 1994.
13. Frymoyer JW: Lumbar disk disease: Epidemiology. Instr Course Lect 41:217–224, 1992.
14. Frymoyer JW: Back pain and sciatica. N Engl J Med 318:291–300, 1988.
15. Gatt CJ, Hosea TM, Palumbo RC, Zawadsky JP: Loads on the lumbar spine during football blocking. Am J Sports Med (in press).
16. Gill K: Percutaneous lumbar diskectomy. J Am Acad Orthop Surg 1:33–40, 1993.
17. Granbed H, Janson Ragnar, Hanson T: The loads on the lumbar spine during extreme weight lifting. Spine 2:146–149, 1987.
18. Herkowitz HN: Spinal stenosis: Clinical evaluation. Instr Course Lect 41:183–185, 1992.
19. Herkowitz HN, Kanwaldeep SS: Lumbar spine fusion in degenerative conditions. J Am Acad Orthop Surg 3:123–135, 1995.
20. Hosea TM, Boland AL: Rowing injuries. Postgrad Adv Sports Med 3:1–17, 1989.
21. Hosea TM, Gatt CJ, Galli KE, et al: Biomechanical analysis of the golfer's back. *In* Cochran AJ (ed): Science and Golf. Proceedings of the First Scientific Congress of Golf. London, E & FN Spon, 1990, pp 43–48.
22. Jackson DW: Low back problems in the runner. *In* Mack RP (ed): AAOS Symposium on the Foot and Leg in Running Sports. St. Louis, CV Mosby, 1982.
23. Jackson DW, Wiltse L, Cirincione R: Spondylolysis in the female gymnast. Clin Orthop 117:68, 1976.
24. Kardong D: Spine tingling. Runner's World Sept:42–48, 1988.
25. Martinelli TA, Wiesel SW: Epidemiology of spinal stenosis. Instr Course Lect 41:179–181, 1992.
26. Matheson GO, Clement DB, McKenzie MC, et al: Stress fractures in athletes: A study of 320 cases. Am J Sports Med 15:46–58, 1987.
27. McKenzie DC, Clement DB, Taunton JD: Running shoes, orthotics and injuries. Sports Med 2:334–337, 1985.
28. Micheli L: Back injuries in gymnasts. Clin Sports Med 4:85, 1985.

29. Miller JAA, Haderspeck KA, Schultz A: Posterior element loads in lumbar motion segments. Spine 8:331–337, 1983.

30. Mooney V: Treating low back pain with exercise. J Musculoskel Med 12:24–36, 1995.

31. Nachemson A: The load on lumbar disks in different positions of the body. Clin Orthop 45:107–122, 1966.

32. Postacchini F: Lumbar Spinal Stenosis. New York, Springer-Verlag Wien, 1989, pp 49–74.

33. Stinson JT: Spondylolysis and spondylolisthesis in the athlete. Clin Sports Med 12:517–528, 1993.

34. White AW: Back to health. Runner's World Dec:56–60, 1986.

================ *CHAPTER SEVEN*

Overview of Leg Injuries in Running

This entire overview chapter is organized into five sections. These include

1. Causes of running injuries
2. Office history and physical examination
3. Treatment plan
4. Specific conditions
5. Case reports

Following is a brief review of the frequency of injuries and the risk/reward ratio concept.

FREQUENCY OF INJURIES

Many epidemiology studies during the past 25 years have been reviewed for this section.[13, 14, 16, 20, 32, 39, 55, 59, 70, 80] Reviewed in the preface of this book are the risks and rewards of running. Briefly restated, aerobic exercise effects a significant 44% reduction in all-cause mortality as measured by the Cooper Aerobic Institute.[8, 23] However, runners pay a price in the form of injuries—four per 1000 hours of running, or one to two injuries per year.[59] (See Chapter 14 for a discussion of arthritis and running.[5, 25, 45, 47, 48, 56, 66–70])

In our sports medicine practice, we find the relative incidence of running injuries similar to that of earlier studies, with two exceptions. What has changed since the 1970s is the age of patients and frequency of running injuries. In the 1990s, we see fewer young runners with problems[62, 69] but more mature runners, especially men with varus alignment of the knees, affected by medial compartment osteoarthritis.

Jacobs's 1986 study of 451 runners in a 10,000-meter race showed the relative incidence of injuries in 210 runners (Fig. 7–1).[40] The incidence of knee pain was very high. A study in 1985 by Lutter analyzed the preva-

Figure 7–1

Incidence of leg running injuries. (From Jacobs S, Berson BL: Injuries in runners. Am J Sports Med 14:153, 1986.)

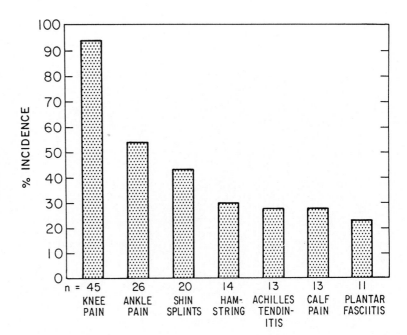

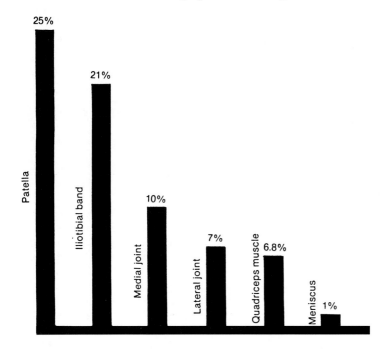

Figure 7–2

Incidence of knee running injuries. (From Lutter L: Running injuries. Instr Course Lect 33:263, 1984.)

lence of knee pain and found patella pain to be the most prevalent (Fig. 7–2).[55] Running injuries were compared with swimming and cycling injuries in a 1986 study by Collins and Wagner at the Seafair Triathlon.[16] Running accounted for 62% of these injuries (Fig. 7–3).

The reason why fewer runners are now being seen in sports medicine clinics may be that

- Education of runners has improved
- The popularity of running is reduced

- Running shoes have improved
- Running intensity has moderated—fewer marathons
- Medical insurance has reduced access
- Injuries are becoming chronic and well tolerated

REWARD/RISK RATIO

The rewards of sports in general and running in particular are numerous (Table 7–1).

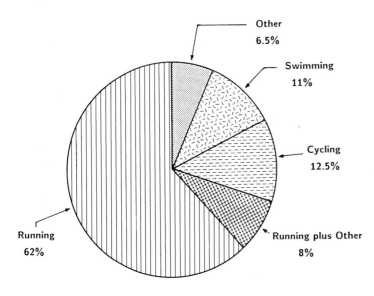

Figure 7–3

Frequency of injuries in a triathlon. (From Collins K, Wagner M, Peterson K, Storey M: Overuse injuries in triathletes. Am J Sports Med 17:677, 1989.)

TABLE 7–1 Rewards of Running

Prevention of musculoskeletal injuries by maintaining muscle tone
Improved flexibility and range of motion
Prolonged physical and mental health
Improved cardiovascular endurance
Improved positive feeling of good health
Opportunity to learn new skills
Opportunities for friendship and socialization
The fun of games
Team membership
For a few, a career, an opportunity to earn high income

From Guten G: Play Healthy, Stay Healthy. Champaign, IL, Human Kinetics Publishers, 1991.

These should be kept in mind by health providers to understand what is motivating runners. The effects of the overuse syndrome[51] are well defined in this book in Chapter 13.

On the other hand, risks may cause a runner to stop running because of injuries. Complications of inactivity and prolonged rest may then develop (Table 7–2). The psychologic aspects of running must always be kept in mind.[35, 72, 77, 78] They are well reviewed in this book in Chapter 16.

Thus, the challenge and goal for those treating runners is to balance the rewards of running with the risks of stopping.[26]

CAUSES OF INJURIES

The first step in treatment of injuries is prevention. Understanding four factors that contribute to sports injuries can be very helpful. To remember these four factors, think of the acronym CATS. The more factors that are combined, the higher the risk for injury.[34]

- Change
- Alignment
- Twisting
- Speed

TABLE 7–2 Complications of Inactivity

Weight gain
Loss of muscle mass
Loss of bone strength (particularly in women who are prone to developing osteoporosis)
Mental inactivity leading to depression
Loss of cardiovascular conditioning

From Guten G: Play Healthy, Stay Healthy. Champaign, IL, Human Kinetics Publishers, 1991.

CHANGE

The human body does not tolerate sudden change. Many biomechanical studies have been conducted and reviewed. Overuse injuries result from a sudden increase or change in training technique. Most injuries occur in spring when the amount and intensity of sports participation dramatically increase. Here is a good rule of thumb: Do not increase the distance, frequency, or duration of the training program by more than 10% per week. The human body has wonderful adaptive power and potential if given enough time to adapt.

Our definition of *change* is related to the concept of training errors, which are the main cause of running injuries. The balance between training errors, surfaces, and malalignment was elucidated in a study by Lysholm and Wiklander in 1987 (Fig. 7–4).[57]

ALIGNMENT

Alignment means "arrangement in a straight line." Well-aligned athletes—those born with straight legs, straight spines, and straight arms—have fewer injuries. People who have slight spine curvatures, bowed legs, or knock-knees are more susceptible to injury. Young women who have wide hips and knock-knees injure their kneecaps more frequently than others. Middle-aged men who become more bowlegged commonly develop knee problems.

Sometimes little can be done for one who is not born with straight alignment. In rare cases, extensive bone surgery can be per-

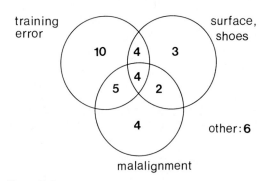

Figure 7–4

Relationship of training error, surface, and malalignment. (From Lysholm J, Wiklander J: Injuries in runners. Am J Sports Med 15:170, 1987.)

formed. A podiatrist can put inserts in running shoes, and these may help manage the alignment problem. The important thing for patients with poor alignment to remember is to be very careful with the intensity in their approach to sports.

TWISTING

The human body evolved primarily as a straight locomotion system for running, not for high-intensity twisting maneuvers like those performed in volleyball, basketball, or gymnastics. We find that runners seem to injure themselves more easily in twisting sports. Running seems to develop the forward propulsive muscles and reduce one's lateral, jumping, and twisting muscle groups. Thus, in twisting sports, runners seem to be more easily injured.

SPEED

As related to speed, the human body can be compared to a car. The more often you drive your car and the faster you drive it, the more likely it is that you will have an accident and that the accident will be serious. The faster you run, bicycle, or swim and the more you do these activities, the more you will stress the musculoskeletal system and the more opportunity you will have for injury.

The worst scenario is a springtime athlete who, after being inactive all winter, suddenly starts exercising and has three or four factors combining to create problems. The athlete may suddenly increase the amount of exercise (change), have bowlegs (alignment), turn suddenly (twist), and then run faster (speed). This athlete is very susceptible to injuries. If runners are aware of these four factors, they can undoubtedly prevent most injuries from happening.

OFFICE HISTORY AND PHYSICAL EXAMINATION

This section emphasizes that a health care provider should have a complete overview of the runner in the office. Many comprehensive articles on biomechanics have been reviewed[3, 12, 36, 43, 57, 63, 64] (see also Chapter 3). Consequently, our office has been constructed with a 100-foot-long corridor to allow running back and forth while we actually view the runner's stride and gait pattern. To fine-tune the view, we adapted a simple treadmill television viewing system to study the dynamics of the leg.

The office evaluation has the three components:

1. History
2. Physical examination
3. Radiographic studies

HISTORY

Runners are questioned about five important aspects of their history to assess their level of running:

1. Shoes
2. Longest run
3. Miles
4. Goals
5. Change

Shoes

It is important to have runners bring their most recent shoes along for the examination to check their wear patterns. We also tell runners to bring running shorts to help facilitate the examination in the office. In general, we find that runners have shoes that are too soft and not stable enough.

Longest Run

Questions about a runner's longest run give the health care provider a quick and easy assessment of the intensity of the running pattern. Runners who say their longest run is 5 miles certainly have different stresses and pressures than do marathon runners.

Miles per Week

A runner who runs 10 miles per week is certainly treated differently than a runner who runs 75 miles per week.

Goals

Questions about a runner's goals give the health care provider insight into the drive and motivation of the runner. Runners who state that their goal is to set a personal best in a 3-

hour marathon are certainly treated differently than runners who want to enter a local community 5-k walk-run.

Change

The key question to ask is "What are you doing differently? What has changed?" This important question about change reveals some of the most common reasons for running injuries:

- Change of speed and friends
- Change of terrain and hills
- Change of shoes
- Change of goal

PHYSICAL EXAMINATION

Although it would be helpful to have an elaborate and expensive biomechanical laboratory to study runners, this is not practical for every runner in a clinic setting. In our sports medicine clinic, three key tests are given:

1. Running longitudinally in our hallway
2. One-leg hopping
3. Running on a treadmill in the office

Hallway Running

After the initial history, patients are observed running in our long office hallway. This gives a general overview of leg alignment, limp, and degree of discomfort (Fig. 7–5).

One-Leg Hopping

Having a patient hop on one leg tends to be the most revealing test for localizing discomfort, pain, and limp (Fig. 7–6).

Office Treadmill

The concept of an office treadmill video system was first seen in the private offices of Lutter and Brody, in the early 1980s. The system used in our office is shown in Figures 7–7 to 7–9. The treadmill is a Sears model 780, which cost about $750 in 1995 (Fig. 7–7). The floor-based video camera is a simple hand-held model with a zoom lens, costing about $600 (Fig. 7–8). These are connected to a simple home model television and video

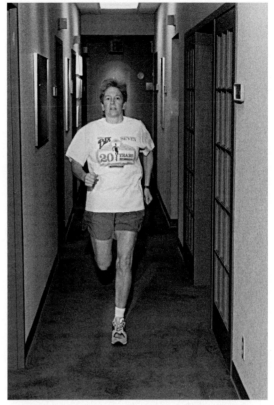

Figure 7–5

Office hallway running.

recorder costing about $500. Thus, the entire office system costs about $2000.

Using this simple office treadmill system, patients and physicians are able to enhance their knowledge of running patterns and shoe dynamics (Fig. 7–9). Foot and shoe dynamics can be studied on the video screen and immediate feedback given to the patient and physician (Figs. 7–10 and 7–11).

RADIOLOGIC STUDIES—FOUR TYPES

Standard

Standard radiographs are very similar to those reviewed by James.[41] Radiographic examination of the knee includes at least four views:

- Weight-bearing anterior and posterior views
- Lateral view in 45 degrees of flexion
- Tangential view of the patella
- Notch view in either weight-bearing or non–weight-bearing positions

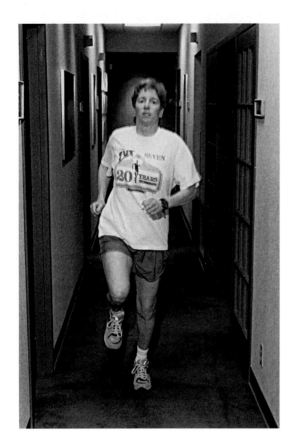

Figure 7–6

One-leg hopping test. Note that all of the force is applied to one leg. The patient will localize the pain.

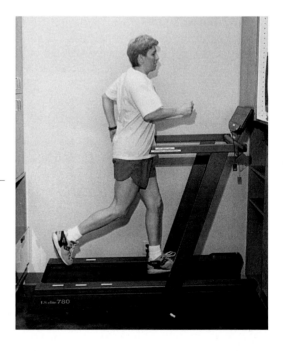

Figure 7–7

Office treadmill with patient.

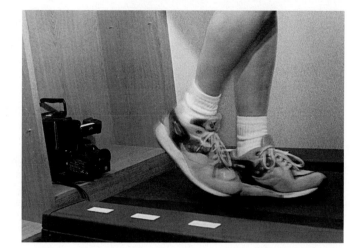

Figure 7–8

Video camera system at surface level. The image is projected on the video screen in front of the patient.

Standing 45-Degree Flexion Radiograph of the Knee

One important knee radiograph we use in our office, especially for patients who are having persistent medial joint line pain, is the 45-degree flexion weight-bearing radiograph of the knee as described by Rosenberg (Fig. 7–12).[76] This shows the amount of wear in the posterior compartment, which is not well seen in the standard anterior view of the knee. Narrowing on the 45-degree flexion view is an unfavorable prognostic sign for return to normal running (see Figs. 7–30 and 7–38 as examples of a 45-degree flexion radiograph).

Bone Scan

We find that a delayed bone scan is an extremely helpful technique for isolating and localizing an inflammatory process of the bone and cartilage.[15, 30] This is based on a research study that was performed in our of-

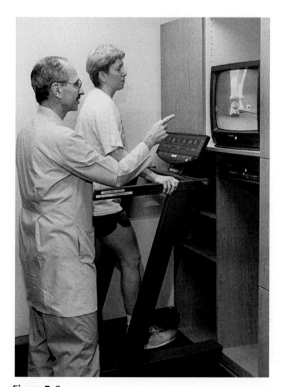

Figure 7–9

Patient and physician reviewing video image of foot and shoe.

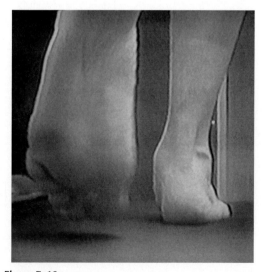

Figure 7–10

Video picture showing normal pronation of the right foot in the stance phase. The left foot is in the swing phase.

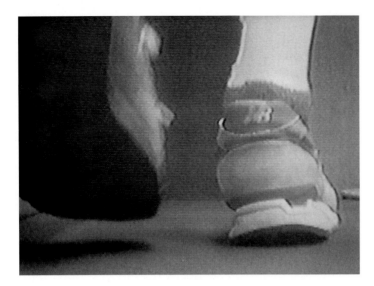

Figure 7–11

Video picture showing excessive pronation of the right foot.

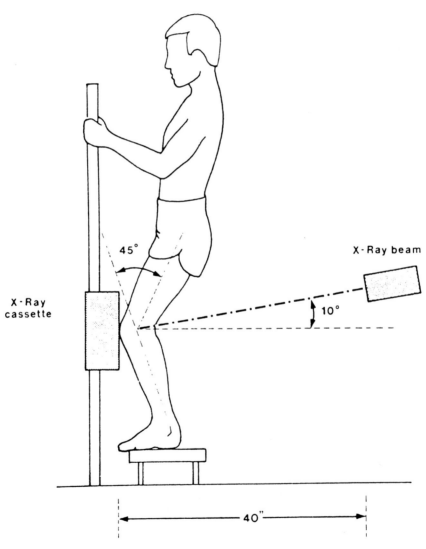

45°

X-Ray beam

X-Ray
cassette

10°

40"

Figure 7–12

Forty-five-degree standing flexion radiograph. (From Rosenberg T: The 45-degree posteroanterior flexion-weight-bearing
radiograph of the knee. J Bone Joint Surg 70-A:1479, 1988.)

fice and that correlated arthroscopic findings and bone scan results.[44] Positive bone scan results localized to one compartment are not a favorable prognostic sign for return to normal running (see Figs. 7–31 and 7–39 for case reports using bone scans).

Magnetic Resonance Imaging

MRI can be extremely helpful in localizing a tear of the meniscus.[38, 41, 75] However, we are finding many false positives, especially in marathon runners (see the later case study section, with Fig. 7–40 as an example of a false-positive MRI scan).

TREATMENT

In this overview of leg injuries due to running, the "Stop and Go" activity program developed in our office is reviewed.[27] The complete 10-point Stop and Go sports medicine program is outlined (Table 7–3).[29]

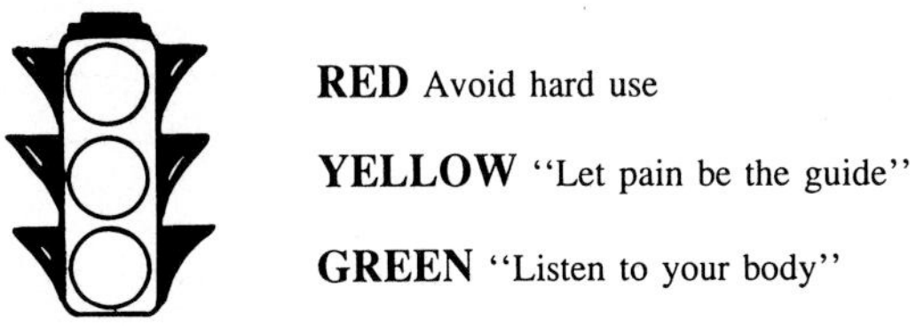

RED Avoid hard use

YELLOW "Let pain be the guide"

GREEN "Listen to your body"

Figure 7–13

Stop and Go sports medicine program. Meaning of red, yellow, and green. (From Play Healthy, Stay Healthy *[pp. 101–152] by Gary N. Guten, Champaign, IL: Human Kinetics Publishers. Copyright 1991 by Gary N. Guten. Reprinted by permission.)*

10-POINT STOP AND GO SPORTS MEDICINE PROGRAM

The Stop and Go system is based on the concept that activities can be classified as follows (Fig. 7–13):

- Red: Minimal activity—allowing "no pain"
- Yellow: Moderate activity—"let pain be the guide"
- Green: Full activity—"listen to your body"

TABLE 7–3 The Stop and Go Sports Medicine Program

● **Stop** ⊗ **Caution** ○ **GO**	
Activity Level	*Surface*
● Minimal use	○ Cement, concrete
⊗ Moderate use: "Let pain be the guide"	⊗ Blacktop streets, indoor tracks (16 turns/mile)
○ Full use: "Listen to your body"	● Blacktop bike paths, indoor tracks (8–10 turns/mile)
Exercise	
● Hard stretch, vigorous bent-joint exercise with weights	*Shoes*
⊗ Moderate stretch, moderate bent-joint exercise with weights	● Soft heel, rigid forefoot
○ Light stretch, straight-joint exercise with weights	⊗ Semisoft heel
	○ Firm heel, soft forefoot
Thermal	*Alternative Exercises*
● Hot packs	○ Hard twist (basketball, volleyball, racquetball, wrestling)
⊗ Lukewarm soaks	⊗ Moderate twist (skiing, dancing, tennis, bowling, golf)
○ Ice packs	● Straight-joint (walking, swimming, biking, jogging, running, cross-country skiing, jumping rope)
Support	
● Cast	*Nutrition (% of fat calories)*
⊗ Elastic sleeve, brace	○ 45% (U.S. diet)
○ Simple elastic wrap	⊗ 30% (heart diet)
Medication	● 10%–20% (Pritikin, Haas diets)
● High-dose vitamins, minerals	*Fluids*
⊗ Nonsteroidal antiinflammatory drugs	● High salt, high sugar, high caffeine
○ Aspirin (with or without antacid), two with each meal	⊗ Low salt, low sugar, low caffeine
	○ Water

From Guten G: A ten-point "stop and go" sports medicine program. J Musculoskel Med 3:24–26, 1986.

TABLE 7–4   Program for Graduated Return to Running

Week	Activity
1	Walk 4 to 8 laps (alternate 50 m fast, 50 m normal)
2	Walk 8 to 12 laps (alternate 100 m fast, 100 m normal)
3	Jog 10 minutes every other day at an easy pace
4	Jog 15 minutes every other day
5	Jog 15 minutes one day, 25 minutes the next
6	Jog 20 minutes one day, 30 minutes the next
7	Jog 20 minutes one day, 35 minutes the next
8	Jog 20 minutes one day, 40 minutes the next
9	Resume training at an appropriate mileage and intensity

From James S: Running injuries to the knee. J Am Acad Orthop Surg 3:309–318, 1995.

The following is a review of the 10 important points of the Stop and Go system, outlining the 10 important items that health providers need to review with an injured runner:

1. Activity level
2. Exercise
3. Thermal
4. Support
5. Medication
6. Surface
7. Shoes
8. Alternative exercises
9. Food
10. Fluids

Activity Level. Whether a patient's problem is overuse or an acute injury, the main recommendation affects the activity level. You cannot tell a vigorous person to stop all exercise. Here, the red zone means minimal use, such as walking or swimming, as long as it causes no discomfort. The yellow zone means moderate use; we tell patients to go with caution and let pain be the guide. The green zone means full activity, yet we caution patients,

"Listen to your body." We do not believe in the philosophy of "no pain, no gain."

Many programs for gradual return to running have been devised. Some runners benefit from a very structured program such as that outlined by James in 1995 (Table 7–4).[41] We find that most runners tolerate simply being told to reduce running by about 50% and let pain be the guide.

Exercise. These recommendations cover the two basic types: exercises that are done with joints straight and with joints bent.[11, 60, 76, 78] The red zone activities (to be avoided) require hard stretching and vigorous bent-knee exercises on the commercial exercise machines. Yellow zone activities involve moderate stretching and moderate bent-joint weightlifting. The green zone exercises, for patients with patellar chrondromalacia, for example, allow light stretching and weightlifting done with the joint straight.

We classify the qualities of muscle by the acronym FESS[29]:

- Flexibility
- Endurance
- Speed
- Strength

It is important for health care providers and athletes to remember that each sport has its unique muscle demands. The flexibility needs of a gymnast are certainly different from the needs of a 100-yard-dash runner who requires speed. Marathon runners need endurance, compared with weight lifters, who need strength (Table 7–5).

Thermal. Patients and physicians alike are frequently confused about when to use heat and when to use ice. Our motto is, "Ice is nice; hot is not." Therefore, hot packs are in the red zone, soaking in a lukewarm tub is in the yellow zone, and ice packs are in the green zone.

TABLE 7–5   Qualities of Muscle in Specific Sports

Sport	Flexibility	Endurance	Strength	Speed
Gymnastics	+	0	0	0
Marathon running	0	+	0	0
Weightlifting	0	0	+	0
100-yard dash	0	0	0	+
Basketball (professional)	+	+	+	+

From Guten G: Play Healthy, Stay Healthy. Champaign, IL, Human Kinetics Publishers, 1991.

Support. Many musculoskeletal injuries require local tissue support.[37] We believe the best support for a joint is the patient's own musculature. Until muscle development is adequate, three types of immobilization may be used. In the red zone is a cast; in the yellow zone, an elastic sleeve or a brace; and in the green zone, an elastic wrap.

Medication. During the healing period, antiinflammatory medication is helpful. The red zone agents are megadoses of supplemental vitamins and minerals, which we consider unnecessary. Yellow zone medications are the nonsteroidal antiinflammatory drugs (NSAIDs), which are occasionally necessary. The green zone medication is aspirin or acetaminophen. Two tablets (plain or buffered) can be taken with each meal during periods of pain.

Surface. Many of our patients are runners and dancers. The red zone surfaces are concrete or cement, which should be avoided. Yellow zone surfaces are blacktop streets or indoor tracks with up to 16 turns to the mile. Green zone surfaces, which are those most recommended, are blacktop bicycle paths or indoor tracks with only 8 to 10 turns per mile.

Shoes. Proper shoes specific for the sport are vital to prevent overuse syndromes.[6, 42, 58] Red zone shoes have a soft heel and rigid forefoot and should be avoided because they do not provide adequate heel control. Yellow zone shoes are moderately priced models that are made with a semisoft heel. Green zone shoes are well-constructed models with a firm, well-stabilized heel and flexible forefoot.

In general, we find that the most common mistake that runners make is buying shoes that are too soft. The basic reason for running shoes is to provide protection and stability. Jokingly, we tell patients that "If Mother Nature wanted you to run on air, she would have put your lungs on your feet."

Alternative Exercises. These exercises consist of twisting or straight activities.[21, 28] The red zone alternative exercises require hard twisting, as in racquetball, soccer, and basketball, and should be avoided during the initial period of rehabilitation. Yellow zone exercises require bent joints with minimal twisting, as in bowling and baseball. Green zone activities are the straight joint activities that can be done in moderation during periods of reha-

bilitation, including walking, biking, light jogging, and cross-country skiing. The following is a summary of the Stop and Go system:

- Red—hard twisting activities such as basketball, volleyball, racquetball, wrestling, football, and soccer (Fig. 7–14)
- Yellow—moderate twisting activities such as dancing, tennis, bowling, golf, and skiing (Fig. 7–15)
- Green—race walking, running, biking, jogging, running in a swimming pool, cross-country skiing, and the balance between running, swimming, and cycling (Fig. 7–16)

Food. Evaluate the patient's food requirement by calculating the percent of fat calories.[33, 71] Athletes need energy for rehabilitation and healing. In the red zone is the so-called standard American diet, of which about 45% is fat. This should be avoided. In the yellow zone is the standard heart diet, which includes 30% fat. The green zone diet has between 10% and 20% fat.[71]

Fluids. Aerobic activity and muscle metabolism necessitate a proper fluid balance.[65] Fluids in the red zone have high salt, sugar, and caffeine content, such as many of the ergogenic drinks, and should be avoided. Yellow zone drinks are low in salt and sugar and have minimal caffeine. The green zone fluid, which is the best, is simply water, which should be drunk liberally.

In summary, we tell most patients to stay in the yellow and green zones: Go with caution.

SPECIFIC LEG INJURIES

The following is a general review of 12 specific conditions of the lower extremity associated with running[33] (see Chapters 4 and 10 for more detailed information).

The tone of this section is rather nontechnical to allow it to be used as a handout for students and patients. Excellent detailed technical articles have been published on specific leg injuries.

Each medical condition is reviewed with six sections:

- Definition
- Cause
- Subjective symptoms
- Objective findings
- Testing procedure
- Prognosis

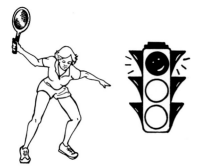

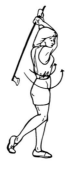

RED Hard twisting activities—basketball, volleyball, racquetball, wrestling, football, soccer

Figure 7–14

Red zone—hard twisting activities. (From Play Healthy, Stay Healthy *[pp. 101–152] by Gary N. Guten, Champaign, IL: Human Kinetics Publishers. Copyright 1991 by Gary N. Guten. Reprinted by permission.)*

Figure 7–15

Yellow zone—moderate twisting activities. (From Play Healthy, Stay Healthy *[pp. 101–152] by Gary N. Guten, Champaign, IL: Human Kinetics Publishers. Copyright 1991 by Gary N. Guten. Reprinted by permission.)*

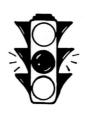

YELLOW Moderate twisting activities—dancing, tennis, bowling, golf, skiing

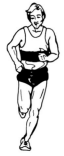

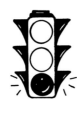

GREEN Straight activities—race walking, swimming, biking, jogging, running, running in a swimming pool, cross-country skiing, jumping rope

Figure 7–16

Green zone—straight activities. (From Play Healthy, Stay Healthy *[pp. 101–152] by Gary N. Guten, Champaign, IL: Human Kinetics Publishers. Copyright 1991 by Gary N. Guten. Reprinted by permission.)*

STRESS FRACTURE OF THE NECK OF THE FEMUR   Figure 7–17

Definition

An overuse condition characterized by a localized weakening and fracture of the femoral neck due to repetitive lower extremity activities such as prolonged running on hard surfaces.[4, 19] Potentially a very serious problem that may require surgery if displacement of the fracture is suspected or imminent.

Cause

A prolonged running program on hard surfaces in a thin person, often a young woman, who is overtraining and losing weight—known as the *female athletic triad* (see Chapter 17).

Subjective Symptoms

- Progressive pain on the lateral side, posterior aspect of the hip, or groin, with radiation into the inner thigh.
- Numbness and tingling usually not present.
- Muscle spasm present in some cases and confused with a simple muscle strain.
- Pain usually brought on by activities and relieved with rest and sitting.

Objective Findings

- Limp is present, especially with hopping and running.
- Motion is guarded on hip flexion and rotation.
- Neurologic findings are normal.
- Local bone tenderness may be present.

Testing Procedure

- Initial radiographs may be normal, but the physician should have a high index of suspicion.
- Repeat radiographs should be performed if pain persists. All persistent pain in the hip should be radiographed to rule out a hip stress fracture because of serious risk of displacement of the fracture.
- Bone scan is very helpful in the early phases.
- MRI test results may be positive and may show the fracture.
- Results of electromyography and nerve testing are normal.

Prognosis

Generally good, if rest is prescribed to allow the bone to heal. It may take 3 months for the fracture to heal. During this period, graduated crutch walking, swimming, and biking are permissible. Some surgeons recommend pinning of the fracture in a highly active individual.

Stress Fracture of the Neck of the Femur

Figure 7–17

Stress fracture of the neck of the femur. (From Play Healthy, Stay Healthy [pp. 101–152] by Gary N. Guten, Champaign, IL: Human Kinetics Publishers. Copyright 1991 by Gary N. Guten. Reprinted by permission.)

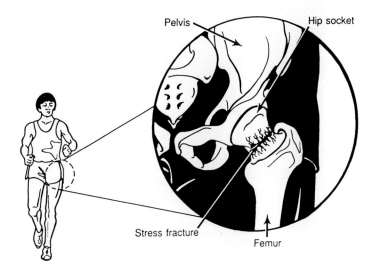

TROCHANTERIC BURSITIS   Figure 7–18

Definition
Localized inflammation on the lateral aspect of the hip, characterized by local pain and limp—common in aerobic sports.

Cause
- Long-distance running and biking cause the muscle tendons to rub over the side of the greater trochanter, leading to irritation of the bursa.
- The athlete may have leg alignment problems (knock-knee), and shoes may have worn excessively on the lateral heel.

Subjective Symptoms
- Localized pain exists on the lateral side of the hip.
- Local swelling may be present.
- Numbness and tingling are not present.
- Pain is relieved with rest.
- Sneezing and coughing are not painful.

Objective Findings
- Slight limp with running.
- Hip motion possibly guarded.
- Local tenderness directly on the lateral side of the hip–greater trochanter.
- Neurologic findings normal.

Testing Procedures
- Radiographs usually appear normal but may show soft tissue calcifications.
- Specialized tests such as MRI, CT scan, myelogram, and EMG are not necessary.
- Bone scan results may be positive.

Prognosis
Healing generally occurs after initial rest. Symptoms may linger for several months. Surgery is rarely necessary; sometimes the bursa has to be excised and the tendon divided surgically, but this is unusual.

Trochanteric Bursitis

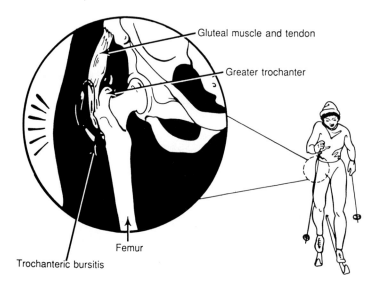

Gluteal muscle and tendon

Greater trochanter

Femur

Trochanteric bursitis

Figure 7–18

Trochanteric bursitis. (From Play Healthy, Stay Healthy [pp. 101–152] by Gary N. Guten, Champaign, IL: Human Kinetics Publishers. Copyright 1991 by Gary N. Guten. Reprinted by permission.)

CHONDROMALACIA PATELLA—PATELLOFEMORAL PAIN SYNDROME Figure 7–19

Definition

A traumatic or degenerative cartilage condition characterized by local breakdown of the undersurface of cartilage, usually at the patella. Can be an early localized form of primary osteoarthritis or degenerative arthritis.

The term *chondromalacia patella* can be subclassified by orthopedic surgeons into the excessive lateral pressure syndrome and patella instability syndrome.[18, 40, 49]

Cause

- Direct local trauma such as that which occurs when the knee hits the dashboard in an automobile accident.
- Repeated bending microtrauma, especially if the lower extremity is not aligned properly.

Subjective Symptoms

- Dull, aching pain leading to sharp localized pain in the front of the knee.
- Grinding sensation frequently.
- Swelling and effusion generally not present.
- Stiffness in squatting, bending, and climbing stairs.
- Sensation of giving way.

Objective Findings

- Motion is intact.
- Stability of ligaments is good.
- Swelling is not present.
- Tenderness is localized to the patella joint.
- Patella maltracking may be present with excessive lateral pressure syndrome and patella instability.
- Crepitation (grinding sensation) is felt.

Testing Procedures

- Gait analysis may show knock-knees or bow legs with pronation of the feet.
- Radiographs may show slight spurring of the patellar joint and malalignment of the patella.
- Bone scan helps to show localized uptake and inflammation.
- MRI is not very helpful.
- Arthroscopy is diagnostic but should be done only after failure of extensive conservative treatment.

Prognosis

Good, but healing can be very prolonged. Some extreme cases progress and may need surgery in the form of arthroscopy or major open patella realignment.

Chondromalacia Patella

Figure 7–19

Chondromalacia patella. (From Play Healthy, Stay Healthy *[pp. 101–152] by Gary N. Guten, Champaign, IL: Human Kinetics Publishers. Copyright 1991 by Gary N. Guten. Reprinted by permission.)*

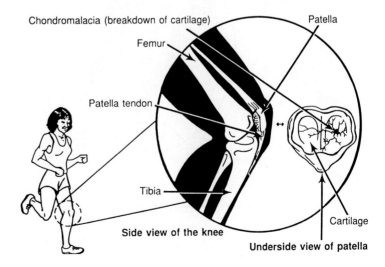

ILIOTIBIAL BAND SYNDROME   Figure 7–20

Definition
An overuse inflammatory condition of the outer (lateral) aspect of the knee, characterized by an ache and burning sensation during or after running.[31, 52] Due to local friction of the tendon band as it rubs over the lateral femoral condyle.

Cause
- Acute, local, direct trauma—a rare cause.
- Chronic overuse microtrauma, usually early in training in sports such as running or biking. Pain usually not disabling.

Subjective Symptoms
- Pain is well localized to the lateral aspect of the femoral condyle. The pain may radiate up the side of the thigh to the hip.
- Swelling is not usually present.
- Motion is normal, but tightness may be perceived.
- Snapping may be present.

Objective Findings
- Tenderness is well localized to the band directly over the lateral condyle.
- Swelling is generally not present.
- Crepitation and noise usually are not present.
- Instability is not present.
- Findings on knee examination are normal.
- Tightness of the lateral muscles may be present.

Testing Procedures
- Radiographs generally appear normal.
- Bone scan may be positive in chronic cases showing bone inflammation.
- MRI is not indicated.
- Arthroscopy is not indicated.

Prognosis
Progressive healing occurs with simple reduction in activity and muscle rehabilitation. The athlete may continue moderate biking and running during this condition. Surgery to split and decompress the tendon may be performed in rare cases.

Iliotibial Band Syndrome

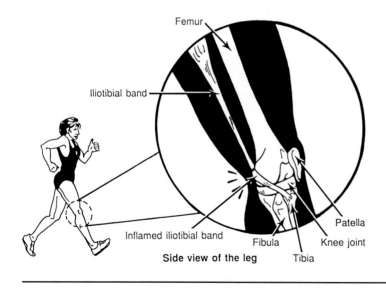

Side view of the leg

Figure 7–20

Iliotibial band syndrome. (From Play Healthy, Stay Healthy *[pp. 101–152] by Gary N. Guten, Champaign, IL: Human Kinetics Publishers. Copyright 1991 by Gary N. Guten. Reprinted by permission.)*

OSTEOARTHRITIS   Figure 7–21

Definition

A traumatic or degenerative condition of the cartilage of the knee joint, characterized by progressive wearing of the articular surface (hyaline cartilage). Progressive pain and stiffness.

Many studies have investigated the relationship of running and osteoarthritis.[5, 25, 45, 47, 48, 56, 66–70] Bone spur formation gives the condition the name *osteoarthritis.* Progressive deterioration may occur because of poor circulation to the cartilage.

Cause

- Acute: traumatic injury to the surface of the joint from an impact or a twisting injury.
- Chronic: years of microtrauma to a joint, especially if malalignment or instability is present, such as with a torn anterior cruciate ligament.
- Other causes: obesity, idiopathic changes, endocrine and hereditary factors.
- See Chapter 14.

Subjective Symptoms

- Pain and ache are present after activity. The pain may be delayed until the next day or night.
- Swelling may be present in or around the joint.

- A sensation of giving way may be felt while climbing stairs.
- Crepitation and noise can be felt and heard by the patient.
- Limp progressively develops.

Objective Findings

- Tenderness is present directly on the joint and along bone spurs.
- Swelling and fluid accumulation can be perceived.
- Crepitation can be felt and heard by the physician.
- Stiffness and loss of motion are detected.
- Limp is present with weight-bearing and jumping.

Testing Procedures

- Initial radiographs appear normal, even though cartilage is wearing. As the condition worsens, radiographs reveal roughness, narrowing of the joint line, and spur formation.
- Bone scan is very helpful for detecting bone inflammation.
- MRI may show tears of the meniscus and wearing of the cartilage. After age 50, MRI loses some of its reliability and may show false-positive meniscus changes even though the meniscus is not torn.
- Arthroscopy definitely shows defects in the

Osteoarthritis

Figure 7–21

Osteoarthritis. (From Play Healthy, Stay Healthy [pp. 101–152] by Gary N. Guten, Champaign, IL: Human Kinetics Publishers. Copyright 1991 by Gary N. Guten. Reprinted by permission.)

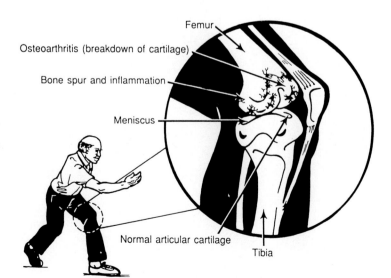

Femur

Osteoarthritis (breakdown of cartilage)

Bone spur and inflammation

Meniscus

Normal articular cartilage

Tibia

hyaline cartilage, but the test generally is not used early to establish the diagnosis. Arthroscopy may be helpful in treating moderate cases by debriding roughened surfaces and removing loose bodies. However, a study by the Mayo Clinic found arthroscopy in a degenerative knee to be effective only 50% to 60% of the time.

Prognosis

Progressive deterioration of the joint occurs if the patient does not listen to his or her body. Pain indicates that progressive wearing is occurring. Reduce the intensity of activities until pain is minimal. Moderation of activity and intensity is very important.

Twisting sports should be minimized. Non-impact activities such as biking, walking, and swimming are satisfactory. Surgery, ranging from arthroscopy to eventual total joint replacement, may be required if the condition is very serious and progresses.

PATELLAR TENDINITIS Figure 7–22

Definition
A traumatic inflammation of the tendon directly below the kneecap (patella), initiated by jumping, running, or climbing sports and resulting in incomplete local tearing of the tendon. Prolonged symptoms are common for many months because of poor blood supply and resulting inflammation. This condition is often called *jumper's knee*. Running can be thought of as a series of one-legged jumps.

Cause
- Acute, violent jumping episode results in pain below the kneecap (patella) and leads to chronic pain and inflammation.
- Chronic repetitive jumping, climbing, and running activities can weaken the tendon. Because running is a jumping sport, jumper's knee is relatively common in runners. Foot imbalance and running up hills are aggravating factors.

Subjective Symptoms
- Pain localized to the inferior pole of the patella.
- Swelling generally not present.
- Motion within normal limits.

- Noise and crepitation generally not present.
- Giving way present with hard jumping.

Objective Findings
- Tenderness directly on the lower tip of the patella.
- Swelling generally not present.
- Crepitation not present.
- Instability not present.

Testing Procedures
- Radiographs appear normal, but a spur may be present in chronic cases.
- Results of bone scan may be positive at the inferior (lower) pole of the patella.
- In chronic cases, MRI may show an incomplete tear and a chronic tendon problem.
- Arthroscopy is rarely indicated.

Prognosis
Expect many months to a year in some cases for complete healing. Some cases in basketball players never heal. Long-term restriction of jumping may be required for 1 or 2 years. Some patients require surgery to remove scarred tendon. This can affect the long-term playing ability of a volleyball or basketball athlete or a very serious runner.

Patellar Tendinitis (Jumper's Knee)

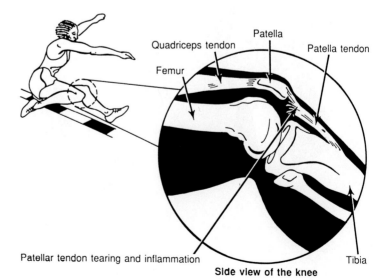

Figure 7–22

Patellar tendinitis. (From Play Healthy, Stay Healthy *[pp. 101–152] by Gary N. Guten, Champaign, IL: Human Kinetics Publishers. Copyright 1991 by Gary N. Guten. Reprinted by permission.)*

TORN MENISCUS   Figure 7–23

Definition
A traumatic fibrocartilage condition associated with wearing and eventual tearing of the fibrocartilage (the meniscus), one of the main shock absorbers of the knee and the structure that provides cushioning between the femur and the tibia. Knee pain and running are the subject of many excellent articles.[1–3, 7, 9, 10, 17, 24, 40, 46, 50, 53, 54, 61, 73]

Cause
- Acute twisting trauma such as hard flexion or rotation injury in basketball or soccer.
- A chronic overuse condition due to repetitive bending and frequent twisting, such as running on a small curved track.

Subjective Symptoms
- Well-localized tenderness on the joint line, leading to progressive pain and swelling.
- Locking of the joint a feature in some cases.
- Good stability, but a sensation of giving way is present in some cases.
- Tenderness well localized at the joint line.

- Limp present, especially with bending and twisting.
- Swelling present.
- Clicking sensation present in some cases.

Testing Procedures
- Routine radiographs generally appear normal; 45-degree flexion radiograph may show narrowing.
- Bone scan shows local inflammation but is not diagnostic.
- MRI is very reliable for a subtle tear, but be cautious about false positives in runners and patients older than 50 years.
- Arthrogram can be helpful and diagnostic.
- Arthroscopy should be performed if conservative treatment fails.

Prognosis
Untreated, the symptoms subside if activities are greatly reduced. Some cases heal spontaneously if the tear is in the outer portion of the meniscus near the blood supply. If activity has to be maintained and symptoms persist, arthroscopic surgery can be performed to remove or repair the torn portion.

Torn Meniscus

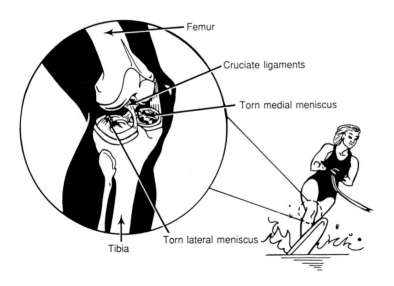

Figure 7–23

Torn meniscus. (From Play Healthy, Stay Healthy [pp. 101–152] by Gary N. Guten, Champaign, IL: Human Kinetics Publishers. Copyright 1991 by Gary N. Guten. Reprinted by permission.)

SHIN SPLINTS Figure 7–24

Definition
An inflammation along the periosteum (outer lining of the bone), characterized by diffuse pain along the front of the shin and due to repetitive stress.

Cause
- Associated with a foot imbalance and repetitive running on hard surfaces.
- If prolonged, may progress to a stress reaction and eventually to a stress fracture.

Subjective Symptoms
- Diffuse pain along the inner side of the shin starts 2 or 3 inches below the knee and radiates to the ankle.
- Thickening of the muscle belly and muscle tenderness can develop.
- Local swelling may be present.
- If swelling increases, nerve symptoms such as numbness and weakness of the foot can develop. This is known as *compartment syndrome.*

Objective Findings
- Diffuse and localized tenderness of the muscle and bone.
- Firmness of the muscle.
- Running with external rotation and a pronated foot.
- Late nerve damage detected in compartment syndrome in some cases.

Testing Procedures
- Routine radiographs generally appear normal.
- Compartment testing, involving placement of a needle in the muscle, may show increased muscle pressure.
- MRI is not helpful.
- Bone scan may show diffuse bone inflammation and may help rule out a fracture.

Prognosis
Healing usually progresses as you reduce training, correct muscle imbalance, and treat inflammation. If symptoms are prolonged, a stress fracture may develop.

Shin Splints

Figure 7–24

Shin splints. (From Play Healthy, Stay Healthy *[pp. 101–152] by Gary N. Guten, Champaign, IL: Human Kinetics Publishers. Copyright 1991 by Gary N. Guten. Reprinted by permission.)*

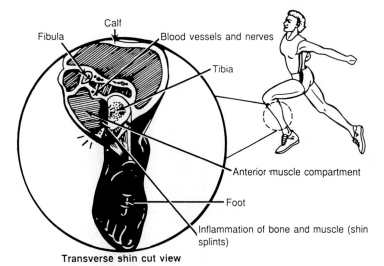

Calf
Fibula
Blood vessels and nerves
Tibia
Anterior muscle compartment
Foot
Inflammation of bone and muscle (shin splints)

Transverse shin cut view

TIBIA OR FIBULA STRESS FRACTURE   Figure 7–25

Definition
A traumatic bone condition characterized by early persistent inflammation due to shin splints, leading to persistent weakening of the bone and actual fracture.[22]

Cause
- Repetitive overuse associated with muscle imbalance and poor alignment of the leg, leading to actual weakening and fracture of the bone.
- Leg malalignment with foot pronation.
- Running on concrete roads with poor shoes.
- Eating disorder with excess weight loss—the female athletic triad.

Subjective Symptoms
- Initial diffuse pain progresses to a well-localized point of pain, generally on the tibia on the inside of the shin or the outer aspect of the leg above the ankle (fibula bone).
- Vague pain and slight limp can progress to severe local pain and limp.
- Swelling is generally not present until late.

- Nerve symptoms are not present.
- Pain with impact and use is relieved by rest.

Objective Findings
- Bone tenderness is well localized.
- Local swelling may occasionally be present.
- Neurologic findings are normal.

Testing Procedure
- Initial radiographs may appear normal, but after several weeks a fracture and healing bone formation may appear.
- Initial bone scan is very helpful in substantiating the diagnosis and in indicating prognosis by the intensity of the scan.

Prognosis
With adequate rest, healing generally occurs after 2 to 3 months. Casting generally is not necessary. Displacement of the fracture is very unusual. With a program of rest and gradual walking, swimming, and biking, progressive healing occurs. Long-term correction with an orthotic is generally very helpful.

Tibia or Fibula Stress Fracture

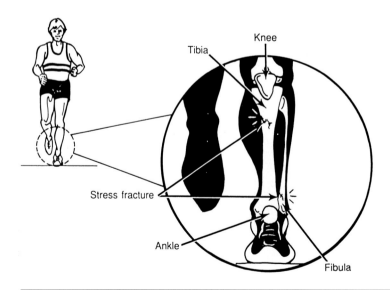

Figure 7–25

Tibia or fibula stress fracture. (From Play Healthy, Stay Healthy [pp. 101–152] by Gary N. Guten, Champaign, IL: Human Kinetics Publishers. Copyright 1991 by Gary N. Guten. Reprinted by permission.)

ACHILLES TENDINITIS   Figure 7–26

Definition

A traumatic or degenerative tendon condition characterized by chronic pain and inflammation on the posterior aspect of the ankle along the Achilles tendon, at the junction where the large muscle group of the calf attaches to the heel bone. Not a complete tear but a partial tendon fiber disruption and inflammation.

Cause

- Acute, sudden jumping or running, causing a microscopic tearing of the muscle group, possibly a previously weakened tendon.
- Chronic repetitive microtrauma to the Achilles tendon, usually associated with muscle imbalance, excessive running up hills, or both. Foot imbalance present in some cases.

Subjective Symptoms

- Localized pain appears behind the ankle along the Achilles tendon.
- Local thickening and swelling of the tendon may be present.
- Stiffness: The ankle may be tight, and pain may be aggravated by walking on the toes.

Objective Findings

- Well-localized tenderness appears directly on the Achilles tendon, either in the mid-substance of the tendon or where it attaches to the bone.
- Local swelling may be present.
- Muscle testing induces pain with plantar flexion of the ankle and on walking on the toes.

Testing Procedures

- Routine radiographs are generally nondiagnostic, but a small spur may be present on the back of the heel.
- Bone scan is not helpful but may show slight bone inflammation.
- MRI test may show tearing of the tendon in acute and chronic stages.

Prognosis

Healing can be prolonged because of poor circulation in the tendon. On a conservative program, slow but progressive healing may occur with incomplete or micro-chronic tears. If pain persists, open surgical removal of scar tissue in the tendon may be necessary. For acute tears, either casting or surgical treatment is indicated, depending on the activity level of the athlete and the philosophy of the surgeon.

Achilles Tendinitis

Figure 7–26

Achilles tendinitis. (From Play Healthy, Stay Healthy *[pp. 101–152] by Gary N. Guten, Champaign, IL: Human Kinetics Publishers. Copyright 1991 by Gary N. Guten. Reprinted by permission.)*

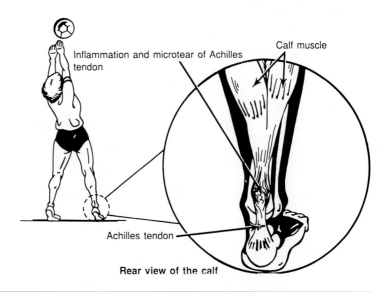

METATARSAL STRESS FRACTURE   Figure 7–27

Definition

An overuse condition in the bone, characterized by a microfracture of the metatarsal bone. An aching pain in the foot during long running.

Cause

- Acute: a sudden pain or snap in a previously weakened bone. Occurs during a jump.
- Chronic: repeat microtrauma in a runner or dancer who has foot imbalance and who performs on hard surfaces. Associated factors: obesity, malnutrition, and in some cases eating disorders.

Subjective Symptoms

- Pain well localized directly over the bone on top of the foot.
- Swelling initially not present.
- Stiffness present after running.
- Crepitation not present.

Objective Findings

- Tenderness is well localized on the bone surface.
- Local swelling may be present as the healing bone forms.
- Loss of motion is not present.

Testing Procedures

- Initial radiographs may appear normal, but radiographs 2 or 3 weeks later show healing bone formation.
- Bone scan is diagnostic.
- MRI is not required.

Prognosis

The most important aspect of this condition is proper recognition and diagnosis; otherwise, many months of bone healing are required. Total rest is not required. Casting generally is not needed. Many alternative activities are available. Proper shoes and orthotics are very helpful. Avoiding obesity and malnutrition is important.

Metatarsal Stress Fracture

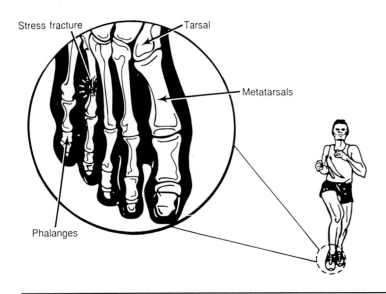

Figure 7–27

Metatarsal stress fracture. (From Play Healthy, Stay Healthy _[pp. 101–152] by Gary N. Guten, Champaign, IL: Human Kinetics Publishers. Copyright 1991 by Gary N. Guten. Reprinted by permission.)_

PLANTAR FASCIITIS (HEEL PAIN)   Figure 7–28

Definition
A traumatic, degenerative process characterized by pain along the inner aspect of the heel and radiating along the arch. May occur in a young runner or a middle-aged person with foot imbalance.

Cause
- Acute: violent jumping and tearing of the plantar fascia (the heavy ligament band along the arch).
- Chronic: microtrauma or overuse of the foot, associated with foot imbalance, muscle imbalance, and tight ligaments in the foot.

Subjective Symptoms
- Pain, especially on awakening in the morning and with first steps.
- Swelling generally not present.
- Stiffness present, especially in the morning with weight-bearing on the rested foot.
- Occasional numbness in the heel.

Objective Findings
- Tenderness is well localized to the inner aspect of the heel.

- Swelling is generally not present.
- Instability of the foot may be present with a pronated foot.
- Results of nerve examination are generally normal.

Testing Procedures
- Radiographs may appear normal, but a spur on the heel may be present.
- Scan may show a positive area on the bone where the ligament attaches.
- MRI is generally not necessary.
- Arthroscopy is not performed.

Prognosis
Chronic pain due to poor healing is usual because of poor circulation to the ligament and stresses on the heel. Referral to a sports podiatrist to fabricate orthotics may be necessary. Surgery is unusual, but chronic cases may require cutting the ligament where it attaches to the heel.

Plantar Fasciitis (Heel Pain)

Figure 7–28

Plantar fasciitis. (From Play Healthy, Stay Healthy *[pp. 101–152] by Gary N. Guten, Champaign, IL: Human Kinetics Publishers. Copyright 1991 by Gary N. Guten. Reprinted by permission.)*

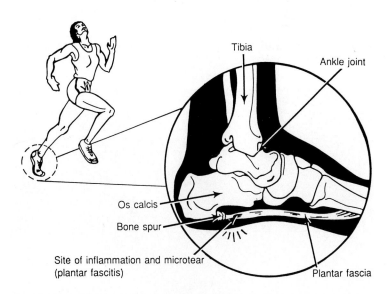

Tibia
Ankle joint
Os calcis
Bone spur
Site of inflammation and microtear (plantar fascitis)
Plantar fascia

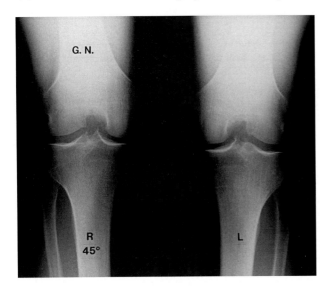

Figure 7–29

Case 1: 45-degree flexion radiograph. Note minimal degenerative changes of the knees.

CASE REPORTS—RADIOLOGIC

"WE TREAT PEOPLE—NOT X-RAYS"

In our sports medicine clinic, we have a sign under every radiography view box that says "We treat people—not x-rays." The following cases are examples of how standard radiologic studies can sometimes lead to incorrect treatment pathways. The history and physical examination are the most important elements of a proper diagnosis and treatment plan—especially for runners. We find the bone scan and the 45-degree flexion radiograph to be helpful adjuncts in the diagnosis and treatment plan.

■ **CASE 1**   This 59-year-old man has run 62 marathons and developed knee pain. His family physician had been treating him for degenerative meniscus problems. Results of flexion radiographs were within normal limits (Fig. 7–29). A tangential patella radiograph showed considerable narrowing and degenerative changes primarily of the right knee (Fig. 7–30). The bone scan showed a dramatic amount of inflammation at the patellofemoral joints (Fig. 7–31). The patient responded to a patella rehabilitation program, light running, and race walking.

■ **CASE 2**   This 65-year-old man has run 250 marathons. His best time, in 1974, was 2 hours and 55 minutes. His last marathon was in 1992, when his time was 4 hours and 22

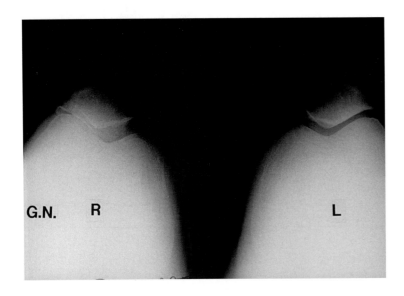

Figure 7–30

Case 1: Tangential patella radiograph. Note extensive degenerative changes of the right patella.

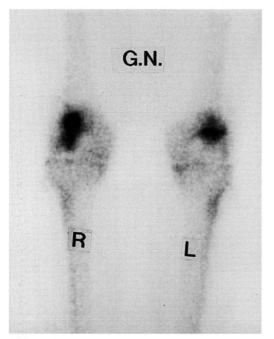

Figure 7–31

Case 1: Bone scan of the knees. Note localized uptake at the patella, right greater than left.

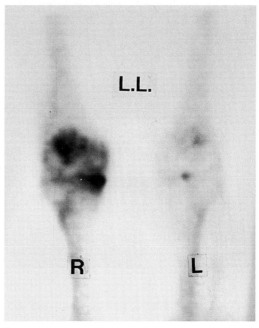

Figure 7–33

Case 2: Bone scan of the knees. Note localized uptake in the right medial compartment and patella.

minutes. He has developed progressive pain on the medial compartment of his right knee. Anteroposterior radiographs showed no significant joint space narrowing or degenerative changes (Fig. 7–32). However, a bone scan showed localization of the inflammation of the medial compartment of the right knee and the patellofemoral joint (Fig. 7–33).

An arthrogram showed only a very ques-

tionable tear of the anterior aspect of the medial meniscus. However, after failure of conservative management, arthroscopy was performed. It revealed a very significant complex tear of the posterior horn of the medial meniscus with very little degenerative joint disease, despite very positive findings on the bone scan.

In our experience, the findings on bone

Figure 7–32

Case 2: Standing radiograph of the knees showing slight degenerative changes.

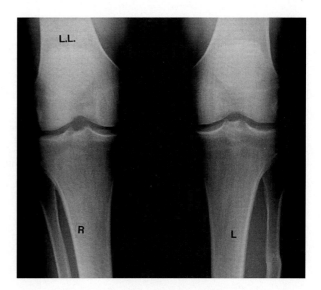

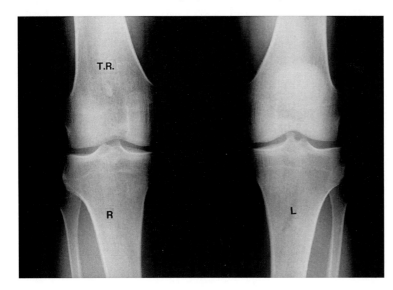

Figure 7–34

Case 3: Standing radiograph of the knees showing patellectomy on the right. All symptoms are in the left knee.

scan and the amount of osteoarthritis normally are closely correlated. In this case, the patient had minimal osteoarthritis. The inflammatory response was related to the torn medial meniscus.

Long-term results of this case are not available, but the patient was encouraged to return to light running and race walking.

■ *CASE 3*   This 37-year-old man had a patellectomy of the right knee after an auto accident. He has been able to run about 15 miles per week and developed vague pain on the opposite left knee. The pain was responding to conservative management. He has no signs or symptoms when running despite the patellectomy of the right knee. An

anteroposterior standing radiograph shows the right knee with the patellectomy has not developed degenerative changes (Fig. 7–34). Although some patients are encouraged not to run with a patellectomy, this patient demonstrates that the knee, in selective cases, can tolerate running without a patella.

■ *CASE 4*   This 41-year-old man runs 15 miles per week. He hit his knee on a power cart and developed progressive pain about the right patella. A standard lateral radiograph of the knee showed minimal spurring and degenerative changes on the inferior pole of the patella (Fig. 7–35). Bone scan showed increased, intense localization of the inflammation to the inferior pole of the patella

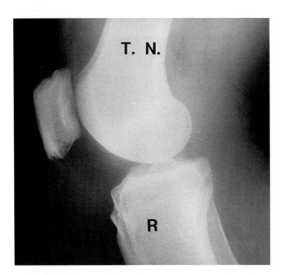

Figure 7–35

Case 4: Lateral radiograph of the right knee showing spurs on the inferior pole of the patella.

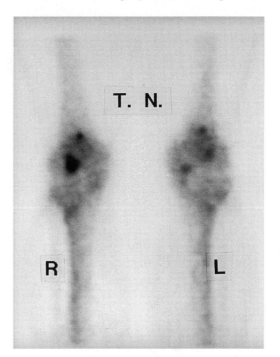

Figure 7–36

Case 4: Bone scan of the knee, anteroposterior view. Note the localized uptake at the right patella, where it was very painful.

(Fig. 7–36). He responded to conservative management and was allowed to return to light running, swimming, and race walking.

▮ *CASE 5* This 61-year-old man currently runs 15 miles per week. He developed slowly progressive medial joint pain without any specific trauma. Anteroposterior standing radiographs show moderate degenerative changes with maintenance of the joint space

(Fig. 7–37). However, a 45-degree flexion radiograph shows complete obliteration of the posterior joint space and the varus alignment in flexion (Fig. 7–38). Bone scan shows well-localized intense inflammation of the medial compartment of the right knee (Fig. 7–39). Despite these findings, the patient is still active and has minimal symptoms while running 15 miles per week, race walking, swimming, and biking. He understands that he will

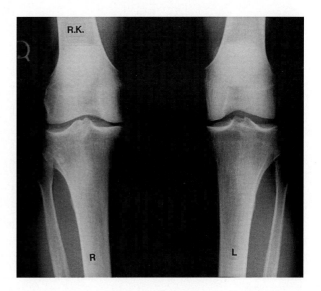

Figure 7–37

Case 5: Standing radiograph of the knees. Note moderate narrowing of the right medial compartment.

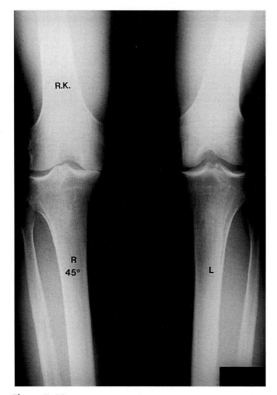

Figure 7–38

Case 5: 45-degree flexion radiograph of the knees. Note the bone-on-bone changes and loss of the medial compartment of the right knee.

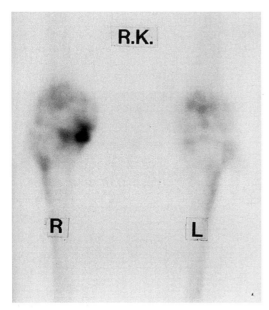

Figure 7–39

Case 5: Bone scan of the knees, anteroposterior view. Note the intense localized uptake at the medial compartment of the right knee.

eventually need a knee replacement or an osteotomy, but at this time his symptoms are minimal.

■ **CASE 6** This 32-year-old, highly competitive triathlete, who usually finishes in the top 5% of his events, developed a workers' compensation injury with trauma to the anterior aspect of the knee. MRI was performed, and results were interpreted as a torn medial meniscus. The patient was referred for arthroscopic menisectomy. Clinical findings, however, revealed tenderness on the patella ligament and no joint line tenderness. The lateral view of the MRI scan showed a horizontal signal in the medial meniscus, most likely on a degenerative basis—not traumatic and not clinically significant (Fig. 7–40).

A bone scan showed intense uptake along the anterior aspect of the knee, corresponding to the tenderness and swelling of the patella ligament (Fig. 7–41). He responded to conservative management and returned to running without any surgery.

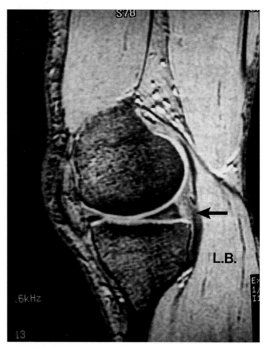

Figure 7–40

Case 6: MRI of the knee. Lateral view of the medial meniscus. Note the horizontal signal read as a tear of the medial meniscus. The patient had no medial joint symptoms.

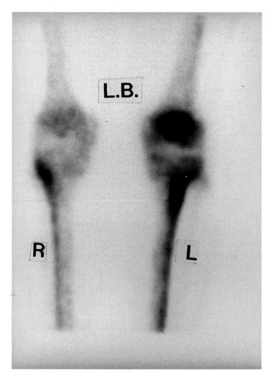

Figure 7–41

Case 6: Bone scan of the knees; anteroposterior view showing intense anterior uptake. Injury occurred along the patellar ligament.

SUMMARY

With this general overview of leg injuries, health care providers can approach the more specific and detailed sections of this book. Discussed were the following areas:

- Causes of injuries
- History and physical examination
- Treatment plan
- Specific injuries (12)
- Case reports

REFERENCES

1. d'Ambrosia R, Drez D: Prevention and Treatment of Running Injuries. Thorofare, NJ, Slack, 1982.
2. Andrews J: Overuse syndromes of the lower extremity. Clin Sports Med 2:137–149, 1983.
3. Apple D: End state running problems. Clin Sports Med 4:657–670, 1985.
4. Atwell EA, Jackson D: Stress fractures of the sacrum in runners; two case reports. Am J Sports Med 19:531–533, 1991.
5. Baker M, Swafford D, Paty JG: Knee effusions in long distance runners. Arthritis Rheum 245:61, 1981.
6. Baxter D, Zingas C: The foot in running. J Am Acad Orthop Surg 3:136–145, 1995.
7. Beck J, Wildermuth B: The female athlete's knee. Clin Sports Med 4:345–366, 1985.
8. Blair S, Kohl III H: Changes in physical fitness and all-cause mortality: A prospective study of healthy and unhealthy men. JAMA 273:1093–1098, 1995.
9. Brody D: Running injuries—prevention and management. Clin Symp 39:1–36, 1987.
10. Brouklin B, Fox J: The synovial shelf syndrome. Clin Orthop Rel Res 142:132–138, 1979.
11. Butts N, Tucker M, Greening C: Physiologic response to maximal treadmill and deep water running in men and women. Am J Sports Med 19:612–614, 1991.
12. Cavanagh P, LaFortune M: Ground reaction forces and distance running. J Biomech 13:397–406, 1980.
13. Clancy W: Runner's injuries: Evaluation and treatment of specific injuries. Am J Sports Med 8:287–289, 1980.
14. Clement D, Taunton J: A survey of overuse running injuries. Physician Sportsmed 9:47–58, 1981.
15. Collier D, Fogelman I: Bone scintigraphy: Orthopedic bone scanning. J Nucl Med 34:22–41, 1993.
16. Collins K, Wagner M: Overuse injuries in triathletes: A study of the 1986 Seafair Triathlon. Am J Sports Med 17:675–678, 1989.
17. Cox J: Patellofemoral problems in runners. Clin Sports Med 4:699–715, 1985.
18. Czerniecki J, Lippert F: Biomechanical evaluation of tibiofemoral rotation in anterior cruciate deficient knees during walking and running. Am J Sports Med 16:327–331, 1988.
19. DeFillippo J, Yu J: Too much exercise. J Musculoskel Med August:61–66, 1994.
20. Fixx J: The Compete Book of Running. New York, Random House, 1977.
21. Foster C, Anholm J, Guten G: World-record rope skipping performance. Physician Sportsmed 8:65–70, 1980.
22. Fredericson M, Bergman AG, Hoffman K, Dillingham M: Tibial stress reaction in runners. Am J Sports Med 23:472–480, 1995.
23. Fries J, Singh G: Running and the development of disability with age. Ann Intern Med 121:502–509, 1994.
24. Grana W, Coniglione T: Knee disorders in runners. Phys Sportsmed 13(5):127–133, 1985.
25. Guten G: Methylene blue staining of articular cartilage during arthroscopy. Orthop Rev 7:59–60, 1977.
26. Guten G: Herniated lumbar disk associated with running: A review of 10 cases. Am J Sports Med 9:155–159, 1981.
27. Guten G: A ten-point "Stop and Go" sports medicine program. J Musculoskel Med 3:24–26, 1986.
28. Guten G: Walking, an excellent alternative to running. Ann Sports Med 5:209, 1990.
29. Guten G: Play Healthy Stay Healthy. Champaign IL, Human Kinetics Publishers, 1991.
30. Guten G, Craviotto D: Bone scan changes in a marathon runner; case report. Wis Med J 68:11, 1985.
31. Guten G, Craviotto D, Maier T: Iliotibial band friction syndrome in runners with bone lesion of lateral femoral condyle. Ann Sports Med 1:79–81, 1983.
32. Guten G, Harvey D: Herniated lumbar disc with leg paralysis associated with jogging—case report. Wis Med J 76:119–120, 1977.
33. Guten G, McGlocklin J: Exercise, Nutrition and Cancer. Milwaukee, WI, Montgomery Media, 1995.

34. Guten G, Pietrocarlo T: Change, alignment, twisting and speed—foot orthotics for knee pain. American Medical Athletic Association Quarterly 6:5–10, 1991.

35. Guyot W: Psychological and medical factors associated with pain running. J Sports Med 31:452–460, 1991.

36. Harrison R, Lees A: A bioengineering analysis of human muscle and joint forces in the lower limbs during running. J Sports Sci 4:201–218, 1986.

37. Highgeboten C, Jackson A: The effect of knee brace wear on perceptual and metabolic variables during horizontal treadmill running. Am J Sports Med 19:639–643, 1991.

39. Ho S, Coel M: Magnetic resonance imaging abnormalities in asymptomatic, older knee. Proceedings of the Annual Meeting of the American Academy of Orthopaedic Surgeons. Orlando, FL, Feb 16–21, 1995.

40. Jacobs SJ, Bernson BL: Injuries to runners: A study of entrants to a 10,000 meter race. Am J Sports Med 14:151–155, 1986.

41. James S: Running injuries to the knee. J Am Acad Orthop Surg 3:309–318, 1995.

42. Jerosch J, Castro W, Halm H, et al: Magnetic resonance imaging findings in the meniscus and asymptomatic subjects. Proceedings of the Annual Meeting of the American Academy of Orthopaedic Surgeons. Orlando, FL, Feb 16–21, 1995.

43. Jorgensen U: Body load in heel-strike running; the effect of firm heel counter. Am J Sports Med 18:177–181, 1990.

44. Kibler B, Goldberg C: Functional biomechanical deficits in running athletes with plantar fasciitis. Am J Sports Med 16:66–71, 1991.

45. Kohn H, Guten G: Chondromalacia of the patella: Bone imaging correlated with arthroscopic findings. Clin Nucl Med 13:96–100, 1988.

46. Kondrasen L, Hansen EM: Long distance running and osteoarthrosis. Am J Sports Med 18:379–381, 1990.

47. Kujala UM, Jaakkola L: Scoring of patellofemoral disorders. J Arthroscopy 9:159–163, 1993.

48. Kujala U, Kettunen Y: Knee osteoarthritis in former runners, soccer players, weight lifters, and shooters. Arthritis Rheum 38:539–546, 1995.

49. Kujala U, Kvist M, Osterman K: Knee injuries in athletes: A review of exertion injuries and retrospective study of outpatient sports clinic material. J Sports Med 3:447–460, 1986.

50. Lane N, Michael B: Risk of osteoarthritis with running and aging: A 5-year longitudinal study. J Rheumatol 20:461–468, 1993.

51. Lane N, Bloch D: Long distance running, bone density, and osteoarthritis. JAMA 255:1147–1151, 1986.

52. Leach R: In d'Ambrosia R, Drez D: Prevention and Treatment of Running Injuries. Thorofare, NJ, Slack, 1982.

53. Lehmann M, Foster C, Keul J: Overtraining in endurance athletes; a brief review. Med Sci Sports Exerc 25:854–862, 1993.

54. Lindenberg G, Pinshaw R, Noakes T: Iliotibial band friction syndrome in runners. Physician Sportsmed 12:119–130, 1984.

55. Lutter L: Runner's knee injuries. Instruct Course Lect 33:253–268, 1984.

56. Lutter L: The knee and running. Clin Sports Med 4:684–698, 1985.

57. Lysholm J, Wiklander J: Injuries in runners. Am J Sports Med 15:168–171, 1987.

58. Marti B, Knobloch M: Is excessive running predictive of degenerative hip disease? Br Med J 299:91–93, 1989.

59. McCaw S: Leg length inequality. Sports Med 14:422–429, 1992.

60. McKenzie D, Clement DB, Taunton JE: Running shoes, orthotics, and injuries. J Sports Med 2:334–347, 1985.

61. Mechelen W: Running injuries: A review of the epidemiologic literature. J Sports Med 14:320–335, 1992.

62. Mechelen W, Hlobil H, Kemper H, et al: Prevention of running injuries by warm-up, cool-down, and stretching exercises. Am J Sports Med 21:711–719, 1993.

63. Messier S, Davis S: Etiologic factors associated with patellofemoral pain in runners. Med Sci Sports Exerc 23:1008–1015, 1991.

64. Micheli L, Fehlandt A: Overuse injuries to tendons and apophyses in children and adolescents. Clin Sports Med 11:713–725, 1992.

65. Montgomery W, Pink M: Electromyographic analysis of hip and knee musculature during running. Am J Sports Med 22:272–278, 1994.

66. Murray M, Guten G: Kinematic and electromyographic patterns of Olympic race walkers. Am J Sports Med 11:68–73, 1983.

67. Newmark S, Toppo F: Fluid and electrolyte replacement in the ultramarathon runner. Am J Sports Med 19:389–391, 1991.

68. Panush R, Schmidt C: Is running associated with degenerative joint disease? JAMA 255:1152–1154, 1986.

69. Paty J: Diagnosis and treatment of musculoskeletal running injuries. Semin Arthritis Rheum 18:48–60, 1988.

70. Paty J: Running injuries. Curr Opin Rheumatol 6:203–209, 1994.

71. Paty J, Swafford D: Adolescent running injuries. J Adolesc Health Care 5:87–90, 1984.

72. Powell KE, Kohn HW, Capersen CJ: An epidemiological perspective on the causes of running injuries. Phys Sportsmed 14:100–114, 1986.

73. Pritikin N: The Pritikin Program for Diet and Exercise. New York, Grosset & Dunlap, 1979.

74. Puffer J, McShane J: Depression and chronic fatigue in athletes. Clin Sports Med 11:327–337, 1992.

75. Rice S, Blasingame S: Anterior knee pain in a 29 year old woman. Physician Sportsmed 17:129–132, 1989.

76. Rosenberg T, Paulos L, Parker R, et al: The forty-five degree posteroanterior flexion weight-bearing radiograph of the knee. J Bone Joint Surg Am 70:1479–1482, 1988.

77. Shellock F, Deutsch A, Mink JH: Do asymptomatic marathon runners have an increased prevalence of meniscus abnormalities? An MR study of the knee and 23 volunteers. AJR Am J Roentgenol 157:1239–1241, 1991.

78. Stamford B: No pain no gain. Physician Sportsmed 15:244, 1987.

79. Verde T, Thomas S: Potential markers of heavy training and highly trained distance runners. Br J Sports Med 26:167–175, 1992.

80. Wilder R, Brennan D: A standard measure of exercise prescription for aqua running. Am J Sports Med 21:45–48, 1993.

GREGG R. FOOS ■ JAMES M. FOX

━━━━━ *CHAPTER EIGHT*

Arthroscopy of the Knee in Runners

Distance running has undergone a dramatic increase in popularity since the early 1970s. The achievements of Frank Shorter in the 1972 Olympics helped draw public attention to the sport. A renewed interest in personal fitness during the late 1970s and 1980s and the realization that running has a significant role as part of a basic fitness program are responsible for increasing the popularity of distance running as a sport. Distance running has become not only a sport of elite athletes but a sport that is enjoyed by the general public. This tremendous increase in the number of runners was followed by a dramatic increase in the prevalence of running injuries. The medical field quickly began to focus more attention on the problem of running injuries. Approximately 30% of serious runners experience an injury in any given year.[62] In 1991, MacIntyre and colleagues surveyed 4173 running injuries and found the knee to be the site most commonly injured.[77] Several other studies have confirmed these findings, recognizing that more than one third of running injuries involve the knee.[63, 115]

Advancements in technology allowed the surgeons of the early 1970s to explore the inner aspects of the knee during the same time as this increased prevalence of running injuries. The arthroscope opened new horizons to surgeons for the diagnosis and treatment of knee injuries, including those commonly due to running. Before the development and refinement of arthroscopic techniques, open knee surgery was the only option available to surgeons. Although the results of knee surgery following arthrotomy were good, the recovery phase after surgery was often prolonged. The arthroscope has provided a minimally invasive approach to diagnose knee injuries accurately and a means to perform sophisticated procedures to treat pathologic disorders. Arthroscopy has been associated with minimal morbidity and quick recovery, allowing expeditious return to training.

The vast majority of injuries to the knee during running are related to overuse. These injuries often can be accurately diagnosed by physical examination and various radiographic studies, including standard radiographs, arthrograms, computed tomography (CT), and magnetic resonance imaging (MRI). Arthroscopy is an important means for diagnosis of disorders not revealed by more conservative means. Arthroscopy provides direct visualization of the intraarticular anatomy and enhances the surgeon's ability to identify lesions of the articular cartilage, meniscus, and ligaments. The arthroscope also allows dynamic assessment of motion of the knee joint for patellofemoral tracking disorders.

Most running injuries involving the knee respond to conservative treatment, but occasionally, when conservative management fails to allow a patient to return to his or her preinjury performance level, surgical intervention may be indicated. The arthroscope allows surgeons to deal with the intraarticular pathology through limited incisions, thereby expediting the return of athletes to their sport. Arthroscopic techniques should not be considered a replacement for open surgery but a means by which the surgeon may approach treatment of the injured joint less invasively.

This chapter reviews development and refinement of the arthroscope and arthroscopic technique. The most common intraarticular pathologies encountered in the sport of running are discussed in detail. Included in this discussion are the latest approaches to treatment of these injuries and the role of the arthroscope in this treatment.

ARTHROSCOPY

The arthroscope was first developed as early as the late 1800s and consisted of a rudimentary cystoscope that used candlelight as a light source. The arthroscope continued to undergo changes, and reports of intraarticular visualization are found in the early 1920s.[11] Burman and colleagues reported their experience with cadaver knee arthroscopy at the Hospital for Joint Disease in 1934.[18] The practical use of the arthroscope for diagnosis of knee pathology did not occur until the 1960s in Japan, where Watanabe and associates published the *Atlas of Arthroscopy* in 1969.[116] The arthroscopic revolution was started in the early 1970s with the advent of fiberoptics, which allowed safe delivery of light into the joint, creating a cold light source that was not damaging to the internal structures of the knee.

Advances in optics have further enabled surgeons to delineate intraarticular pathology. In 1975, O'Connor introduced the operative arthroscope, which provided direct visualization along with a channel for placement of operative instruments.[90] The need for this has largely been replaced by the development of triangulation techniques and use of oblique lenses. These techniques involve placement of instruments through separate operative portals that are visualized by the arthroscope. This allows the surgeon to gain greater perspective of the operative field. Modern technology has introduced video capabilities that allow surgeons to operate comfortably while viewing the knee structures at significant magnification, thereby providing precise visualization of the operative field (Fig. 8–1). Small, flexible arthroscopes have been introduced to enable arthroscopists to perform diagnostic arthroscopy in an office setting.

Paralleling the advancement of visualization is the development of operative instruments for dealing with the pathology at hand (Fig. 8–2). A large array of probes, basket forceps, and small scalpel blades are available to help reach within the confines of the joint. Motorized shavers and abraders also expedite removal of meniscal and synovial tissue. Electrocautery was introduced in the 1980s and has proved effective for intraarticular hemostasis and ablation of material within the knee. Laser technology has also been implemented as a tool for ablation of synovial and meniscal tissue where operative instruments prove to be difficult to manipulate.

RUNNING INJURIES

The arthroscope is a tool that allows a less invasive means by which to diagnose and manage the intraarticular pathology of the

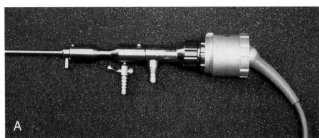

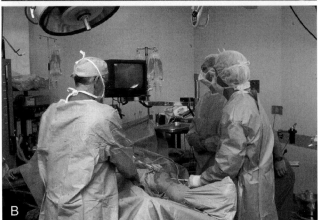

Figure 8–1

A: *The modern arthroscope.* **B:** *The operating room setup with video monitor capabilities.*

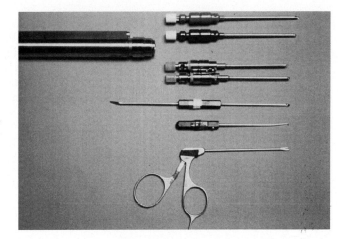

Figure 8–2

Arthroscopic instruments including motorized shavers, an arthroscopic probe, and meniscal basket forceps.

knee joint. The majority of knee injuries in runners are extraarticular and are not accessible to arthroscopic treatment. Intraarticular pathology that occurs in runners usually includes symptomatic plica, chondral lesions, patellofemoral alignment problems, and meniscal tears. Although the arthroscope renders these problems accessible to a surgeon, it must be emphasized that surgery is often the last resort. Technique modifications and conservative treatment options are primary approaches to these problems. Surgery is used as an early treatment in certain conditions that are effectively treated only arthroscopically, such as loose bodies and entrapped meniscal lesions. Surgery may also be indicated when conservative treatment fails to allow a runner to return to his or her premorbid level of training.

SYMPTOMATIC PLICA

A plica is a normal fold of synovium in the knee. These folds represent mesenchymal septa that are found embryologically during knee development and have undergone incomplete degeneration. The plica performs no known function in the human knee.

Plica can occur at four locations in the knee, and each bears a descriptive name (Fig. 8–3). *Plica synovialis patellaris (ligamentum mucosum)* occurs in the intracondylar notch, often connecting the fat pad to the contents of the notch. The ligamentum mucosum is the most commonly occurring plica but the least commonly symptomatic. The *plica synovialis suprapatellaris (suprapatellar plica)* is the second most common and varies in shape and width. The *plica synovialis mediopatellaris (medial plica)*

creates a shelf of synovium along the medial compartment of the knee in the coronal plane. The *plica synovialis lateropatellaris (lateral plica)* is uncommon but has been reported.[68]

Symptomatic plica syndrome represents a thickened, hypertrophic plica that causes pain on flexion of the knee (Fig. 8–4). The prevalence of plica syndrome is 2% to 5.5%.[15, 29, 89, 97] There is no consensus on the pathophysiology of symptomatic plica. Approximately half of the cases involve a blow to the knee, supporting a trauma theory of origin. This theory proposes that trauma causes inflammation and hemorrhage within the plica,

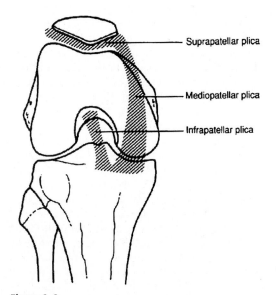

— Suprapatellar plica

— Mediopatellar plica

— Infrapatellar plica

Figure 8–3

The three most commonly occurring locations for synovial plica. (From Aglietti P, Windsor RE, Kelly MA, et al: Disorders of the patellofemoral joint. In Insall J [ed]: Surgery of the Knee 2nd ed. New York, Churchill Livingstone, 1993.)

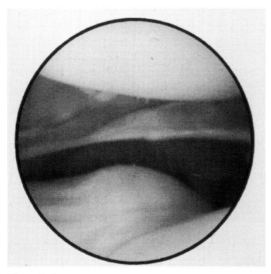

Figure 8–4

Arthroscopic picture of a symptomatic plica. Notice the thickened, hypertrophic appearance of the synovial fold. (From Johnson L: Arthroscopic Surgery—Principles and Practice. St. Louis, CV Mosby, 1986.)

eventually leading to the pathologic thickening. A second theory, the impingement theory, proposes that strenuous activity creates impingement of the plica between the patella and medial femoral condyle.

Plica syndrome results in chronic anteromedial knee pain and tightness in the suprapatellar region on full flexion. An effusion usually is not present.[89] Symptoms also include snapping, buckling, and pain with strenuous activity or prolonged sitting. In runners, pain may occur gradually with distance running or may be associated with sudden changes in training routine. The nonspecific nature of this disorder makes it a diagnosis of exclusion. Medial meniscal tear and patellofemoral malalignment/chondromalacia are the most common misdiagnoses.[15, 47] Also included in the differential diagnosis are jumper's knee, bipartite patella, and degenerative joint disease. Physical findings most commonly include tenderness over the medial femoral condyle or a palpable snap along the medial joint line with flexion of the knee. Diagnostic studies such as double-contrast arthrography and MRI may demonstrate a plica but are unable to determine a causative association with the symptoms.

Conservative treatment of symptomatic plica includes rest, nonsteroidal antiinflammatory medications, hamstring stretching, and moist heat. Progressive rehabilitation

after symptoms are relieved may return the patient to running activities. Intraplical steroid injection has been reported as treatment for symptomatic plica.[99] Iontophoresis and phonophoresis are also advocated as means to decrease swelling and pain associated with this diagnosis.

The arthroscope has an important role in diagnosis of a symptomatic plica. The plica is best observed with the arthroscope placed through the superolateral portal.[14, 66] A symptomatic medial plica usually appears wide (<12 mm), thickened, and avascular through the arthroscope.[32] While viewing from an arthroscope, a symptomatic plica may be found to impinge between the medial patellar facet and the medial femoral condyle. Advanced cases demonstrate grooving of the articular cartilage secondary to impingement. A symptomatic suprapatellar plica is also thickened and can be seen to impinge on the femur as the knee is brought into full flexion. Arthroscopic treatment is accomplished by resection of the entire plica with use of basket forceps, electrocautery, or motorized shavers. Simply dividing the plica is inadequate, because symptoms may recur during the healing process.[47, 61]

The results of treatment of symptomatic plica are good when other causes of pain are first precluded. Ewing reports good or excellent results with resection of symptomatic plica by arthroscopic technique in 77% of patients.[32] Arthroscopy allows diagnosis and treatment of symptomatic plica without the need for a formal arthrotomy. This means of treatment is minimally invasive and benefits runners in that it allows a fast return to training activities after a short rehabilitation period of usually 4 to 6 weeks.

CHONDROMALACIA PATELLAE

The breakdown of articular cartilage involving the patellofemoral joint was first noted by Budinger in 1906 when he drew attention to softening and fissuring of the normally smooth articular cartilage.[17] In 1917, Aleman began to use the term *chondromalacia* in his clinical work to describe these articular cartilage changes.[3, 64] The term *chondromalacia* first appeared in the literature in a report by Koenig in 1924.[92] Since that time, chondromalacia has been a subject of much controversy. Although *chondromalacia* is a descriptive term for softening and fissuring of articular cartilage, it has been used synonymously with *patellofemoral pain syndrome.* No mechanism for production of pain has ever been conclusively associated with these articular cartilage changes. The correlation between the presence and severity of chondromalacia and the clinical symptoms associated with patellofemoral pain syndrome seems poor.[8, 21, 22, 44, 45, 56, 58, 59, 67, 70, 72, 75, 81, 84, 94, 112]

The patellofemoral joint is a unique articulation. The patella increases the moment arm of the quadriceps mechanism while protecting the knee from direct blows. The patella centralizes the extensor mechanism in the trochlear groove. The articular cartilage decreases the coefficient of friction across the joint, thereby increasing the efficiency of the quadriceps mechanism. Normal articular cartilage relies on compressive forces but has a threshold for injury. Disuse causes articular

cartilage changes mainly on the odd facet of the patella, and these changes are usually reversible.[44] Overuse and abnormally large compressive forces produced by maltracking syndromes cause surface degeneration of the articular cartilage.

Outerbridge provided a classification for breakdown of the articular cartilage (Fig. 8–5).[91] Grade 0 is normal articular cartilage. Grade 1 represents swelling and softening of the cartilage with minimal surface disruption. Grade 2 involves fibrillation and fragmentation of the most superficial layers of cartilage. Grade 3 is marked by fibrillation extending into the deeper zones and is described as having a "crabmeat" appearance. Grade 4 is represented by destruction of the articular cartilage with exposure of the subchondral bone.

Chondromalacia occurs with a higher incidence in adolescents and young adults, in

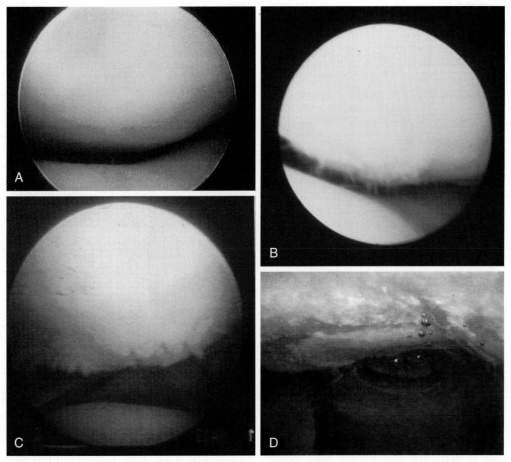

Figure 8–5

*Outerbridge classification of chondromalacia. **A:** Grade 1 involvement including softening of the articular cartilage. **B:** Superficial fibrillation marks grade 2 changes. **C:** Grade 3 changes with deep fibrillation and fragmentation. **D:** Complete cartilage erosion with exposed subchondral bone indicative of grade 4.*

particular females. A history of trauma or an underlying patellar malalignment is commonly reported. Patella alta, vastus medialis obliquus atrophy, or tight hamstrings often accompany this condition. Symptoms include pain, swelling, and stiffness. Pain often occurs with prolonged sitting or stair climbing and is often localized to the patellofemoral joint but may be more generalized. Crepitus and giving way of the knee are often reported by patients. Provocative tests consistent with diagnosis of chondromalacia include a positive compression sign and pain associated with extension of the knee against resistance.[41] It should again be emphasized that chondromalacia commonly occurs with advancing age and may be completely asymptomatic.

The underlying cause of chondromalacia must be sought through history taking and physical examination. Axial radiographs and special studies such as CT scan and MRI are often helpful in determining the underlying cause of cartilage breakdown. Trauma is frequently an inciting factor. A blow to the knee or dislocation of the patella oftens cause cartilage breakdown in the area of the medial ridge and medial patellar facet. As previously stated, disuse alters the normal compressive forces needed for normal cartilage matrix production, leading to chondromalacia, usually limited to the odd facet.[44] This is found to be reversible in the early stages. Overuse tends to cause cartilage breakdown in the region of the central patellar ridge and extending medially and laterally. Tightness of the lateral retinaculum causes tilt of the patella known as *lateral compression syndrome*. This increases the forces across the lateral facet and causes cartilage breakdown. If no other underlying cause is found, the condition is classified as idiopathic. The underlying cause must be pursued because the prognosis depends on elimination of the incipient factors responsible for the cartilage injury.

Arthroscopes have enabled surgeons to determine the exact location of the cartilage damage and to classify the extent of the lesion adequately. Probing the cartilage surface reveals any softening of the cartilage and may also reveal the depth of fibrillation or the presence of exposed bone.

The efficacy of debridement of the damaged cartilage is controversial. In the past, open articular cartilage shaving was associated with poor results. Merchant points out that these results may have been secondary to failure to recognize underlying patellofemoral mal-tracking.[23] Also, the importance of axial radiographs for diagnosis of maltracking was not recognized at this time. Furthermore, the medial parapatellar incision used may have worsened the problem by weakening the medial stabilizers of the patella. Arthroscopic shaving with basket forceps or motorized shavers allows smoothing of the articular surface. This theoretically eliminates catching of these articular flaps during knee flexion and extension. Loose cartilage flaps within the joint have been implicated as the source of protease production, which may be responsible for a reactive synovitis and the pain.[25]

Debridement alone does not correct the underlying mechanical forces that may be responsible for the cartilage breakdown. Any maltracking must be evaluated arthroscopically and corrected to avoid further articular damage. This approach is now recommended for grade 2 and grade 3 chondromalacia. The prognosis depends on the extent of the lesion and whether the underlying cause is identified and corrected.

Grade 4 articular lesions involve complete articular cartilage loss and exposed subchondral bone. Management of these lesions is the subject of significant controversy. The chondral surfaces lack the ability to regenerate normal hyaline cartilage in these regions. Abrasion arthroplasty involves the removal of the bony surface of the lesion with an arthroscopic bur. This removes the surface of dead osteons exposed by the full-thickness cartilage loss. Vascular ingrowth can then promote fibrocartilage formation to fill the void left by articular cartilage loss. Fibrocartilage is not as functionally resilient as normal hyaline cartilage, and this procedure is indicated mainly for low-activity patients experiencing rest and night pain. A period of deferred weight-bearing is suggested for approximately 6 to 8 weeks after abrasion arthroplasty to allow fibrocartilage ingrowth. The success and usefulness of abrasion arthroplasty in severe chondromalacia remain open to debate.

Although lesser degrees of chondral injury are adequately treated through arthroscopy, advanced chondromalacia in runners is a particularly difficult problem. Debridement or abrasion chondroplasty may provide relief of symptoms associated with chondral lesions, but no long-term solution is yet available. The future may hold some promise for articular cartilage replacement through cloning and culturing of chondrocytes, but no long-term studies have been conducted to support use of such techniques.

MALALIGNMENT OF PATELLOFEMORAL MECHANISM

Anterior knee pain occurring in runners may commonly be due to malalignment of the extensor mechanism. The bony configuration of the patellofemoral joint, the balanced retinaculum, and the muscular pull of the quadriceps all act together to center the patella in the trochlear groove. In a normally aligned patellofemoral articulation, the compressive forces are distributed across the surface of the patella and trochlea. Disorders of bony alignment, imbalance of muscle pull, or retinacular tightness can disrupt the normal tracking of the patella in the femoral groove. The result is tilting or subluxation of the patella. When the normal compressive forces are disrupted, the result is abnormally high loads applied to the cartilage surface. This commonly manifests as chondromalacia. Pain in the malaligned knee may also arise from the retinacular structures as they are stretched to accommodate the maltracking patella.[42]

The concept of patellofemoral malalignment and its contribution to anterior knee pain began evolving in the late 1960s. Hughston described chondromalacia of the medial patellar facet, which he believed was secondary to relocation of the laterally subluxated patella.[53] Merchant and colleagues were the first to classify chondromalacia into two types, those with normal alignment and those with abnormal alignment of the patellofemoral mechanism.[83] This work demonstrated the importance of axial radiographs in the evaluation of patellofemoral alignment. Insall recognized patella alta and excessive quadriceps (Q) angle to be associated with recurrent patellar subluxation.[57] The concept of excessive lateral pressure syndrome was introduced by Ficat and associates in 1975.[34] They suggested that the tightness of the lateral retinaculum caused the patella to tilt, creating an increased contact pressure along the lateral patellar facet. Fulkerson and coworkers described neuromatous degeneration of the small nerves of the tight lateral retinaculum; this was implicated as a source of retinacular pain in this syndrome.[42]

The contribution of these researchers has allowed us to classify the malalignment syndromes further. Malalignment may be separated into subluxation and tilt. Subluxation represents shifting of the patella (most commonly laterally) away from the center of the femoral groove (Fig. 8–6). Bony configuration of the trochlea, imbalanced quadriceps pull, and abnormal femorotibial relationships contribute to maltracking of the patella within the trochlea. Patellar tilt, on the other hand, represents a well-centered patella that is tethered laterally by a tight lateral retinaculum (Fig. 8–7). This substantially increases the lateral facet contact forces. Patellar subluxation and tilt may coexist in the same patient, and both may lead to chondromalacia and eventual osteoarthrosis of the patellofemoral joint.

The pain associated with patellofemoral malalignment may present in various ways. Acute patellar dislocation secondary to a blow to the knee may expose an underlying component of chronic malalignment, but this is uncommon in the running population. More commonly in runners, a long-standing mal-

Figure 8–6

Radiograph of a laterally subluxating patella.

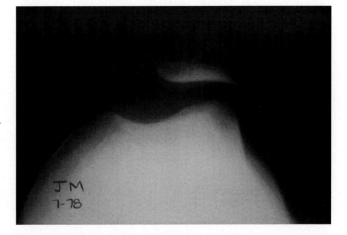

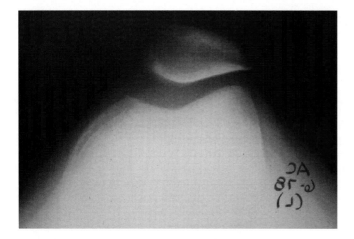

Figure 8–7

Axial radiograph showing lateral tilting of the patella secondary to tightness of the lateral retinaculum.

alignment is responsible for an insidious onset of anterior knee pain. This pain may be associated with changes in the training routine, such as an increase in distance and intensity or the addition of hill training.

Physical examination further helps differentiate malalignment from other causes of anterior knee pain. Flexion and extension of a normal knee reveal that the patella engages the trochlea in approximately 30 degrees of flexion. Visual assessment of the subluxated patella shows that the patella shifts medially or laterally to center in the trochlea. Hypermobility, quadriceps atrophy, and patella alta may be signs of a subluxating patella. Subluxation is also suspected when apprehension is produced by a laterally directed force applied to the patella within the femoral groove.

Tilting of the patella may also be seen on examination. Manual correction of tilt by depressing the medial facet and elevating the lateral facet gives an indication of tightness of the lateral retinaculum.[38] The knee should be evaluated for tenderness, paying particular attention to the lateral patellar margin and lateral retinaculum. Tenderness in the lateral retinaculum may help substantiate the diagnosis of patellar tilt.[41]

Documentation of chondromalacia is important in further classifying the malalignment but alone is not diagnostic of malalignment. A positive compression test of the patella within the trochlea may represent articular damage, particularly when present with effusion and crepitus. Limb alignment needs to be assessed for femoral anteversion, tibial torsion, and foot pronation, all of which may contribute to malalignment of the extensor mechanism.

Radiographic evaluation is essential for the diagnosis of malalignment syndromes. Axial radiographs of the patellofemoral joint may differentiate tilt and subluxation. Merchant and colleagues described the angle of congruence obtained from an axial radiograph of the patella taken with the knee in 45 degrees of flexion and the x-ray beam angled 30 degrees from the horizontal.[83] The angle of congruence defines the position of the apex of the patella in relation to the bisected sulcus angle (Fig. 8–8). An angle greater than 16 degrees defines subluxation of the patella. Laurin and associates used a similar axial radiograph with the knee in 20 degrees of flexion to evaluate patellar tilt.[71] Patellar tilt is represented by the angle created by the lateral facet of the patella and a line drawn across the most prominent aspects of the anterior portions of the femoral trochlea (Fig. 8–9). This angle should normally open laterally, and if it is less than 7 degrees, it may represent tightness of the lateral retinaculum. CT and MRI may also be used to evaluate patellofemoral alignment when midpatellar transverse cuts are taken at various degrees of knee flexion.[102, 103, 107] The angle of congruence and tilt angle may be measured using CT and MRI scans in a similar way as standard radiographs.

The arthroscope has proved invaluable for assessment of patellar malalignment and associated arthrosis. An arthroscope, particularly when placed in the proximal portal, allows evaluation of the patella as it engages the trochlea and tracks through the range of motion. Distension of the joint with saline and removal of the dynamic muscular pull of the quadriceps secondary to anesthesia slightly alter the normal patellar track such that surgical experience and knowledge of the patient's clinical exam should be considered along with

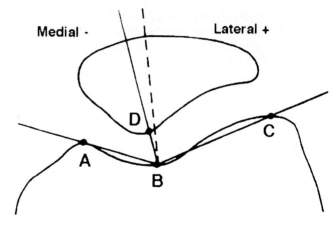

Figure 8–8

Angle of congruence. Line BD is drawn from the deepest point of the sulcus to the central ridge of the patella and compared with the bisected sulcus angle ABC. (Modified from Merchant AC, Mercer RL: Roentgenographic analysis of patellofemoral congruence. J Bone Joint Surg 56A:1391, 1974).

the arthroscopic findings. Both tilt and subluxation may be observed arthroscopically. The arthroscope also allows proper grading of the articular damage present before any realignment. This helps to guide the surgeon in decision making because the prognosis after certain operative procedures is linked to the condition of the articular surface.[40, 74]

Nonoperative management is the mainstay of treatment for all patellofemoral pain syndromes. Reports of success with conservative management range from 50% to 80% for patellofemoral problems, but no studies include only malalignment disorders.[19, 51, 55] The importance of a well-structured rehabilitation program cannot be overemphasized. Treatment should focus on stretching of the deforming structures, such as the retinaculum, hamstrings, and iliotibial band. Strengthening of the quadriceps with isolation of the vastus medialis and retraining of the firing order of the quadriceps muscles is important.[79] External support including patellar tracking braces and patellar taping techniques are advocated to help centralize the extensor mechanism.

Antiinflammatory medications are considered an adjunct to rehabilitation efforts and are used to inhibit inflammation caused by articular degradation within the knee joint. Orthotic correction of foot deformity such as hyperpronation may benefit a runner by correcting tibial rotation as it affects the extensor mechanism alignment. Most cases of patellar malalignment occur in overuse situations and activity modification to eliminate this as an aggravating cause may be necessary.

Operative treatment is considered for only those patients who fail to respond to an organized rehabilitation effort. Operative treatment must be aimed at correcting the underlying malalignment and must also take into account the degree of articular cartilage damage that may be present. Surgical options include lateral release, proximal realignment, distal realignment, or combinations of these.

Lateral release involves sectioning the lateral retinaculum and patellofemoral ligament to allow the patella to seek a more medial position within the femoral groove. Open lateral release was originally introduced by Mer-

Figure 8–9

The patellar tilt angle is formed by a line drawn across the most prominent anterior point of both the medial and lateral condyle and a line drawn along the lateral facet of the patella. This angle should open laterally in a normal knee.

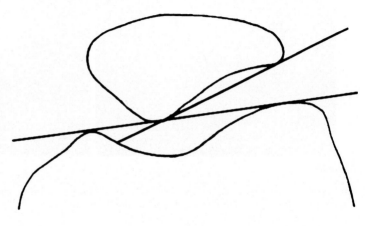

chant and Mercer and has produced varied results.[82] The open technique does not allow the surgeon to assess the patellar tracking from the articular standpoint before disruption of the retinaculum. Arthroscopic lateral release offers many advantages over the open technique. The patellar tracking may be observed before and after the lateral retinaculum is released, thereby allowing the surgeon to assess not only the need for the release but also the immediate results of realignment. This guides decision making in determining whether further balancing of the extensor mechanism is required after the lateral release. Use of an arthroscope also enables a surgeon to adequately grade the condition of the articular surface. This information not only helps determine the prognosis after lateral release but may also guide decision making intraoperatively. In cases of advanced articular damage, a tibial tubercle elevation procedure may be combined with lateral re-

lease. The tibial tubercle elevation acts to decrease the contact forces in the areas of the patella that are damaged. The contact forces are shifted more proximally along the patellar surface when the tibial tubercle is elevated from its normal position.

Arthroscopic lateral release is performed by viewing the lateral retinaculum from a medial suprapatellar portal (Fig. 8–10). Instruments are then placed through either an inferior lateral portal or a superior lateral portal. The synovium and lateral retinaculum are divided from within the joint using one of several instruments. A scalpel blade or scissors may be introduced through a cannula, but excessive bleeding may obscure visualization unless a tourniquet is used. The use of electrocautery for division of the lateral structures is helpful and decreases the occurrence of hematoma postoperatively. Regardless of the instrument used, the synovium and lateral retinaculum must be released entirely to re-

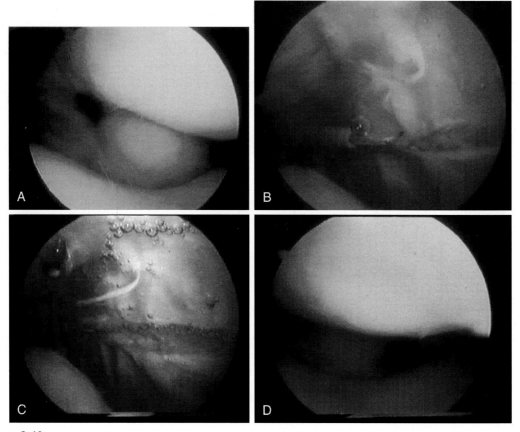

Figure 8–10

*Arthroscopic lateral release. **A:** Subluxated patella before release. **B** and **C:** Electrosurgical tool being used to divide the capsule and lateral retinaculum. **D:** Patellar position after release.*

move the lateral tether and allow the patella to track normally. Care should be taken to avoid injury to the overlying dermal layers when using electrocautery or sharp dissection. The release is performed approximately 1 cm lateral to the patella and should extend from the joint line proximally to the vastus lateralis. Although some researchers recommend division of the most oblique fibers of the vastus lateralis, this has the propensity to weaken the muscle and may lead to overcorrection of the malalignment and medial subluxation of the patella.

Lateral release is indicated for both subluxation and tilt of the patella, when minimal articular cartilage involvement is noted. In cases of tilt, division of the tight lateral retinaculum relieves the excessive pressure on the lateral facet. The patella achieves normal alignment, with the contact forces more evenly distributed across the articular cartilage of both the patellar and trochlear surfaces. Division of the retinaculum may also relieve the pain caused by degeneration of small nerves in the retinaculum that have been stretched. Lateral release is indicated in cases of subluxation in which the patella tracks laterally in the trochlear groove. Division of the lateral structures theoretically allows the patella to become centered within the groove, again better distributing the contact forces across the articular surfaces of both the patella and trochlea.

After arthroscopic lateral release, correction of the malalignment should be viewed arthroscopically as the knee is flexed and extended. In cases of subluxation, lateral release alone may not completely realign the extensor mechanism. The arthroscope guides surgical decision making about whether further realignment procedures are required to balance the patella. If the patella continues to track laterally after lateral release, proximal or distal realignment should be performed. Proximal realignment involves reefing of the medial retinaculum or advancement of the vastus medialis obliquus insertion distally. Arthroscopic techniques have been reported for medial reefing of the patella, but open realignment may allow a surgeon to visualize better the degree of tightening necessary.[114] Distal realignment procedures involve movement of the tibial insertion of the patellar tendon to a more medial position to centralize the patella within the trochlea. Many techniques have been reported to accomplish this. Distal realignment may be best indicated when advanced articular damage is present, requiring tibial tubercle elevation. Fulkerson has described an open procedure in which the tibial tubercle is shifted anteriorly and medially, providing not only correction of malalignment but also a shift of patellar contact forces more proximally on the patellar articular surface, thereby unloading areas of cartilage damage.[39]

The results of both arthroscopic and open realignment procedures for malalignment of the patellofemoral mechanism vary. The factors that affect the prognosis after surgery are the preoperative indications, the degree of articular cartilage damage, and the amount of correction of the malalignment that is achieved during surgery. The indiscriminate use of lateral release for anterior knee pain when normal alignment is present has been associated with poor results, whether done open or arthroscopically. Cadaver studies have shown that lateral release has no effect on tracking when the lateral retinaculum is essentially normal.[96] The results of arthroscopic lateral retinacular release vary among studies and are difficult to compare because of varying techniques and differing indications. Most studies report satisfactory results more than 70% of the time.[1, 9, 10, 22, 24, 26, 30, 31, 45, 48, 52, 67, 69, 70, 78, 81, 83–85, 108, 110] Good or excellent results in cases of knee pain associated with mild tilt or subluxation approach 90% when the malalignment is associated with mild articular cartilage damage (grade 1 or grade 2).[96]

Arthroscopic lateral release is a safe procedure, but complications do occur. A complication rate of 7.2% was reported in a multicenter study.[111] Hemarthrosis is the most common complication, regardless of technique used, but was not shown to compromise the ultimate result.[45, 69, 78, 81, 83, 84, 86, 101, 110] Other complications include skin burns from electrocautery use,[36, 76] deep vein thrombosis,[13, 22] pulmonary embolus,[12] reflex sympathetic dystrophy,[12, 19] infection,[65, 111] adhesions,[36, 108] and medial patellar subluxation.[9, 54] A higher complication rate has been reported with the use of a tourniquet, subcutaneous technique, and the use of postoperative drains.[111]

Runners who have malalignment of the patellofemoral mechanism and who require surgical intervention may return to their running activities. The amount of chondral damage ultimately determines their prognosis. Patients who are well motivated and active in postoperative rehabilitation can expect return to running activities at 6 to 12 weeks postoperatively. The decision to allow return to running should be made only when a patient has completed a progressive running program in therapy without evidence of increased pain, swelling, or limping.

MENISCAL TEARS

The meniscus of the knee was originally thought to have minimal functional significance. Clinical and experimental studies during the past 50 years have shown the important role of the meniscus as it protects the articular surface of the knee by redistributing forces as they are transmitted from the femur to the tibia. Our present understanding of the role of the meniscus stems from experience with knees that have undergone total meniscectomy. Fairbanks observed the radiographic changes that occurred after total meniscectomy and described changes that we now recognize as early radiographic signs of degenerative joint disease: joint space narrowing, squaring of the femoral condyle, osteophyte formation, and subchondral sclerosis.[33]

The menisci consist of fibrocartilaginous discs that are interposed between the femur and tibia. The lateral and medial meniscus vary slightly in shape, but both have a triangular cross section with a thick peripheral border that gradually thins as it progresses centrally to a free edge. Both menisci attach to the tibial plateau at the anterior and posterior horn and attach to the joint capsule by coronary ligaments peripherally. These attachments provide the vascular supply to the meniscus.

The vascular supply to the meniscus has a vital role in healing of the meniscus after meniscal injury. The blood supply to the meniscus originates from the superior and inferior geniculate arteries, both medially and laterally. These form the plexus of vessels within the capsule and synovial tissue attached to the meniscus. The perimeniscal vessels are oriented in a circumferential pattern predominantly, with smaller radial vessels branching toward the center of the knee. Vascular injection studies demonstrate that these vessels penetrate approximately 10% to 30% of the width of the medial meniscus and 10% to 25% of the width of the lateral meniscus.[5] The synovium makes only a minor contribution to the vascular supply of the meniscus.

The meniscus plays an important part in load transmission from the femur to the tibia. Biomechanical studies have shown that the meniscus transmits approximately 50% of the load across the knee in full flexion and up to 85% during flexion.[2] When a total meniscectomy is performed, the contact area between the tibia and the femur is decreased by approximately 50%.[2] This leads to much higher force per unit area placed on the articular cartilage and is responsible for the early degenerative changes noted in meniscectomized knees.

The meniscus has other proposed functions that appear to be important to the normal function of the knee. The meniscus is thought to contribute to the stability of the knee by increasing the congruity between the condyles of the femur and the tibia. This conformity has a role in stability when the primary stabilizers of the knee are injured, such as the anterior cruciate ligament.[73] The viscoelastic nature of the meniscus helps in the role of shock absorption. This dampening of the forces transmitted across the knee joint protects the articular cartilage from damage. Loss of this shock absorber due to meniscectomy has been implicated in the development of osteoarthritis.[95]

Meniscal tear is a common intraarticular cause of knee pain in the general population. Although more than one third of meniscal injuries are associated with sporting activities, distance running is associated with a low incidence of this lesion. Young runners are unlikely to experience a meniscal tear. Sporting activities requiring jumping and twisting have a much higher occurrence of meniscal tear than does running. Young runners with healthy menisci seem fairly well protected from tears of the menisci, barring any misstep or twisting fall. Meniscal lesions are more commonly encountered in middle-aged and older runners. As the menisci age, the fibrocartilage becomes dehydrated and stiff. The normal collagen orientation within the menisci changes, losing the oblique and radially oriented fibers that help convert compressive loads to tensile strain within the menisci. The menisci become susceptible to shearing forces, which tend to split the tissue horizontally.[6, 35] These degenerative, horizontal cleavage tears occur in middle-aged and older runners and become a source of knee pain as flaps catch within the joint.

Meniscal lesions in runners typically present with an insidious onset of pain. The patient is unlikely to report an inciting event, unless a twisting injury occurred. History of a joint effusion or catching is common, but actual locking episodes are rarely reported with these degenerative-type tears. Pain is often present for weeks to months before medical care is sought by the patient.

Physical signs of a meniscal tear are often present on clinical examination. Quadriceps atrophy may accompany any knee injury. A small joint effusion is present in approximately 50% of patients with meniscal tear.[4] Joint line tenderness is the most useful clinical test for a torn meniscus and is present in 77% to 86% of cases.[4, 106] Posterior joint line tenderness is more specific for meniscal tear than that localized anteriorly, which may be found in conjunction with patellofemoral dysfunction. Many provocative tests attempt to cause subluxation of the torn fragment, thereby re-creating the patient's symptoms. Of these tests, the McMurray and Apley grind tests are most clinically helpful.

Clinical examination may be supplemented by use of plain radiography, arthrography, or MRI. Plain radiography is helpful to rule out fracture, bony lesion, and advanced degenerative changes but is rarely diagnostic for meniscal lesion. Double-contrast arthrography was the medium most commonly used in the past for diagnosis of meniscal tears, with a reported accuracy of 60% to 97%.[28, 43, 87, 93] MRI has surpassed arthrography as the medium of choice for evaluation of meniscal pathology because of its noninvasive nature and high specificity, sensitivity, and accuracy. Present technology with enhanced resolution has reported accuracy of 90% to 98% for meniscal tear.[60, 93]

Arthroscopy is still considered to be the best available tool for diagnosis and treatment of meniscal tear. Visualization of the meniscus with the arthroscope, along with probing of potential tears, provides the definitive diagnosis and allows treatment (Fig. 8–11). Arthroscopy is associated with very low morbidity and cosmetically acceptable incisions. Although meniscal pathology can easily and effectively be managed through arthrotomy, the advantages listed, along with a short rehabilitation phase before return to activity, have clearly shown arthroscopy to be the method of choice for treatment of meniscal tears in the running population.

The initial treatment for meniscal tears is generally conservative. A trial of rest and protected weight-bearing is typically indicated

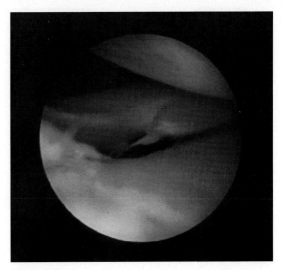

Figure 8–11

Arthroscopic picture of a lateral meniscal tear.

before arthroscopy, and only patients who fail nonoperative treatment are considered candidates for surgical intervention. Patients who experience a locked knee secondary to a displaced meniscal fragment, such as with bucket-handle meniscal tears, are considered early candidates for surgical intervention to restore range of motion of the knee. Even repairable meniscal lesions are amenable to a delay of 8 weeks before treatment with no effects seen on the healing rate of the meniscal tear.[50, 104, 113]

Arthroscopic options for treatment of meniscal tears include total meniscectomy, partial meniscectomy, or meniscal repair. Total meniscectomy has been shown to alter the tibiofemoral contact area significantly, thereby increasing contact stresses.[7, 16, 37, 109] Evidence has clearly associated the occurrence of degenerative changes with resection of the meniscus. Nevertheless, in cases of complex tears that are not amenable to repair, this may be the only option. In this case, patients should be warned of the potential harmful effects of increased stress placed across the knee, such as that caused by high-impact activities including running.

Partial meniscectomy involves removal of only the torn portion of the meniscus, with preservation of any remaining meniscal rim (Fig. 8–12). Less is known about the changes in contact pressures with partial meniscectomy, but these should occur to a lesser degree than with total meniscectomy. The late sequelae of arthritis including pain, effusion,

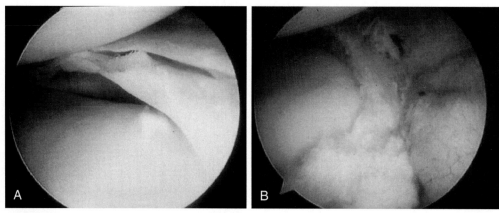

Figure 8–12

A: Meniscal tear. B: Meniscus after partial meniscectomy.

and radiographic changes occur less frequently after partial meniscectomy.[20, 80, 88] For these reasons, partial meniscectomy has supplanted total meniscectomy for treatment of nonrepairable meniscal lesions. Most researchers recommend resection of complex tears and tears involving the inner two thirds of the meniscal rim that have minimal healing potential because of the avascular nature of the meniscus in this region. The goal of the meniscal resection is to remove any portion of torn fibrocartilage that is unstable and may cause catching within the joint. While the tear is visualized arthroscopically, an array of instruments such as scalpel blades, basket forceps, and motorized shavers are used to resect the torn tissues and taper the remaining free edge of the meniscus while leaving the peripheral rim intact.

The realization that the meniscus performs an important functional role within the knee joint has prompted the advent of advanced arthroscopic techniques to allow repair of torn meniscal tissue. The concepts of meniscal repair are based on the premise that the menisci are capable of healing. In order for meniscal healing to occur, a reparative response must be produced by the peripheral blood supply of the menisci. In a peripheral meniscal tear, the normal sequence of events that leads to healing is similar to that in other connective tissues. A fibrin clot that is rich in inflammatory cells first forms, creating a scaffold for vascular proliferation and ingrowth. Undifferentiated mesenchymal cells then create a fibrovascular scar that reconnects the meniscal edges. Remodeling of this fibrovascular scar into normal-appearing

fibrocartilage requires several months. Many peripheral lesions do not heal spontaneously because the initial tear is unstable and the early repair response is too weak to resist the destabilizing forces of knee motion on the meniscus.

Meniscal repair attempts to provide the best environment for local healing of the meniscal tear. Sutures placed into the meniscus anchor the meniscal fragment to the remaining meniscus and capsule, providing the stability needed for healing. Furthermore, the blood supply in the region of the meniscal tear can be maximized through the creation of vascularized access channels and synovial abrasion. Exogenous fibrin clot may be placed into the tear to attempt to create an environment conducive to the reparative process.

Many factors are considered important to the success of meniscal repair. These include the location, type, and chronicity of the tear; the patient's age; and knee stability. Location of the tear within the vascularized portion of the meniscus greatly affects the ability of the tear to heal. Tears occurring in the avascular inner two thirds of a meniscus fail to provide the blood supply necessary for repair. Techniques have been developed to create a better healing environment for these tears, such as creation of vascular access channels, synovial abrasion, and placement of exogenous fibrin clot. Still, the incidence of meniscal healing is much greater for peripheral lesions, and the best rationale for treating lesions in the avascular zone may be partial meniscectomy.

The type of tear also affects results of meniscal repair. Longitudinal tears are easier to stabilize with sutures and have a greater propensity to heal than do radial, flap, and degenerative horizontal cleavage tears. Therefore, the degenerative-type tears common in middle-aged and older runners would probably best be managed by means other than meniscal repair.

No consensus exists about how soon after injury a meniscal repair should be pursued. Many meniscal tears probably spontaneously heal, and yet chronic tears probably lose the capacity to heal with time. Several studies have shown that a delay of up to 8 weeks from time of injury does not affect the ability of the meniscus to heal.[104, 113]

The age of a patient has been considered an important factor regarding indications for meniscal repair. The reparative response is stronger in younger patients, but other factors such as the type and position of tear probably have as great a role in the capacity of the meniscus to heal as does age.

Knee stability has been shown to influence meniscal healing rates. Tears of the cruciate ligaments bring the secondary stabilizing role of the menisci into play. This increased strain placed on the menisci puts any meniscal repair at risk. Follow-up studies of meniscal repair in anterior cruciate ligament–deficient knees have revealed high retear rates.[46, 49, 98, 100, 104, 105]

Several techniques are available for meniscal repair. Open meniscal repair involves repair of the meniscus through a longitudinal incision. Only the most peripheral lesions

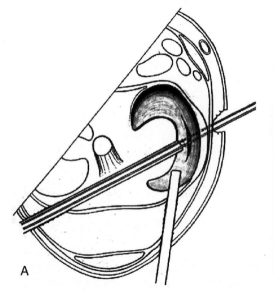

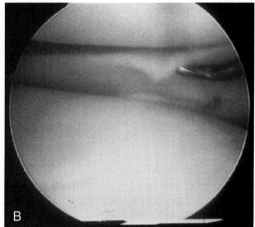

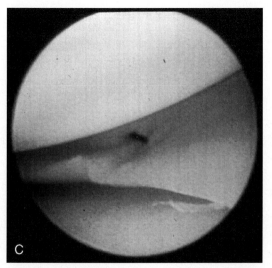

Figure 8–13

A: Inside-out technique for meniscal repair. (From Warren R, Healey S, Bach BR: Chronic anterior cruciate ligament injury. In Paresian JS (ed): Arthroscopic Surgery. New York, McGraw-Hill, 1988.) *B:* Arthroscopic picture of meniscal tear. *C:* Meniscus after repair.

may be repaired using this technique, because visualization of the inner meniscus becomes difficult. The arthroscope allows visualization and manipulation of the entire meniscus. Using instrumentation while viewing the tear arthroscopically, the surgeon can address tears peripherally and at the vascular/avascular junction. Synovial abrasion and trephination can improve results and allow placement of fibrin clots into the tear. Most importantly, the arthroscope allows the surgeon to determine whether the tear is stable or whether suture is required.

Arthroscopic techniques for meniscal repair include outside-in, inside-out, and all-inside techniques. The outside-in technique involves placement of curved needles through the skin and across the tear, carefully avoiding neurovascular structures. The suture is then placed through the needle, grasped within the knee, and brought outside the knee through a separate cannula, where a knot is tied in the suture. The knot is then retracted up against the edge of the tear to resist movement of the fragment. Subsequent sutures are tied together outside the joint capsule. The inside-out technique involves placement of needles and sutures through cannulas placed within the knee joint and passed across the tear and out the capsule (Fig. 8–13). The sutures are again tied outside the joint capsule. A mini-incision is usually used to avoid injury to neurovascular structures. All-inside techniques have been made available with the advent of specialized suture passers and fixation devices.

The results of arthroscopically assisted meniscal repair are promising. Second-look arthroscopy has been performed to classify the healing of a torn meniscus. If healing has occurred, it should be noted whether the meniscus is partially or completely healed. When meniscal repair is performed in properly selected patients, complete healing is documented in 75% to 80% of lesions. Fifteen percent undergo partial healing, and 5% to 10% fail to heal.[27] One factor that improves healing rates is the concomitant reconstruction of the anterior cruciate ligament, which suggests that the presence of hemarthrosis improves healing rates.

Rehabilitation after meniscal repair varies from that after simple meniscectomy. Many surgeons recommend limited range of motion and no weight-bearing to protect the repair. The need for this has been challenged, particularly when concomitant cruciate surgery is performed. With the knowledge that complete healing of meniscal repairs takes several months, most researchers recommend restricted athletic participation for 3 to 4 months after meniscal repair.

CONCLUSION

The development and refinement of the arthroscope and arthroscopic techniques have had an important role in the treatment of knee injuries in the runner. The arthroscope has allowed surgeons to explore the inner aspects of the knee joint with minimal disruption of the surrounding tissues. This has greatly improved the ability to diagnose and treat intraarticular knee pathology. Arthroscopic techniques developed for treatment of chondromalacia, symptomatic plica, patellofemoral malalignment, and meniscal tear have been outlined in this chapter. The arthroscope has also proved to be an asset for disorders less common to the running population, such as ligament reconstruction and intraarticular fracture.

The minimally invasive nature of arthroscopic techniques has proved to be beneficial for patients with knee injuries requiring surgery. The small incisions prove to be cosmetically acceptable. Arthroscopic techniques have changed most knee procedures into outpatient surgery. Most importantly, the use of arthroscopic technique avoids surgical trauma to the surrounding normal tissues of the knee, allowing immediate institution of rehabilitation and hastening an expeditious return to athletic activity.

REFERENCES

1. Aglietti P, Pisanesch A, Buzzi R, et al: Arthroscopic lateral release for patellofemoral pain or instability. Arthroscopy 5:179, 1989.
2. Ahmed A, Burke D: In vivo measurement of static pressure distribution in 70 synovial joints. I. Tibial surface of the knee. J Biomech Eng 105:201, 1983.
3. Aleman O: Chondromalacia post-traumatica patellae. Acta Chir Scand 63:149, 1928.
4. Anderson A, Lipscomb A: Clinical diagnosis of meniscal tears. Description of a new manipulative test. Am J Sports Med 14:291, 1986.
5. Arnoczky S, Warren R: Microvasculature of the human meniscus. Am J Sports Med 10:90, 1982.
6. Aspden R: A model for the function and failure of the meniscus. Eng Med 14:119, 1985.
7. Baratz M, Fu F, Mengato R: Meniscal tears: The

effect of meniscectomy and of repair on intraarticular contact areas and stress in the human knee. Am J Sports Med 14:270, 1986.

8. Bentley G, Dowd G: Current concepts of etiology and treatment of chondromalacia patellae. Clin Orthop 189:209, 1984.

9. Betz R, Lonegran R, Patterson R, et al: The percutaneous lateral release. Orthopedics 5:57, 1982.

10. Bigos S, McBride G: The isolated lateral retinacular release in the treatment of patellofemoral disorders. Clin Orthop 186:75, 1984.

11. Bircher E: Beitrag zur Pathologie und Diagnose der Meniscus Verletzungen (Arthueudoskopie). Bruns Beitr Klin Chir 127:239, 1922.

12. Blumensaat C: Die lageabweichongen und verrenkungen der kniescheibe. Ergeb Chir Orthop 31:149, 1988.

13. Bray R, Roth J, Jacobsen R: Arthroscopic lateral release for anterior knee pain: A study comparing those patients who are claiming worker's compensation and those who are not. Arthroscopy 3:327, 1987.

14. Breif L, Laico J: The superolateral approach: A better view of the mediopatellar plica. Arthroscopy 3:170, 1987.

15. Broom M, Fulkerson J: The plica syndrome: A new perspective. Orthop Clin North Am 17:279, 1986.

16. Brown T, Shaw D: In vitro stress distributions on the femoral condyles. J Orthop 2:190, 1984.

17. Budinger K: Uber ablosung von gelenkteilen und verwadte prozesse. Dtsch Zeitschr Chir 84:311, 1906.

18. Burman M, Finkelstein H, Mayer L: Arthroscopy of the knee joint. J Bone Joint Surg 16:255, 1934.

19. Busch M, DeHaven K: Pitfalls of the lateral retinacular release. Clin Sports Med 8:279, 1989.

20. Cargill A, Jackson J: Bucket-handle tear of the medial meniscus. J Bone Joint Surg Am 57:1116, 1975.

21. Cascells S: The arthroscope in the diagnosis of disorders of the patellofemoral joint. Clin Orthop 144:45, 1979.

22. Ceder L, Larson R: Z-plasty lateral retinacular release for treatment of the patellar compression syndrome. Clin Orthop 144:110, 1979.

23. Chapman M, Merchant A: Patellofemoral disorders. In Chapman M: Operative Orthopaedics. Philadelphia, JB Lippincott, 1988, pp 1699–1707.

24. Chen S, Ramanathan E: The treatment of patellar instability by lateral release. J Bone Joint Surg Br 66:344, 1984.

25. Chrisman O: The role of articular cartilage in patellofemoral pain. Orthop Clin North Am 17:231, 1986.

26. Christensen F, Soballe K, Snernum L: Treatment of chondromalacia patellae by lateral retinacular release of the patella. Clin Orthop 234:145, 1988.

27. Cooper D, Arnoczky S, Warren R: Meniscal repair. Clin Sports Med 10:529, 1991.

28. Daniel D, Daniels E, Aronson D: The diagnosis of meniscal pathology. Clin Orthop 163:218, 1982.

29. Dorchak J, Barrack R, Kneisl J, et al: Arthroscopic treatment of the symptomatic synovial plica of the knee: Long term follow-up. Am J Sports Med 19:503, 1991.

30. Dzioba R: Diagnostic arthroscopy and longitudinal open lateral release. A four year follow-up study to determine predictors of surgical outcome. Am J Sports Med 18:343, 1990.

31. Dzioba R, Stroken A, Mulbry L: Diagnostic arthroscopy and open longitudinal lateral release. A safe and effective treatment for "chondromalacia patellae." Arthroscopy 1:131, 1985.

32. Ewing J: Plica: Pathologic or not? J Am Acad Orthop Surg 1:117, 1993.

33. Fairbanks T: Knee joint changes after meniscectomy. J Bone Joint Surg Br 30:664, 1948.

34. Ficat P, Ficat C, Bailleux A: Syndrome d'hyperpression externe de la rotule (S.H.P.E.) Son interet pour la connaisance de l'arthrose. Rev Chir Orthop 61:39, 1975.

35. Fithian D, Kelly M, Mow V: Material properties and structure-function relationships in the meniscus. Clin Orthop 252:19, 1990.

36. Fox J, Ferkel R, DelPizzo W, et al: Electrosurgery in orthopedics. II. Applications to arthroscopy. Contemp Orthop 8:37, 1984.

37. Fukubayashi T, Kurosawa H: The contact area and pressure distribution pattern of the knee. Acta Orthop Scand 51:871, 1980.

38. Fulkerson J: Awareness of the retinaculum in evaluation of patellofemoral pain. Am J Sports Med 10:147, 1982.

39. Fulkerson J: Anteromedialization of the tibial tuberosity for patellofemoral malalignment. Clin Orthop 177:176, 1983.

40. Fulkerson J, Schulzer S, Ramsby G, et al: Computed tomography of the patellofemoral joint before and after lateral release or realignment. Arthroscopy 3:19, 1987.

41. Fulkerson J, Shea K: Disorders of the patellofemoral joint. J Bone Joint Surg Am 72:1424, 1990.

42. Fulkerson J, Tennant R, Jaivan J, et al: Histologic evidence of retinacular nerve injury associated with patellofemoral malalignment. Clin Orthop 197:196, 1986.

43. Gillies H, Seligson D: Precision in the diagnosis of meniscal lesions: A comparison of clinical evaluation, arthrography and arthroscopy. J Bone Joint Surg Am 61:343, 1979.

44. Goodfellow J, Hungerford D, Woods C: Patello-femoral joint mechanics and pathology. 2. Chondromalacia patellae. J Bone Joint Surg Br 58:291, 1976.

45. Grana W, Hinkley B, Hollingsworth S: Arthroscopic evaluation and treatment of patellar malalignment. Clin Orthop 186:122, 1984.

46. Hamberg P, Gillquist J, Lysholm J: Suture of new and old peripheral meniscal tears. J Bone Joint Surg Am 65:193, 1983.

47. Hardacker W, Wipple J, Barrett F: Diagnosis and treatment of the plica syndrome of the knee. J Bone Joint Surg Am 62:211, 1980.

48. Harwin S, Stern R: Subcutaneous lateral retinacular release for treatment of chondromalacia patellae: A preliminary report. Clin Orthop 156:207, 1981.

49. Henning C, Lynch M, Clark J: Vascularity for healing of meniscal repairs. Arthroscopy 3:13, 1987.

50. Henning C, Lynch M, Tearout K, et al: Arthroscopic meniscal repair using exogenous fibrin clot. Clin Othop 252:64, 1990.

51. Henry J: Conservative treatment of patellofemoral subluxation. Clin Sports Med 8:261, 1989.

52. Henry J, Goletz T, Williamson B: Lateral retinacular release in patellofemoral subluxation: Indications, results and comparison to open patellofemoral reconstruction. Am J Sports Med 14:121, 1986.

53. Hughston J: Subluxation of the patella. J Bone Joint Surg Am 50:1003, 1968.

54. Hughston J, Deese M: Medial subluxation of the patella as a complication of lateral retinacular release. Am J Sports Med 16:383, 1988.

55. Hughston J, Walsh W, Puddu G: Patellar Subluxation and Dislocation. Philadelphia, WB Saunders, 1984.

56. Hvid I, Andersen L, Schmidt H: Chondromalacia patellae: The relationship to abnormal patellofemoral mechanics. Acta Orthop Scand 52:661, 1981.

57. Insall J: Chondromalacia patellae: Patellar malalignment syndrome. Orthop Clin North Am 10:117, 1979.

58. Insall J, Aglietti P, Tria A: Patellar pain and incongruence. II. Clinical application. Clin Orthop 176:225, 1983.

59. Insall J, Falvo K, Wise D: Chondromalacia patellae: A prospective study. J Bone Joint Surg Am 50:1, 1976.

60. Jackson D, Jennings L, Maywood R, et al: Magnetic resonance imaging of the knee. Am J Sports Med 16:29, 1988.

61. Jackson R, Marshal D, Fujisawa Y: The pathologic medial shelf. Orthop Clin North Am 13:307, 1982.

62. James S: Running injuries to the knee. J Am Acad Orthop Surg 3:309, 1995.

63. James S, Jones D: Biomechanical aspects of distance running injuries. In Cavanagh PR (ed): Biomechanics of Distance Running. Champaign, IL, Human Kinetics, 1990, 249.

64. Karlson S: Chondromalacia patellea. Acta Chir Scand 83:347, 1939.

65. Kaufer H: Patellar biomechanics. Clin Orthop 144:51, 1979.

66. Koshino T, Okamoto R: Resection of painful shelf (plica synovialis mediopatellaris) under arthroscopy. Arthroscopy 1:136, 1985.

67. Krompinger W, Fulkerson J: Lateral retinacular release for intractable lateral retinacular pain. Clin Orthop 179:191, 1983.

68. Kurosaka M, Yoshiya S, Yamada M, et al: Lateral synovial plica syndrome: A case report. Am J Sports Med 20:92, 1992.

69. Lankenner P, Micheli L, Clancy R, et al: Arthroscopic percutaneous lateral patellar retinacular release. Am J Sports Med 14:267, 1986.

70. Larson R, Cabaud H, Slocum D, et al: The patellar compression syndrome: Surgical treatment by lateral retinacular release. Clin Orthop 134:158, 1978.

71. Laurin C, Levesque H, Dussault R, et al: The abnormal lateral patellofemoral angle: A diagnostic roentgenographic sign of recurrent patellar subluxation. J Bone Joint Surg Am 60:55, 1978.

72. Leslie I, Bentley G: Arthroscopy in the diagnosis of chondromalacia patellae. Ann Rheum Dis 37:540, 1978.

73. Levy M, Torzilli P, Warren R: The effect of meniscectomy on anterior-posterior translation of the knee. J Bone Joint Surg Am 64:883, 1982.

74. Lindberg U, Hamberg P, Lysholm J, et al: Arthroscopic examination of the patellofemoral joint using a central, one-portal technique. Orthop Clin North Am 17:263, 1986.

75. Lindberg U, Lysholm J, Gillquist J: The correlation between arthroscopic findings and the patellofemoral pain syndrome. Arthroscopy 2:103, 1986.

76. Lord M, Maltry J, Shall L: Thermal injury resulting from arthroscopic lateral retinacular release by electrocautery: Report of three cases and review of the literature. Arthroscopy 7:33, 1991.

77. MacIntyre J, Jaunton J, Clement D, et al: Predicting lower extremity injuries in habitual runners. Arch Intern Med 149:2565, 1989.

78. Malek M: Arthroscopic lateral retinacular release: Functional results in a series of 67 knees. Orthop Rev 14:55, 1985.

79. McConnel J: The management of chondromalacia patellae: A long term solution. Aust J Physiother 2:215, 1986.

80. McGinty J, Geuss L, Marvin R: Partial or total meniscectomy. J Bone Joint Surg Am 59:763, 1977.

81. McGinty J, McCarthy J: Endoscopic lateral retinacular release: A preliminary report. Clin Orthop 158:120, 1981.

82. Merchant A, Mercer R: Lateral release of the patella—a preliminary report. Clin Orthop 103:40, 1974.

83. Merchant A, Mercer R, Jacobsen R, et al: Roentgenographic analysis of patellofemoral congruence. J Bone Joint Surg Am 56:1391, 1974.

84. Metcalf R: An arthroscopic method for lateral release of the subluxating or dislocating patella. Clin Orthop 167:9, 1982.

85. Micheli L, Statinski C: Lateral patellar retinacular release. Am J Sports Med 9:330, 1981.

86. Miller G, Dickason J, Fox J: The use of electrosurgery for arthroscopic subcutaneous lateral release. Orthopedics 5:309, 1982.

87. Nicholas J, Freiberger R, Killoran P: Double-contrast arthrography of the knee. Its value in the management of 225 knee derangements. J Bone Joint Surg Am 52:203, 1970.

88. Northmore-Ball M, Dandy D: Long term results of partial meniscectomy. Clin Orthop 167:34, 1982.

89. Nottage W, Sprague N, Auerbach B, et al: The medial patellar plica syndrome. Am J Sports Med 11:211, 1983.

90. O'Connor R: Arthroscopy. Philadelphia, JB Lippincott, 1977.

91. Outerbridge R: The etiology of chondromalacia patellae. J Bone Joint Surg Br 43:752, 1961.

92. Owre A: Chondromalacia patellae. Acta Chir Scand 77(Suppl):41, 1936.

93. Polly D, Callaghnan D, Sikes R, et al: The accuracy of selective MRI compared with the findings of arthroscopy of the knee. J Bone Joint Surg Am 70:192, 1988.

94. Radin E: A rational approach to the treatment of patellofemoral pain. Clin Orthop 144:107, 1979.

95. Radin E, Rose R: Role of subchondral bone in the initiation and progression of cartilage damage. Clin Orthop 213:34, 1986.

96. Reider B, Marshall J, Ring B: Patellar tracking. Clin Orthop 157:143, 1981.

97. Richmond J, McGinty J: Segmental arthroscopic resection of the hypertrophic mediopatellar plica. Clin Orthop 178:185, 1983.

98. Rosenberg J, Scott S, Coward D, et al: Arthroscopic meniscal repair evaluated with repeat arthroscopy. Arthroscopy 2:14, 1986.

99. Rovere G, Adair D: Medial synovial shelf plica syndrome: Treatment by intraplical steroid injection. Am J Sports Med 13:382, 1985.

100. Ryu R, Dunbar W: Arthroscopic meniscal repair with two year follow-up: A clinical review. Arthroscopy 4:168, 1988.

101. Schonholz G, Zahn M, Magee C: Lateral retinacular release of the patella. Arthroscopy 3:269, 1987.

102. Schutzer S, Ramsby G, Fulkerson J: Computed to-

mography classification of patellofemoral pain patients. Orthop Clin North Am 17:235, 1986.

103. Schutzer S, Ramsby G, Fulkerson J: The evaluation of patellofemoral pain using computed tomography: A preliminary report. Clin Orthop 204:286, 1986.
104. Scott G, Jolly B, Henning C: Combined posterior incision and arthroscopic intraarticular repair of the meniscus. J Bone Joint Surg Am 68:847, 1986.
105. Seedholm B, Hargreaves D: Transmission of the load on the knee joint with special reference to the role of the meniscus. II. N Engl J Med 8:220, 1979.
106. Shakespeare D, Rigby H: The bucket-handle tear of the meniscus. A clinical and arthroscopic study. J Bone Joint Surg Br 65:383, 1983.
107. Shellock F, Mink J, Fix J: Patellofemoral joint: Kinematic magnetic resonance imaging to assess tracking abnormalities. Radiology 168:551, 1988.
108. Sherman O, Fox J, Sperling H, et al: Patellar instability: Treatment by arthroscopic electrosurgical lateral release. Arthroscopy 3:153, 1987.

109. Silva I, Silver D: Tears of the meniscus as revealed by MRI. J Bone Joint Surg Am 70:199, 1988.
110. Simpson L, Barrett J: Factors associated with poor results following arthroscopic subcutaneous lateral retinacular release. Clin Orthop 186:165, 1984.
111. Small N: An analysis of complications in lateral retinacular release procedures. Arthroscopy 5:282, 1989.
112. Sojbjerg J, Lauritzen J, Hvid I, et al: Arthroscopic determination of patellofemoral malalignment. Clin Orthop 215:283, 1987.
113. Tapper E, Hoover N: Late results after meniscectomy. J Bone Joint Surg Am 51:517, 1969.
114. Tucker J, Corsetti J, Gregg J: Arthroscopically assisted proximal quadroplasty for patellar instability. Clin Sports Med 12:81, 1993.
115. Van Mechelen W: Running injuries: A review of the epidemiological literature. Sports Med 14:320, 1992.
116. Watanabe M, Takeda S, Ikeuchi H: Atlas of Arthroscopy, 2nd ed. Tokyo, Igaku-Shoin, 1969.

BRIAN P. H. LEE ▪ FRANKLIN H. SIM ▪ MICHAEL J. STUART

CHAPTER NINE

Reconstructive Surgery of the Hip and Knee in Runners

The success of reconstructive procedures of the hip and knee (osteotomy, knee and hip arthroplasty) has prompted many patients to resume or initiate various sports activities after such operations. Although it is well recognized that successful results of osteotomy generally allow participation in most sports, including running, the guidelines for recommended or acceptable activity after hip and knee arthroplasty are less clearly defined. This issue is of importance because more than 200,000 hip and knee replacements are performed annually in the United States.[36]

The indication for total joint replacement has traditionally been relief of pain. However, the desire for improved functional outcome and higher activity levels is increasing. In addition, the number of young patients undergoing joint replacement is increasing, as is the expected longevity of these patients. Thus, the expectations of both surgeons and patients after joint replacement procedures are becoming increasingly unrealistic. This trend may in part be due to medical advertising and media coverage of professional athletes who continue high-impact activities after arthroplasty. The emphasis on health and participation in recreational sports activities such as jogging, walking, and cycling in the older population has also stimulated interest in activities after joint arthroplasty.[30, 35]

OVERVIEW OF HIP AND KNEE RECONSTRUCTION IN ATHLETES

Several factors need to be considered when formulating guidelines on activity participation after hip and knee reconstruction. The available reconstructive options, individual surgeon knowledge and preference, and re-

sults of risk-to-benefit analysis must be considered. In addition, the particular sport, level and intensity of participation, proficiency in the involved sport, and physical characteristics of the patient (e.g., weight, limb alignment, and presence of other diseased joints) have to be evaluated.

The expectations after hip and knee reconstruction also need to be considered. For most patients, the primary goal of operation is pain relief; in others, functional limitations are the main problem. The expectations postoperatively must be clearly explained to patients.

Current data on which to base recommendations about activity guidelines after hip and knee arthroplasty are sparse. Despite this drawback, with a clear understanding of the issues and a review of the relevant recent literature, general guidelines can be made with respect to participation in sports after hip and knee arthroplasty. However, some degree of individualization may be needed in each case because of the inherent variables.

CURRENT CONCEPTS AND REVIEW OF THE LITERATURE

OSTEOTOMY

Osteotomy of the hip and knee is a viable reconstructive option, especially in patients who are younger than 60 years and who have a mechanical cause of arthritis. Osteotomy enables restoration of more normal mechanical loading and alignment, preservation of the involved joint, a functional range of motion, and general return to full activities after recovery. A successful osteotomy delays any subsequent hip or knee arthroplasty and allows return to sports.

In a retrospective review of hip osteotomies by Boehler,[8] 66% of patients remained pain free 25 years postoperatively, and a significant number of patients returned to alpine skiing. Coventry and associates[14] reported similar success with knee osteotomy. However, the results of osteotomy do deteriorate with time, and participation in high-intensity impact-loading activities may accelerate the process.

HIP AND KNEE ARTHROPLASTY

Total hip or knee arthroplasty provides excellent and reliable pain relief and allows improvement in functions such as walking and climbing stairs. Macnicol and colleagues[27] showed an increase in walking speed, stride length, and cadence in patients after total hip arthroplasty. Oxygen consumption was more normal and mean power output doubled during stair climbing. Several other studies also demonstrated an increase in the proportion of patients participating in regular cycling after hip arthroplasty.[40, 44] Visuri and Honkanen[44] noted increased participation in regular walking and in skiing, but Ritter and Meding[40] noted decreased participation in regular walking, running, and golfing. Running was not addressed in the former study, but fewer than 3% of patients returned to high-impact activities such as running and tennis in the latter study. The differences between the groups are in part related to a variation in guidelines postoperatively (patients were specifically instructed in the study by Ritter and Meding but not in the study by Visuri and Honkanen) and illustrate the diversity of opinions about activity after arthroplasty.

Similar studies have yet to be performed for knee arthroplasty. However, given the similar relevant aspects of hip and knee arthroplasty, the results described for hip arthroplasty can be extrapolated to include knee arthroplasty.

BIOMECHANICAL ISSUES

Biomechanical forces need to be considered when decisions are made about what activities are advisable after hip or knee arthroplasty. The peak resultant contact forces after total hip arthroplasty range from 2.5 to 3.5 times body weight during level walking at a freely selected speed, and peak out-of-plane forces vary from 0.6 to 0.9 times body weight.[9] Contact forces increase up to 43% during easy running.[41, 42] In the knee, the peak resultant contact forces range from two to four times body weight during level walking. They increase up to 25% with ascending and descending ramps.[33]

These forces can be modified. Muscular training after arthroplasty may dampen constant active peak forces during sports activity. Passive peak forces, which increase linearly with running speed, can be reduced with viscoelastic heel pads.[18]

Thus, significant contact forces occur in joint arthroplasties with running. Although they can be modified with muscular conditioning and use of proper equipment, they still remain well above the levels experienced with low-impact activities.

PROSTHESIS DESIGN AND SURGICAL TECHNIQUES

There are two main risks with sports participation after hip and knee arthroplasty. The first, dislocation of the joint or fracture of the prosthesis or periprosthetic bone, is rare as a result of sports participation, but it has been observed.[31] This risk is increased during high-impact sports activities. The second and more significant risk is wear of the weight-bearing surfaces. Repetitive loading activities are more frequent during sports participation. They can result in accelerated wear of the prosthetic materials and the need for early revision of worn parts. The biologic responses to the wear particles generated, particularly osteolysis and bone resorption, can severely jeopardize the survival of the joint replacement. The combination of weakened bone due to osteolysis and high-impact loading also increases the risk of periprosthetic fracture. In addition, the lack of sensory feedback from an artificial joint eliminates self-protective monitoring of at-risk maneuvers.

In hip arthroplasty, prosthesis design and materials can affect the joint stresses and durability. These are especially important in young patients who are active in sports. Forged stems of contemporary design are imperative in young patients.[15] The femoral offset should be adequately reproduced to restore the moment arm, abductor strength, range of motion, and stability.[30] Head size should be a balance between joint stability and optimal wear characteristics. A 28-mm head is currently recommended.[26] Surface treatment of the head may reduce wear but is costly.

Materials used in hip arthroplasties include titanium and cobalt-chrome alloy metals, ceramics, and ultra-high-molecular-weight polyethylene. The modulus of elasticity of the material in the stem should be optimal with bone in order to reduce the incidence of thigh pain when using an uncemented prosthesis. Various combinations of these materials have been used and are in use today, including metal on polyethylene, metal on metal, ceramic on ceramic, and ceramic on polyethylene. The most widely used combination is a metal alloy stem (titanium alloy or cobalt-chrome) with a modular cobalt-chrome head articulating with a polyethylene socket (all polyethylene or metal backed). A minimum of 6 to 8 mm of actual polyethylene should be present.[5, 45]

Similarly, prosthesis design also affects joint stresses and durability in knee arthroplasties.[16] The minimally constrained condylar design has the best record for durability and certainly is the design of choice for active young patients. Early hinged designs, which were constrained, have had unacceptably high rates of loosening. The metal-on-polyethylene articulation with metal backing of the tibia currently is the recommended choice for young patients. At least 6 to 8 mm of actual polyethylene should be present.[7, 10, 19, 23]

Another consideration is preservation of the posterior cruciate ligament. Some studies suggest that preservation of this ligament may reproduce more normal biomechanics, particularly with stair climbing.[3] This finding may indicate that posterior-cruciate-preserving designs should be used in active young patients. However, this advantage relies on perfect soft tissue balancing, which is difficult to achieve in every patient. The designs that sacrifice the posterior cruciate ligament (or posterior stabilized designs), however, more easily allow for correction of severe flexion contractures or joint malalignment. Excellent long-term durability with survival rates of more than 90% at 10 to 12 years can be achieved with either design.[13, 37–39]

The surgical technique of joint replacement must also be considered in young patients who expect to return to sports activity. A posterior approach in hip arthroplasty may allow restoration of abductor strength earlier, although no significant difference has been noted at 1 year postoperatively when compared with the anterolateral[30] or direct lateral[32] approach. Use of the subvastus approach in knee arthroplasty can limit disruption of the extensor mechanism perioperatively and enhance earlier recovery.[21] Restoration of anatomic characteristics such as femoral offset in hip arthroplasty and joint line location and patellar thickness in knee arthroplasty optimizes strength and stability.[30, 38]

In hip arthroplasty, fixation of the prosthesis to bone may be cemented or may use cementless ingrowth designs. Cementless ingrowth designs have been advocated in younger, active patients, but problems of wear and osteolysis are significant.[6] Modern cementing techniques have also significantly improved cemented fixation of the femoral component.[4] Aseptic loosening of cemented acetabular components, particularly in young patients, remains to be resolved.[11, 24] Cementless fixation of the acetabular component may produce better results in this group of patients.

Cemented fixation in knee arthroplasty remains the standard approach, and results are predictable.[37, 39] When compared with total knee arthroplasty performed without resurfacing, resurfacing of the patella may improve relief of pain and the ability to climb stairs. However, this is done at the risk of complications of wear and loosening of the implant and fracture of the patella. The issue of patellar resurfacing remains controversial.[1, 34] An unresurfaced patella may be considered in young, active patients, provided cartilage wear on the patella is relatively minimal and proper patellar tracking can be obtained with a femoral component that is designed for nonresurfacing. This approach is contraindicated in cases of inflammatory cause.

PATIENT CHARACTERISTICS

Patients who undergo hip replacement have significant abductor weakness in comparison with age-matched controls even at 1 year postoperatively. Analogous data are not available for knee replacement, but general and activity-specific strengthening are recommended after joint replacements. In some cases, strength testing should be considered before recommending a return to sports activity.

The longevity of hip and knee arthroplasty is also related to the age of the patient and the diagnosis. Older and less active patients have better prosthesis survival, presumably because of lower demands.[12, 17, 20, 22, 43] Prosthesis survival is better in female patients than in male patients, perhaps because of differences in weight and activity levels.[24]

LEVEL AND EXTENT OF ACTIVITY

The issue of participation in sports after total hip arthroplasty has been addressed in several studies.[18, 25, 28, 40, 44] The duration of follow-up in each study exceeds 4 years, but the effects of increased patient activity are not evident early after arthroplasty. The long-term risk for revision as a result of loosening is usually apparent only 10 years or more postoperatively. Kilgus and colleagues[26] showed that the long-term risk of surgical revision in a conventional prosthesis was twice as high in patients participating in sports activity as in less active patients. In addition, the polyethylene wear rates have

been calculated in active patients, the average being 0.39 mm/year at a mean follow-up of 7 years.[18] This rate is significantly more than the acceptable wear rate of 0.1 mm/year in patients after hip arthroplasty[26] and signifies a potential long-term problem with osteolysis and loosening. In another group of active patients, Ritter and Meding[40] reported a dislocation rate of 3% and pain in 2% postoperatively. These rates are comparable to those in less active patients.

Thus, although sports activity may have no early deleterious effect on total hip arthroplasty, it does have an adverse effect on the long-term survival of conventional hip arthroplasty, although this can be minimized by intelligent participation in low-impact activities, including walking and cycling but not running.

To date, little has been reported on sports after total knee arthroplasty. In one survey of golfers who underwent total knee arthroplasty, the majority of active golfers reported

TABLE 9–1 Recommendations for Resumption of Various Sports Activities After Total Hip Arthroplasty*

Sport	Recommendation (%)			Status†
	Yes	*No*	*Depends*	
Golfing	100.0	0	0	Recommended
Swimming laps	96.4	0	3.6	Recommended
Cycling	96.4	3.6	0	Recommended
Bowling	89.3	0	10.7	Recommended
Sailing	78.6	3.6	17.9	Recommended
Scuba diving	78.6	7.1	14.3	Recommended
Hiking	64.3	3.6	32.1	Intermediate
Cross-country skiing	60.7	14.3	25.0	Intermediate
Speed walking	60.7	25.0	14.3	Intermediate
Backpacking	35.7	32.1	32.1	Intermediate
Ice skating	35.7	32.1	32.1	Intermediate
Doubles tennis	32.1	28.6	39.3	Intermediate
Ballet	21.4	57.1	21.4	Intermediate
Aerobics	17.9	14.3	67.9	Intermediate
Volleyball	14.3	67.9	17.9	Intermediate
Softball	10.7	57.1	32.1	Intermediate
Alpine skiing	10.7	64.3	25.0	Intermediate
Singles tennis	10.7	64.3	25.0	Intermediate
Handball	10.7	78.6	10.7	Not recommended
Racquetball	7.1	78.6	14.3	Not recommended
Running	3.6	89.3	7.1	Not recommended
Hockey	3.6	92.9	3.6	Not recommended
Baseball	0	82.1	17.9	Not recommended
Water-skiing	0	89.3	10.7	Not recommended
Karate	0	92.9	7.1	Not recommended
Basketball	0	96.4	3.6	Not recommended
Soccer	0	96.4	3.6	Not recommended
Football	0	100.0	0	Not recommended

*Based on questionnaire responses of 28 orthopedic surgeons at the Mayo Clinic, Rochester, MN.
†Based on three fourths of the respondents allowing or disallowing return to the sport activity.
From McGrory BJ, Stuart MJ, Sim FH: Participation in sports after hip and knee arthroplasty: Review of the literature and survey of surgeon preferences. Mayo Clin Proc 70:342–348, 1995. By permission of Mayo Foundation for Medical Education and Research.

TABLE 9–2   Recommendations for Resumption of Various Sports Activities After Total Knee Arthroplasty*

Sport	Recommendation (%)			Status†
	Yes	*No*	*Depends*	
Golfing	100.0	0	0	Recommended
Swimming laps	96.4	0	3.6	Recommended
Cycling	96.4	0	3.6	Recommended
Sailing	89.3	0	10.7	Recommended
Bowling	85.7	3.6	10.7	Recommended
Scuba diving	85.7	3.6	10.7	Recommended
Cross-country skiing‡	78.6	10.7	10.7	Recommended
Speed walking	67.9	17.9	14.3	Intermediate
Hiking	64.3	3.6	32.1	Intermediate
Ice skating	50.0	21.4	28.6	Intermediate
Backpacking	35.7	35.7	28.6	Intermediate
Doubles tennis	28.6	32.1	39.3	Intermediate
Ballet	28.6	50.0	21.4	Intermediate
Aerobics	21.4	14.3	64.3	Intermediate
Alpine skiing	14.3	60.7	25.0	Intermediate
Softball	10.7	53.6	35.7	Intermediate
Volleyball	10.7	60.7	28.6	Intermediate
Handball	14.3	78.6	7.1	Not recommended
Racquetball	14.3	78.6	7.1	Not recommended
Hockey	10.7	89.3	0	Not recommended
Water-skiing	10.7	78.6	10.7	Not recommended
Singles tennis	7.1	67.9	25.0	Intermediate
Karate	3.6	85.7	10.7	Not recommended
Soccer	3.6	92.9	3.6	Not recommended
Baseball	0	82.1	17.9	Not recommended
Running	0	92.9	7.1	Not recommended
Basketball	0	96.4	3.6	Not recommended
Football	0	100.0	0	Not recommended

*Based on questionnaire responses of 28 orthopedic surgeons at the Mayo Clinic, Rochester, MN.
†Based on three fourths of the respondents allowing or disallowing return to the sport activity.
‡Residents and fellows were significantly less likely than consultant orthopedic surgeons to allow return to this sport (*P* = 0.037; Mann-Whitney *U* test, corrected for ties).
From McGrory BJ, Stuart MJ, Sim FH: Participation in sports after hip and knee arthroplasty: Review of literature and survey of surgeon preferences. Mayo Clin Proc 70:342–348, 1995. By permission of Mayo Foundation for Medical Education and Research.

significant increases in their handicaps and decreased length of drives postoperatively.[29] Golf carts were used by 87%, and 16% experienced a mild ache while playing golf. Pain was more evident in patients with left knee replacements than in those with right knee replacements. Radiolucency was noted in 54% of 54 knees at a mean follow-up of 4.6 years.

CURRENT OPINIONS AND RECOMMENDATIONS

Most surgeons concur that a successful osteotomy allows many patients to return to sports activities, including high-impact activities such as running. This result is due to preservation of the joint and to restoration of more normal biomechanics. However, osteotomy results do deteriorate with time, and pre-existing wear on the joint may be accelerated by regular participation in high-demand activity. This possibility has to be clearly explained to patients who want to return to high-impact sports, including running.

Although many variables need to be considered when recommendations are made for activity after hip and knee arthroplasty, some efforts have been made toward defining guidelines more clearly. In a survey of 30 orthopedic surgeons, fellows, and fifth-year residents,[31] opinions were evaluated regarding participation in 28 common sports after total hip and total knee arthroplasty. The results are summarized in Tables 9–1 and 9–2. High-impact activities such as running, water-skiing, football, baseball, basketball, hockey, handball, karate, soccer, and racquetball were not recommended after hip or knee arthroplasty. In contrast, low-impact sports such as sailing, swimming laps, scuba diving, cycling, golfing, and bowling were considered recommended sports after hip or knee arthroplasty. Cross-country skiing was recommended after knee arthroplasty but not hip arthroplasty.

The study provided a collective opinion about participation in a fairly comprehensive group of sports. Running was regarded as a high-impact loading activity and was therefore not recommended after hip or knee arthroplasty.

On the basis of these findings and the literature review, the following general recommendations can be made[31]:

1. The goals and expectations for osteotomy, including return to participation in sports, should be discussed with patients and agreed on preoperatively. High-impact activity may be permitted, but the potential risk of accelerated deterioration of results with time should be clearly explained to patients.

2. The goals and expectations for joint arthroplasty, including return to participation in specific sports, should be discussed with patients and agreed on preoperatively.

3. Surgeons should explain to patients the benefit of aerobic activity and encourage fitness in agreement with the current guidelines established by the American College of Sports Medicine.[2]

4. Surgeons should explain the risks of high-impact activities on the longevity of a joint prosthesis—the theoretic increased risk of fracture and dislocation and the previously demonstrated risk of accelerated surface wear in conjunction with the consequences of aseptic loosening, osteolysis, and increased need for revision.

5. For patients who have expressed interest in returning to sports after hip or knee arthroplasty, the surgeon should carefully consider prosthesis design, techniques of implantation, and postoperative rehabilitation options.

6. Intelligent participation in no-impact (swimming laps, cycling, sailing, scuba diving) or low-impact (golfing, bowling) sports should be encouraged after joint replacement.

7. Use of viscoelastic shoe inserts and sport- and joint-specific therapy should be considered, in addition to modifications in sports technique for patients who want to return intermittently to moderate-impact sports (cross-country skiing, speed walking, backpacking, ice skating, tennis, ballet, aerobics, volleyball, softball, and alpine skiing).

8. High-impact sports (running, handball, racquetball, hockey, baseball, water-skiing, karate, basketball, soccer, and football) should be prohibited.

9. Close clinical and radiographic follow-up and early intervention for impending failure of the joint prosthesis are of utmost importance in patients who return to sports activities after arthroplasty.

CONCLUSION

Participation in sports activity such as running is an increasingly relevant issue after hip or knee reconstructive procedures. Numerous benefits can be derived from a regular exercise program. However, the choice of activity is important for patients who undergo hip or knee reconstruction. Most activities, including running, can usually be resumed or commenced after an osteotomy. However, patients who have hip or knee joint replacements should be selective in their activity participation, avoiding high-impact activities such as running. Low-impact activity such as walking or cycling can be as beneficial from a health standpoint as running, but they minimize the long-term risk of wear problems with the prosthesis. The choice of activity should be made in consultation with the surgeon, and in some cases it may need to be individualized. Periodic physical examination and radiographic follow-up are essential.

REFERENCES

1. Abraham W, Buchanan JR, Daubert H, et al: Should the patella be resurfaced in total knee arthroplasty? Efficacy of patellar resurfacing. Clin Orthop 236:128, 1988.
2. American College of Sports Medicine Position Stand: The recommended quantity and quality of exercise for developing and maintaining cardiorespiratory and muscular fitness in healthy adults. Med Sci Sports Exerc 22:265, 1990.
3. Andriacchi TP, Galante JO, Fermier RW: The influence of total knee-replacement design on walking and stair-climbing. J Bone Joint Surg Am 64:1328, 1982.
4. Barrack RL, Mulroy RD Jr, Harris WH: Improved cementing techniques and femoral component loosening in young patients with hip arthroplasty. A 12-year radiographic review. J Bone Joint Surg Br 74:385, 1992.
5. Berry DJ, Barnes CL, Scott RD, et al: Catastrophic failure of the polyethylene liner of uncemented acetabular components. J Bone Joint Surg Br 76:575, 1994.
6. Berry DJ, Cabanela ME: Primary uncemented total hip arthroplasty in patients less than 40 years of age (abstract). Orthop Trans 17:601, 1993–1994.

7. Berry DJ, Rand JA: Isolated patellar component revision of total knee arthroplasty. Clin Orthop 286:110, 1993.

8. Boehler M: Cited by McGrory BJ, Stuart MJ, Sim FH: Participation in sports after hip and knee arthroplasty: Review of literature and survey of surgeon preference. Mayo Clin Proc 70:342, 1995.

9. Brand RA, Pedersen DR, Davy DT, et al: Comparison of hip force calculations and measurements in the same patient. J Arthroplasty 9:45, 1994.

10. Buechel FF, Pappas MJ: New Jersey low contact stress knee replacement system. Ten-year evaluation of meniscal bearings. Orthop Clin North Am 20:147, 1989.

11. Callaghan JJ: Results of primary total hip arthroplasty in young patients. J Bone Joint Surg Am 75:1728, 1993.

12. Chandler HP, Reineck FT, Wixson RL: Total hip replacement in patients younger than thirty years old. A five-year follow-up study. J Bone Joint Surg Am 63:1426, 1981.

13. Colizza WA, Insall JN: Posterior-stabilised total knee prostheses with metal-backed tibial component: 10 to 12 years follow up. Presented at the 61st Annual meeting of the American Academy of Orthopaedic Surgeons, New Orleans, LA, February 24 to March 1, 1994.

14. Coventry MB, Ilstrup DM, Wallrichs SL: Proximal tibial osteotomy. A critical long-term study of eighty-seven cases. J Bone Joint Surg Am 75:196, 1993.

15. Crowninshield RD, Brand RA, Johnston RC, et al: The effect of femoral stem cross-sectional geometry on cement stresses in total hip reconstruction. Clin Orthop 146:71, 1980.

16. Dorr LD, Ochsner JL, Gronley J, et al: Functional comparison of posterior cruciate-retained versus cruciate-sacrificed total knee arthroplasty. Clin Orthop 236:36, 1988.

17. Dorr LD, Takei GK, Conaty JP: Total hip arthroplasties in patients less than forty-five years old. J Bone Joint Surg Am 65:474, 1983.

18. Dubs L, Gschwend N, Munzinger U: Sport after total hip arthroplasty. Arch Orthop Trauma Surg 101:161, 1983.

19. Engh GA, Dwyer KA, Hanes CK: Polyethylene wear of metal-backed tibial components in total and unicompartmental knee prostheses. J Bone Joint Surg Br 74:9, 1992.

20. Ewald F, Christie MJ: Results of cemented total knee replacement in young patients (abstract). Orthop Trans 11:442, 1987.

21. Hofmann AA, Plaster RL, Murdock LE: Subvastus (Southern) approach for primary total knee arthroplasty. Clin Orthop 269:70, 1991.

22. Hungerford DS, Krackow KA, Kenna RV: Cementless total knee replacement in patients 50 years old and under. Orthop Clin North Am 20:131, 1989.

23. Jones SM, Pinder IM, Moran CG, et al: Polyethylene wear in uncemented knee replacements. J Bone Joint Surg Br 74:18, 1992.

24. Joshi AB, Porter ML, Trail IA, et al: Long-term results of Charnley low-friction arthroplasty in young patients. J Bone Joint Surg Br 75:616, 1993.

25. Kilgus DJ, Dorey FJ, Finerman GA, et al: Patient activity, sports participation, and impact loading on the durability of cemented total hip replacements. Clin Orthop 269:25, 1991.

26. Livermore J, Ilstrup D, Morrey B: Effect of femoral head size on wear of the polyethylene acetabular component. J Bone Joint Surg Am 72:518, 1990.

27. Macnicol MF, McHardy R, Chalmers J: Exercise testing before and after hip arthroplasty. J Bone Joint Surg Br 62:326, 1980.

28. Mallon WJ, Callaghan JJ: Total hip arthroplasty in active golfers. J Arthroplasty 7 (Suppl):339, 1992.

29. Mallon WJ, Callaghan JJ: Total knee arthroplasty in active golfers. J Arthroplasty 8:299, 1993.

30. McGrory BJ, Cahalan TD, Morrey BF, et al: Correlation of femoral offset and abductor muscle strength following total hip arthroplasty. Presented at the 61st Annual Meeting of the American Academy of Orthopaedic Surgeons. New Orleans, LA, February 24 to March 1, 1994.

31. McGrory BJ, Stuart MJ, Sim FH: Participation in sports after hip and knee arthroplasty: Review of literature and survey of surgeon preferences. Mayo Clin Proc 70:342, 1995.

32. Minns RJ, Crawford RJ, Porter ML, et al: Muscle strength following total hip arthroplasty. A comparison of trochanteric osteotomy and the direct lateral approach. J Arthroplasty 8:626, 1993.

33. Morrison JB: Bioengineering analysis of force actions transmitted by the knee joint. Biomed Eng 3:164, 1968.

34. Picetti GD III, McGann WA, Welch RB: The patellofemoral joint after total knee arthroplasty without patellar resurfacing. J Bone Joint Surg Am 72:1379, 1990.

35. Pollock ML, Wilmore JH: Exercise in Health and Disease: Evaluation and Prescription for Prevention and Rehabilitation, 2nd ed. Philadelphia, WB Saunders, 1990, p 1.

36. Praemer A, Furner S, Rice DP: Musculoskeletal Conditions in the United States. Park Ridge, IL, American Academy of Orthopaedic Surgeons, 1992, p 127.

37. Ranawat CS, Flynn WF Jr, Saddler S: Long-term results of the Total Condylar knee arthroplasty. A 15-year survivorship study. Clin Orthop 286:94, 1993.

38. Rand JA, Ilstrup DM: Survivorship analysis of total knee arthroplasty. Cumulative rates of survival of 9200 total knee arthroplasties. J Bone Joint Surg Am 73:397, 1991.

39. Ritter MA, Herbst SA, Keating EM, et al: Long-term survival analysis of a posterior cruciate-retaining total condylar total knee arthroplasty. Clin Orthop 309:136, 1994.

40. Ritter MA, Meding JB: Total hip arthroplasty. Can the patient play sports again? Orthopedics 10:1447, 1987.

41. Rydell N: Biomechanics of the hip-joint. Clin Orthop 92:6, 1973.

42. Rydell NW: Forces acting on the femoral head-prosthesis. A study on strain gauge supplied prostheses in living persons. Acta Orthop Scand 37 (Suppl 88):1, 1966.

43. Stuart MJ, Rand JA: Total knee arthroplasty in young adults who have rheumatoid arthritis. J Bone Joint Surg Am 70:84, 1988.

44. Visuri T, Honkanen R: Total hip replacement: Its influence on spontaneous recreation exercise habits. Arch Phys Med Rehabil 61:325, 1980.

45. Wright TM, Rimnac CM: Ultra-high-molecular-weight polyethylene. In Morrey BF (ed): Joint Replacement Arthroplasty, New York, Churchill-Livingstone, 1991, p 37.

========= **CHAPTER TEN**

Shin Pain and Compartment Syndromes in Running

The shin is defined in Webster's Dictionary as "the front part of the leg below the knee." Although commonly associated with the tibia, shin pain is more broadly defined in this chapter to include more pervasive discomfort from the knee to the ankle in runners.

Recreational runners have been a large part of our practice during the past 15 years, because the senior partners themselves are avid runners. We encounter many recreational running injuries and have developed a conservative philosophy in their treatment. In our practice, most of these problems can be solved with conservative treatment and with resetting of reasonable running goals. This is especially true of recreational athletes. Surgery is occasionally necessary for more competitive runners to correct lower leg injuries that have not responded to conservative management.

Distance runners (who run 25 miles or more per week) soon learn to differentiate discomfort associated with a hard workout from nagging leg pain. The former rapidly diminishes by the time of the next workout, whereas the latter lingers on, necessitating a change in duration and intensity of workouts. My running experience has been remarkably paralleled by that of my patients. In the 1970s, during the height of "mileage mania" in intensive workouts, I was also training for marathons and running more than 60 miles per week. Runners' athletic lives, in retrospect, appeared less controlled than today—that is, there were fewer options for running surfaces, shoes were either light and cushiony or heavy and supportive, and information about appropriate workouts and running injuries was less advanced.

Consequently, as soon as an injury (new pain) developed, the runner sought orthope-

dic counseling and care. In the 1990s, ample information can be gained from running magazines, health club newsletters, athletic shoe stores, and other runners and coaches, so runners make initial decisions on their own. Only after trying a period of modified running activities, selective rest, shoe changes, and so on is orthopedic care now sought.

Patients are much more knowledgeable about their injuries and consequently are more receptive to recommendations of running program modifications. My own running activities now include a more manageable 30 miles per week.

Ten to 15 years ago, a sure way to alienate a patient was to tell a runner to stop running. Today, however, cross-training is not only well received but commonly practiced routinely. NordicTrack, exercise bikes, and pool running are not only widely accepted but embraced by the majority of injured runners.

Lower leg running problems are difficult to quantify in an office setting. Unlike other office orthopedic presentations, those due to running are stress-related phenomena that initially have a paucity of physical and radiographic findings. The diagnosis depends on a well-taken history and the location of the runner's pain and is confirmed by ancillary tests such as bone scans, magnetic resonance imaging (MRI) scans, compartment pressure examinations, and so on.

A classification of lower leg pain is important not only to decide the best course of treatment for runners to return to activities but to give patients a working diagnosis that they can relate to for a better understanding of the problem. In our office practice, runners more than the other athletes like to be intimately involved in their treatment plan and options.

A *shin pain* classification traditionally includes shin splints, stress fracture, and compartment syndrome in a somewhat arbitrary diagnostic manner. I have found the classification by location in the lower leg to be most helpful in my practice in developing a treatment plan.

CLASSIFICATION

The classification of shin pain is as follows:
I. Lateral shin pain
   1. Nerve entrapment
   2. Peroneal tendinitis
   3. Anterior and lateral compartment syndrome
II. Medial shin pain
   1. Shin splints (medial tibial stress syndrome or medial tibial syndrome)
   2. Stress reaction
   3. Stress fracture
      a. Clinical
      b. Subclinical
   4. Posterior tibial tendinitis
   5. Posterior compartment syndrome
   6. Rhabdomyolysis (rare)

RUNNING EVALUATION

Each runner is examined in our clinic after an appropriate history is taken. Our clinic's individual sports evaluation sheet for runners includes (1) number of years of running; (2) types of running surfaces; (3) shoe information: types, how often changed, and so on; (4) average weekly mileage; (5) history of previous injuries; and (6) description and location of pain (on a lower leg diagram). A pattern is sought for possible overuse syndrome with respect to mileage and intensity buildup.

This history taking is followed by a physical examination in which the location of the patient's pain is ascertained and a complete lower extremity examination is carried out, beginning with the back. This includes flexibility examination, alignment, range of motion of the lower extremities, and muscle strength with any imbalances. A supine, sitting, and standing examination is carried out in a lower extremity evaluation. Running shoes are examined, and a biomechanical gait analysis on the treadmill with a video camera projected with a television monitor is effected with the individual's running shoes. Wear patterns on the shoes are noted, and any supports or orthotic devices in the shoes are evaluated. Specific alignment abnormalities are noted, such as genu varum or valgum, tight heel cords, or increased foot pronation or supination. Radiographs are taken in two planes of the lower leg at the first visit.

In evaluating causes of lower leg pain syndrome, in our practice, training errors are more common than malalignment. Improper footwear was formerly a significant cause of runners' problems in our clinic, but running shoes have dramatically improved and can accommodate most runners' individual needs.

If alignment problems are noted, a recommendation for orthotics is made and any leg length discrepancies are corrected (to within 1/4 inch). Shoe recommendations are made, if applicable.

TREATMENT

PHYSICAL THERAPY

Physical therapy is recommended only to correct muscle imbalances, such as use of the Magic Six of Sheehan for strengthening the extensors of the leg and increasing the flexibility of the flexors of the foot and ankle (Fig. 10–1).[22] If tendinitis is suspected, ultrasound and electric galvanic stimulation may be included in treatment modalities.

MEDICATION

Nonsteroidal antiinflammatory drugs (NSAIDs) are prescribed for any residual inflamed areas for a short course until symptoms have sufficiently resolved to allow a return to painless running. Alternate athletic activities are prescribed, including Nordic-Track, exercise bike, rowing machines, and pool running with an Aqua-Jogger.

Recommendations for a change of running surfaces from concrete to macadam (more forgiving) are made. For indoor runners, avoiding either clockwise or counterclockwise banking of the track is suggested, depending on which leg is involved.

CONDITIONS

For organizational purposes, shin pain is described as (1) tendinitis, (2) stress-related

Lower Leg Rehabilitation Program

The following exercises are recommended for rehabilitation and to prevent injury.

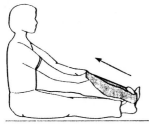

▲1 Calf Stretching

- Hold a towel in both hands, looping the middle of the towel around the ball of your foot.
- Pull towel toward you, moving the foot upward until a stretch is felt in the calf.
- Hold 20-30 seconds. Relax.
- Perform ___ sets, ___ repetitions, ___times/day.

2 Resistive Exercises with Theraband

Dorsiflexion:

- Tie theraband around a stationary object.
- Place theraband over top of foot. Pull up against it toward face.
- Return slowly to starting position.
- Perform ___ set, ___ repetitions, ___ times/day.

Plantarflexion:

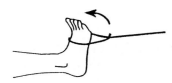

- Hold theraband in both hands, looping the middle of the theraband around the ball of your foot.
- Push foot in a downward direction against the theraband.
- Return slowly to starting position.
- Perform ___ set, ___ repetitions, ___ times/day.

Inversion:

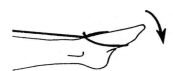

- Tie theraband around a stationary object.
- Place theraband around inside of foot. Pull inward against the theraband. Do not twist hip/knee.
- Return slowly to starting position.
- Perform ___ set, ___ repetitions, ___ times/day.

Eversion:

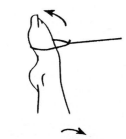

- Tie theraband around a stationary object.
- Place theraband around outside of foot. Push outward against the theraband. Do not twist hip/knee.
- Return slowly to starting position.
- Perform ___ set, ___ repetitions, ___ times/day.

Figure 10–1

Strength and flexibility exercises of the lower leg. (Adapted from Sheehan G: Make '76 the year of the Magic Six. Running wild. Phys Med Sports Med 4:29, 1976.)

Illustration continued on following page

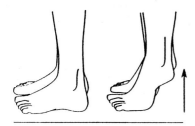

❸ Toe Raises

- Stand with both feet flat on the floor.
- Raise up on both toes. Slowly lower to starting position.
- Progress to one foot on flat surface.
- Progress to both feet off edge of step, then one foot off edge of step.
- Perform ___ set, ___ repetitions, ___ times/day.

▲ Gastroc-Soleus Stretch

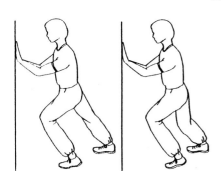

- Face a wall and stand about 2 feet away. Place palms flat against the wall and step forward with one foot and place the leg to be stretched straight behind you.
- Bend opposite leg and place flat on the floor in front of you.
- Keep heel of back leg down and slowly move your hips forward toward the wall, keeping your back straight until a stretch is felt in the calf.
- Hold 20-30 seconds. Relax.
- Repeat the exercise with back leg slightly bent at the knee.
- Perform ___ set, ___ repetitions, ___ times/day.

▐5 Balance Exercise

- Stand on one leg with your eyes open.
- When able to do this without difficulty for 1 minute, progress to standing on one leg with eyes closed for 1 minute.
- Perform ___ set, ___ repetitions, ___ times/day.

Figure 10–1

Continued

disorders, or (3) compartment syndromes (Table 10–1).

TENDINITIS

Posterior tibial tendinitis occurs in the distal one fourth of the lower leg, where the posterior tibial tendon can be palpated for areas of tenderness, fullness, and thickening.[3] Acute problems relate to increased mileage on unforgiving surfaces; the tendon appears normal. Runners prone to these problems have increased pronation on gait. In chronic posterior tibial tendinitis, the tendon is abnormal on palpation and has a thickened sheath.

Acute problems are managed with physical therapy modalities of ultrasound and electric galvanic stimulation, NSAIDs, diminution of intensity and duration of running activities, change of surfaces, supportive shoes, and soft

TABLE 10–1   Injuries to Runners: Sports Medicine Knee Surgery Center (254 Consecutive Patients)

Tendinitis, 44
Tibial stress fracture, stress reaction, 52
Compartment syndrome, 8
Medial tibial stress syndrome, 147
Superficial peroneal nerve entrapment, 3
Rhabdomyolysis, 1

inserts. For more chronic problems, modalities are less effective and require use of orthotics and modification of running activities on a day-to-day basis. MRI for a recurrent or recalcitrant situation may show a tendinopathy with chronic tearing, which may be amenable to surgical debridement and possibly tendon transfer. If this latter procedure is performed, distance running is not advisable afterward.

Posteromedial tibial tenderness is not in our clinic believed to be synonymous with posterior tibial tendinitis in the distal quarter of the leg and is discussed in more detail later in this chapter.

Peroneal tendinitis is noted on examination in the posterolateral third, behind the fibula.[3] This entity requires differentiation from fibular stress fractures (pain over the fibula) and lateral compartment syndromes as well as nerve entrapment. It is associated with increased foot pronation or occasionally with increased supination at heel strike, with excessive wearing of the outer sole of the runner's shoes. Treatment is directed to modification of running workouts, updated running shoes, appropriate shoe inserts, NSAIDs, and physical therapy modalities until symptoms are controlled. An MRI scan for more recalcitrant cases in a runner rarely identifies a longitudinal overuse tear of the peroneus brevis or longus tendon, which is amenable to surgical repair.

STRESS-RELATED DISORDERS AND NERVE ENTRAPMENT

Medial Tibial Stress Syndrome

Numerous citations in the literature have attempted to define medial leg pain. The term *shin splints* has been used descriptively to characterize the painful condition of the middle to distal third of the posteromedial tibial region with normal radiographic findings.[2, 10, 11] Stress fractures and stress reaction, which are disruptions in the integrity of the bone, can be confirmed by discrete pinpoint pain on the posteromedial aspect of the tibia. However, shin splints are best thought of as medial tibial stress syndrome, which occurs at the junction of the periosteum and fascia.[12, 23, 26]

This has been variously described by Mubarek and associates as a periostitis and by Michael and Holder as disruption of the tibial attachment of the soleus.[16, 17] Posterior com-

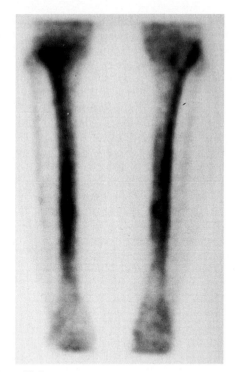

Figure 10–2

Stress reaction, positive bone scan. Note transverse uptake pattern.

partment syndrome with a similar clinical presentation is described later. The best treatment for this condition is prevention.[4] The condition usually occurs in distance runners logging 20 to 30 miles per week and is invariably due to training errors—too much speed work, as well as hill and distance work, too soon. Improper footwear can compound the situation, but gross malalignment has not been directly correlated with this entity. However, we have seen more subtle malalignment in runners presenting in our office and have found this to be correlated with tight Achilles tendon complex.

Physical examination of runners with a *stress fracture* or *stress reaction* reveals pinpoint tenderness on examination of the posteromedial tibia over a very discretely defined area, whereas medial tibial syndrome (shin splints) has an area of more diffuse tenderness of the posteromedial tibia corresponding to the soleus attachment. The radiographs for medial tibial syndrome are nondiagnostic and may be initially nondiagnostic for a stress fracture. A bone scan (phase 3) shows a horizontal discrete area in the posteromedial tibia (Fig. 10–2).[3, 9, 12] A *stress reaction* by definition, however, has no radiographic abnormalities but positive findings on a bone scan, similar to the stress fracture pattern.[9, 29] A stress fracture ultimately reveals positive radiographic findings, but a *stress reaction* is manifested by positive findings only on a bone scan (Fig. 10–3). The medial tibial syndrome has negative radiographic results by definition and either a nondiagnostic bone scan or a diffusely positive longitudinal bone scan pattern at the distal middle/third of the tibia in the area of the attachment of the soleus (Fig. 10–4).[3, 4] *Asymptomatic tibial stress phenomena* are subclinical stress manifestations that can be demonstrated on a bone scan or radiograph in an otherwise asymptomatic area of the tibia and are of no clinical significance.[10]

Symptoms of medial tibial stress syndrome may vary from mild to significant with respect to activities (grades 1 to 4).[10] A runner initially having grade one may only have pain that resolves after a run and does not affect performance. With grade 2, this may progress to pain that lingers until the next workout.

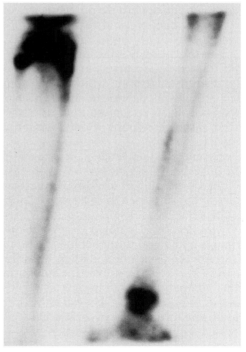

Figure 10–4

Positive bone scan for medial tibial syndrome (shin splints). Note the longitudinal pattern of uptake.

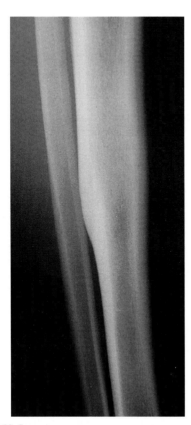

Figure 10–3

Chronic healed stress fracture.

With grade 3, the pain affects performance. Grade 4 pain affects the activities of daily living. In the literature and at our clinic, attempts have been made to correlate the various grades with degrees of intensity of objective data such as bone scan findings.[12]

Treatment for *tibial stress reaction syndrome* includes selective rest for up to 10 weeks with a break from full or vigorous training.[4] This is coupled with correction of any muscle imbalance or malalignment, and recommendations are made for aerobic activities substituted for running to prevent deconditioning.

Tibial stress fractures are managed in similar fashion in our clinic, with up to 12 to 16 weeks of abstention from running, depending on the extent of the patient's symptoms and radiographic bone reaction changes.

Treatment for *medial tibial syndrome* is similar to the foregoing, with the addition of modalities in physical therapy such as the Magic Six and NSAIDs to decrease any inflammation that has been noted on biopsy of the periosteum in this condition as described in the literature.[4, 17, 22]

Orthotics are recommended for any problems with chronic conditions of distinct pronation on running gait. Velcro shin aids and compressive shin supports have occasionally been of benefit in our practice (Fig. 10–5).[28] Modification or cessation of running activities is made commensurate with symptoms, as described previously.

In the past 15 years in our clinic, we have not found it necessary to perform a release of the investing fascia of the posteromedial tibial for chronic medial tibial syndrome to return runners to full activities. The results of the surgery were found to be dismal in one literature review, although the soleus bridge was not specifically released from the distal third of the tibia in this series.[1]

Series with a release of the posterior compartment fascia, along with the soleus bridge along the area of the patient's symptoms, have yielded more acceptable results.[4] If a surgical approach is taken, a bone scan can be used to delineate the extent of the surgical release.

The literature has described *lateral shin splints* resulting from inflammation of the tibialis anterior and extensor digitorum communis due to overuse.[3] This can theoretically be due to malalignment of the lower extremity and excessive pronation, and it is linked to excessive hill running with poor, unsupportive running shoes.[3]

If these symptoms are easily controlled by arch supports, shoe modification, NSAIDs, and selective rest with return to running, the actual diagnosis and etiology are relatively immaterial. If these symptoms persist, in our experience, a compartment pressure measurement should be performed to rule out anterior compartment syndrome.

The literature has mentioned posteromedial pain secondary to overuse of the flexor digitorum longus with intrinsic muscle weakness of the foot. We have not noted this entity in our own running practice in the past 15 years, but the literature notes that a medial arch support with a metatarsal pad usually suffices for improvement.[18]

Nerve Entrapment

Entrapment of the superficial peroneal nerve is usually associated with chronic compartment syndrome and fascia hernias. However, symptoms for isolated superficial peroneal nerve involvement can be insidious, with lateral leg pain out of keeping with the patient's level of activity, and can be of gradual onset. Minor trauma such as an ankle sprain or direct trauma from a fall affecting the anterolateral compartment of the leg in a runner has been noted in our clinic. Physical findings are suggestive of entrapment, with tenderness in the area at the intermuscular septum and at the distal third of the anterolateral lower leg, and a positive Tinel sign is noted. Electromyograms (EMGs) and nerve conduction tests may be confirmatory. Compartment pressure should be tested as part of the diagnostic workup.

Treatment for recalcitrant symptoms includes release of the nerve in the lateral compartment at the distal third of the leg and release of the anterolateral compartment or any residual fascial hernias, if necessary.[7] This is discussed more fully later.

For completion of differential diagnosis of lower leg pain in runners, exertional *rhabdomyolysis* is included.[6] This is quite rare with respect to runners' injuries, and only one case has been treated and monitored in our clinic. The entity is more likely in untrained runners exercising too vigorously for their level of training. However, it can also affect more highly trained runners after a significantly difficult intensive training session. Symptoms of muscle soreness and swelling of the lower

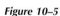

Figure 10–5

Shin aid for chronic shin splints.

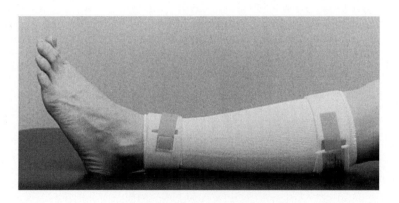

leg are noted within a few hours of vigorous exercising.

Physical examination is remarkable for decreased range of motion of the affected contiguous joints, soft tissue swelling, and exquisite tenderness over the affected muscle group or groups. This should be differentiated from the "normal" soreness and stiffness after a vigorous early season workout.

The hallmark of the diagnosis is an elevated creatine phosphokinase (CPK) level (>10 times normal) and the presence of myoglobinuria on urine testing. The risk of renal compromise is quite real in these patients; therefore, this condition is treated as a medical emergency.

Rapid hydration, the use of diuretics, and acute compartment syndrome with affected muscle should be ruled out in a tense, swollen leg by measuring compartment pressure, and appropriate fasciotomy should be carried out immediately if warranted.[18, 20] Blood urea nitrogen (BUN) and creatinine measurements are monitored closely, and with appropriate treatment the CPK level should return to normal within a 2-week period. Athletic workout should be avoided with affected muscle groups until laboratory results and function of activities of daily living have returned to normal levels.

COMPARTMENT SYNDROMES

The lower leg is anatomically divided into four compartments—anterior, lateral, superficial posterior, and deep posterior.[27] Each is a closed compartment containing muscles, tendons, and neurovascular structures (Fig. 10–6). These compartments are deemed to be closed because of unyielding bony and inelastic fascial coverings.

Small changes in volume in a compartment thus may cause increased pressure. This is considered irreversible in an acute situation or acute compartment syndrome (ACS) and reversible in chronic compartment syndrome (CCS).

ETIOLOGY

ACS is caused by increased tissue compartment pressures due to either an increase in volume of the compartment contents (swelling—*internal*) or *external* factors such as tight casts or dressings.[7] *Internal* compression is

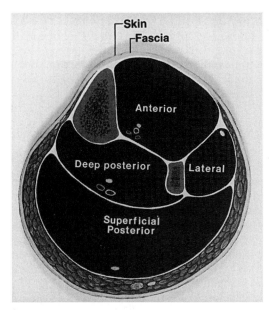

Figure 10–6

The four compartments of the lower leg, midportion. (By special permission from Mubarak SJ [ed]: Operative Techniques in Sports Medicine 3[4], 1995.)

more common and may follow an episode of intense running or military marching. When fluid pressure exceeds capillary perfusion pressures, local flow is restricted and ischemia occurs. Fortunately, the situation is encountered rarely in running injuries.

CCS has been estimated to occur in as many as 15% of runners.[2] It was previously thought to be due to reversible local ischemia secondary to increased muscle swelling leading to increased compartment volume. This has not been borne out by local MRI scans.[25]

Our clinic experience has found an incidence of CCS closer to 5% in our population of recreational runners (see Table 10–1).

Nonetheless, an exercise-induced pain syndrome occurs in a compartment and can be measured. Several methods have been used to measure compartment pressures. These include the wick catheter and slit catheter, both indwelling catheter systems, as well as handheld digital monitor systems. The former two are *dynamic assessments* performed during exercise, and the latter is a *static* examination performed before and after exercise. Both the slit and wick catheters monitor intermuscular tissue pressure by using microscopic fibers at the tip of a catheter, whereas the hand-held system has a needle with multiple side holes.[15, 21]

We have used the *Stryker* hand-held digital

monitor with the updated needle for the past 8 years at our clinic for measuring compartment pressures. Because dynamic compartment pressure readings are not necessary to make the diagnosis of a compartment syndrome, we therefore prefer the simplicity and reproducibility of this device (Fig. 10–7).

The diagnosis of CCS is usually one of exclusion in a runner. By history, in CCS, the pain is reproducible by a certain level of running, respective distance, and intensity, and it dissipates after the workout. It is unusual for pain to be present 24 hours later, and it is unlikely that the chronic condition threshold will be exceeded and converted to an irreversible ACS.

An affected runner may complain of muscle tightness, fatigue or numbness of the foot occurring during exercise, and decreased muscle power or weakness in certain muscle groups while running. The symptoms may be bilateral but are usually more intense in one extremity, in our experience.[5] In recreational runners, the symptoms may persist for several months to years before a diagnosis is made. Runners therefore learn to self-limit their activities.

Physical examination in the office setting invariably yields no findings of tenderness in CCS. In the literature, fascia hernias are noted in as many as 50% of these patients.[7] This may be specious, however, because another condition such as medial tibial syndrome may be the main problem. For example, a history of pain at rest between running activities, with tenderness on palpation of the leg on static examination, suggests another diagnosis.[4]

Appropriate radiographs are ordered at the initial office visit. Most patients with an unconfirmed diagnosis (i.e., by compartment pressure) of CCS undergo physical therapy with exercises, possible shoe and orthotic modification, and NSAIDs. No scientific evidence shows that these will be beneficial for CCS once it is established.[13, 14]

The diagnosis of CCS is confirmed by intracompartment pressure measurement. Normal compartment pressures at rest should be less than 10 mm Hg. Our clinic's criterion for diagnosis of CCS is a resting pressure of greater than 15 mm Hg and immediate postexercise pressure greater than 30 mm Hg. Other confirmatory pressure measurement findings are a 5-minute postexercise value of greater than 20 mm Hg and a 15-minute value greater than 15 mm Hg.[21] Compartment pressures are measured in either one or both legs at the same appointment, as symptoms warrant.

The compartments tested are also dictated by the patient's symptoms, with the anterior and posterior compartments tested according to the patient's symptom complex.

Runners are instructed to bring running shoes at the time of pressure measurement for exercise on the treadmill until symptoms are confirmed in the lower leg. This is immediately followed by DuraPrep preparation of the lower leg and the use of Stryker pressure apparatus. After infusion with a small amount of saline into a self-contained well, the needle is placed under local anesthesia into the ap-

Figure 10–7

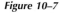

Stryker static compartment pressure device used in our clinic. No elaborate setup is required.

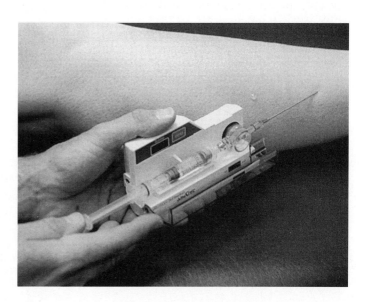

propriate compartment or compartments parallel to the tibia. The literature recommends a relatively acute angle for needle insertion directed to the muscle, allowing for more accurate pressure readings.[24] However, this appears to be theoretically more important in obtaining correct pressure measurements with the wick and slit catheters than with the stouter side-hole metal needle used in our clinic's measuring device. The anterior compartment, as well as the posterior compartment, are tested when appropriate. The lateral compartment and superficial posterior compartment are not routinely tested but are released when the respective adjacent compartments require treatment.

If compartment pressures confirm CCS, treatment modalities of activity modification versus surgery are discussed. For runners who wish to continue running at or near their present desired level, surgery is recommended. We do caution patients who are prospective surgical candidates that our results for anterior and lateral compartment releases are greater than 90%, with expectations to return to appropriate running activities. Posterior compartment releases do not have nearly this level of success, however, either in the literature or formerly in our clinic. Therefore, a description of our modified posterior compartment release is described later, with the intention of improving the clinical results of posterior compartment releases.

Patients are advised that a diagnosis of compartment syndrome is not mutually exclusive of other diagnoses such as medial tibial syndrome. For example, appropriate testing and therapy modalities to treat such an entity, such as a bone scan, are recommended when appropriate. Surgery is performed on an outpatient basis for anterior and lateral compartment releases and as a 24-hour stay for posterior compartment releases. For the latter, a postoperative drain is used and a vascular surgeon assists in dissecting out the proximal neurovascular bundle in hopes of improving the clinical success in posterior compartment releases.

Until 1990, the anterior and lateral compartment releases for CCS were performed through a series of small transverse incisions (after Detmer).[5] Because of a clinical recurrence, however, we now perform these compartment releases through a single vertical incision.[7, 19] This is fashioned halfway between the tibia and fibula in the middle third of the lower leg over the intermuscular sep-

tum. The superficial peroneal nerve is exposed and dissected out when thought to be clinically entrapped. The superficial peroneal nerve is dissected out to facilitate exposure if there is a fascial hernia, with the incision made through the herniated area and extended to the lateral and anterior compartments as appropriate. A fascial release is performed along the fibula proximally and distally for the lateral compartment release. A release is carried out to the ankle extensor retinaculum distally and toward the lateral tibial plateau proximally for the anterior compartment (Fig. 10–8).

For the anterior compartment release, a tourniquet is not used and local anesthesia with epinephrine is infiltrated into the skin and fascial tissue for hemostasis. A pressure dressing is applied after the compartment release, and cold therapy coils are placed over the dressing to diminish swelling during the next week. The patient is discharged on crutches in the outpatient department.

For the posterior compartment, a single incision is made 2 cm posterior to the medial

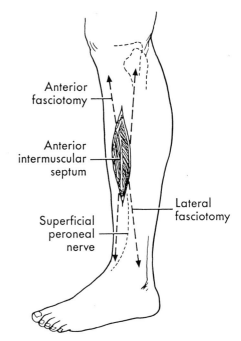

Figure 10–8

Fasciotomy of the anterior and lateral compartments through a single incision. (From Campbell's Operative Orthopedics. St. Louis, CV Mosby, 1992; as redrawn from Mubarak SJ, Owens CA: Double incision fasciotomy of the leg for decompression in compartment syndrome. J Bone Joint Surg 59A:184, 1977.)

tibial flare. The incision extends proximally from the soleus bridge toward the distal third of the lower leg. The saphenous nerve and vein are retracted anteriorly, and the superficial gastrocnemius/soleus complex is released first. With a vascular surgeon, the deep posterior compartment is entered and a fasciotomy is performed of all individual compartments, releasing the posterior tibia and flexor digitorum areas. The soleus bridge is released, freeing up the neurovascular bundle (Figs. 10–9 and 10–10). This procedure is not performed under tourniquet control as in the anterior compartment; thus, all bleeders are meticulously clamped and coagulated to leave a dry field at the time of primary skin closure over a J-Vac. A compression dressing is applied, and cold therapy coils are placed over the dressing. Patients are admitted overnight, because the degree of postoperative discomfort for posterior compartment releases is much greater.

Crutches are used postoperatively until patients are seen for their first office visit at 8 to 10 days. Formal physical therapy begins after the sutures are removed at the first postoperative visit. Range of motion of the ankle, use of Isoflex tubing, and early return to biking, swimming, or pool running with a flotation device are recommended as soon as the wounds are healed primarily. In our experience, return to a former level of running activity takes longer than suggested in the literature.

Our patients generally do not return to full running activities for 8 to 10 weeks for anterior compartment release and for 3 to 4 months for posterior compartment release.

In our practice, 80% of compartment releases are for the anterior and lateral compartments and 20% include a posterior compartment release also. In the past 10 years, we have found it necessary to perform only 15 compartment releases. The remainder of the runners have modified their activities and have been able to accommodate their running schedules (25 runners).

The last three patients with the modified posterior compartment releases were able to return to their former running activities. We believe that this is because of meticulous release of all individual muscular compartments as well as release of the proximal neurovascular bundle with a vascular surgeon; this had not been performed earlier in our clinic.

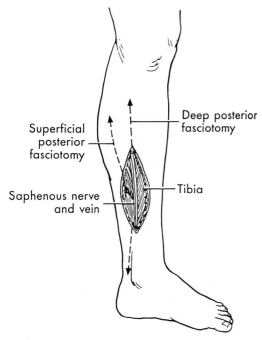

Figure 10–9

Fasciotomy at the superficial and deep posterior compartments through a 15-cm incision. (From Campbell's Operative Orthopedics. St. Louis, CV Mosby, 1992; as redrawn from Mubarak SJ; Owens CA: Double incision fasciotomy of the leg for decompression in compartment syndrome. J Bone Joint Surg 59A:184, 1977.)

CASE REPORTS

■ *CASE 1* C.M., a 15-year-old female high school cross-country runner, presented in March 1987 with anterior right leg pain with numbness of her foot after cross-country practice runs of 2 miles. Examination was essentially unremarkable, and radiographs of the tibia and fibula appeared normal. The patient was placed on a physical therapy program and given orthotics; she improved dramatically with cessation of running activities. Problems recurred when she returned to running the following season, at which time she developed symptoms of pain in her right lower leg after 15 minutes and numbness of the dorsum of her foot.

Compartment pressures at this time revealed a lateral compartment pressure of 29 mm Hg and an anterior compartment pressure of 37 mm Hg after running on the treadmill. A compartment release of both the anterior and lateral compartments was carried out

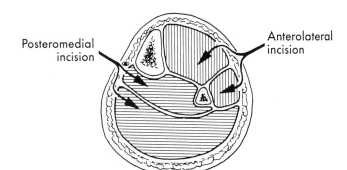

Posteromedial incision   Anterolateral incision

Figure 10–10

Cross section of compartment releases. (From Campbell's Operative Orthopedics. St. Louis, CV Mosby, 1992; as redrawn from Mubarak SJ; Owens CA: Double incision fasciotomy of the leg for decompression in compartment syndrome. J Bone Joint Surg 59A:184, 1977.)

in October of 1987 through two small transverse incisions. After appropriate physical therapy, the patient returned to running and in the winter of 1988 was able to run up to 3 to 4 miles. The patient's numbness on the dorsum of her foot and the pain in her right lower leg gradually returned and included not only the anterior but also the posterior aspect of her right lower leg.

EMGs and bone scans were unremarkable, and repeat compartment pressures were 34 mm Hg posteriorly and 24 mm Hg anteriorly on the right side. The patient wished to defer surgery. She dramatically reduced her running activities and began biking.

In 1992, the patient attempted to return to running activities, with recurrent symptoms. Repeat compartment pressures were unchanged from 1989, and the patient underwent a four-compartment release. At the time of surgery, which was performed through two longitudinal incisions, 4 inches for the anterior lateral release and 6 inches for the posterior release, the anterior lateral compartment fascia was found to be reformed. This was rereleased, and with a vascular surgeon, the deep posterior compartment was released from the soleus bridge over the neurovascular bundle to just superior to the ankle retinaculum. The superficial posterior compartment was released at the same time.

Postoperatively, the patient slowly brought up her mileage to 5 miles over a year's period of noncompetitive running after appropriate rehabilitation. She also integrated cross-training and was encouraged to wear her orthotics for sports activities and to continue on a lower extremity strength and flexibility program. Her numbness and aching after running were essentially gone at her last visit in 1994.

This case illustrates the possibility of recurrence of ACS after releases through small in-

cisions, as well as the appearance of new symptoms in the posterior compartment of the same leg.

We no longer use a series of transverse incisions for the anterior and lateral compartment releases because of the recurrence in this patient.

∎ *CASE 2* E.C., an 18-year-old female college track athlete, presented with a 1-year history of increasing bilateral anterior leg pain with competitive running. Physical examination was unremarkable, with no significant tenderness noted in either leg. Alignment was normal, and radiographs were unremarkable. The patient had been given orthotics and a course of NSAIDs by her college trainer and had been told to ice the leg after competition. Compartment pressure testing of both legs revealed left anterior compartment pressure of 56 mm Hg and a right anterior compartment pressure of 44 mm Hg. Both posterior compartment pressures were less than 10 mm Hg.

During the patient's summer vacation, anterior compartment releases of both legs were carried out through two 6-inch incisions. Postoperatively, the patient completed a rehabilitation program and was able to return to running by the end of the summer, up to 30 minutes, and to participate in full varsity sports when returning to school. She has remained asymptomatic with the latest follow-up in early 1996, and has successfully completed her college athletic career.

∎ *CASE 3* C.V., a 42-year-old competitive tennis player and jogger, fell onto her right leg with her ankle directly beneath her while running, sustaining direct trauma. Despite several months of physical therapy following casting at another clinic, the patient presented with no resolution of her symptoms—pain, weakness, and giving way of her right lower extremity.

Physical examination revealed a distinct limp with tenderness generalized to the patient's anterior and lateral compartment areas of her right lower leg with a questionable Tinel sign over her superficial peroneal nerve. Because of the patient's presentation, thermography was ordered to rule out reflex sympathetic dystrophy, and the results of this test were negative. EMGs and nerve conduction tests suggested a superficial peroneal nerve involvement. Compartment pressures tested after walking on the treadmill revealed right anterior compartment pressure of 37 mm Hg and right lateral compartment pressure of 34 mm Hg.

Surgery was performed through a 15-cm incision over the intermuscular septum and revealed a small fascia hernia, as well as scarring of the superficial peroneal nerve. The nerve was freed up, and a fasciotomy was performed of the anterior and lateral compartments, which included the patient's herniated muscular area.

Postoperatively, the patient had immediate relief of her aching and weakness and within 6 weeks was able to return to aerobic activities. After 3 months, the patient still had some residual lower leg stiffness in the morning after exercise.

This case illustrates the difficulty in diagnosing some lower extremity injuries that involve nerve entrapments and in which symptoms may even point to a possibility of reflex sympathetic dystrophy. Symptoms may appear to be disproportionate to the patient's injury and clinical presentation. However, once a proper diagnosis or diagnoses are made, good relief can be anticipated with appropriate surgical releases.

■ **CASE 4** G.P., a 37-year-old man, presented with significant bilateral calf pain after a vigorous aerobic workout at a health club. The patient was noted to be quite muscular and was unable to walk with a plantigrade gait, owing to calf pain, walking instead on his tiptoes. He was exquisitely tender over both calf areas.

Radiographs were nondiagnostic, and the patient was placed on NSAIDs, crutches, and ice. CPK determination was ordered and was 32,000; myoglobinuria was noted in the patient's urine. Anterior and posterior compartment pressures were less than 10 mm Hg. A diagnosis of rhabdomyolosis was made.

Hospitalization with comanagement with a nephrologist was carried out; treatment consisted of intravenous hydration and alkalization of the patient's urine.

Within 2 weeks, the patient's CPK level was less than 200 and his gait was normal. He was begun on a progressive fitness program and, when last seen 3 months after his initial presentation, had normal results on examination and was engaged in a "sensible" aerobic exercise program.

This case illustrates the importance of making the correct diagnosis, because rhabdomyolysis is rare and when not treated expeditiously may result in significant renal as well as musculature changes.

■ **CASE 5** R.L., a 16-year-old male high school cross-country runner, was involved in a motor vehicle accident at 11 years of age in 1987 and fractured his left tibia. He was treated in another clinic with a long leg cast for 3 months and then rehabilitated, returning to normal activities of daily living within 6 months. At age 16, in 1992, he was participating in cross-country running 50 miles per week when, over a period of 2 weeks, he developed progressive burning, numbness, and coldness in his left shin and foot.

Physical examination in 1992 at our clinic revealed tenderness over his entire left shin area and paresthesias over the dorsal area of his left foot after he ran on the treadmill for 10 minutes. Radiographs revealed a well-healed fracture of the left tibia with extensive remodeling (Fig. 10–11). Compartment pressures after treadmill running revealed 37 mm Hg in the anterior compartment and 48 mm Hg in the posterior compartment.

Findings of EMGs were within normal limits. Laboratory workup revealed a CPK level markedly elevated at 977. The patient's workup for his elevated CPK concluded that this was a marker for malignant hyperthermia, and the family therefore wished to postpone any surgical procedures when informed of the possible risks.

However, the patient's symptoms progressed so that any running whatsoever became out of the question. Therefore, the family decided to proceed with surgery under epidural block, 1 year after his initial presentation to our clinic.

Surgery proceeded uneventfully, with release of the patient's anterior/lateral compartment without use of a tourniquet and

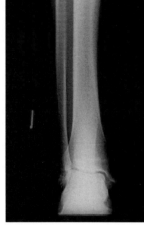

Figure 10–11

Old posttraumatic tibial fracture.

without any unusual scarring. However, the posterior compartment release, performed with a vascular surgeon, revealed extensive scarring between the fracture callus and the soleus in the superficial posterior compartment as well as between the individual compartments of the deep posterior compartment. Fasciotomies were carried out of both the superficial and deep posterior compartments, and a branch of the posterior tibial artery that was irretrievably encased in scar and lacerated was suture ligated. The incisions were closed primarily, and a posterior splint applied. The patient was kept overnight for pain control and neurovascular observation. The patient was kept on crutches for 2 ½ weeks, and his wounds healed primarily.

He was begun in physical therapy with use of the Aquaciser (walking tank) at 2 ½ weeks, with progression through sports cords and exercises for strength and flexibility. Exercise on the treadmill and stair-climber was added at 7 weeks.

Ten months after surgery, the patient was running 3 miles without symptoms in his left lower extremity. He redirected himself from competitive to recreational running activities. His physical examination was unremarkable; incisions of his left lower extremity were well healed.

This case illustrates a rather unusual circumstance of a compartment syndrome in a runner—that resulting from remote tibial fracture with consequent scarring due to extensive callus formation. The patient's symptoms were borne out at the time of surgery; extensive adhesions were noted, even of the patient's posterior tibial artery, which required meticulous dissection by a vascular surgeon. The patient's increased CPK level ultimately was found to have no relationship to his compartment syndrome per se.

CONCLUSION

Running injuries of the shins are a virtual certainty for those who exceed their threshold of mileage and intensity in workouts. Logic would therefore dictate "listen to your body" and keep running under this level. Nonetheless, early recognition of any injury is key to treatment in prevention of recurrences. Muscular imbalances and malalignment can be corrected and a sensible running program prescribed. A range of diagnostic modalities in the 1990s can enhance the running evaluation, and surgical correction should be confined to only those recalcitrant patients who absolutely insist on returning to their respective running activity programs.

Options for aerobic activity and cross-training are available and are well received in today's sports market. We have found it necessary to perform very few surgical procedures for painful shin conditions in runners in our practice, including compartment syndrome.

REFERENCES

1. Abramowitz AJ, Schepsis A, McArthur C: The medial tibial syndrome. The role of surgery. Orthop Rev 23:875–881, 1994.
2. Bates P: Shin splints, a literature review. Br J Sports Med 19:132–137, 1985.
3. Brody D: Running injuries. Ciba Clin Symp 32:2–33, 1980.
4. Detmer DE: Chronic shin splint classification and

management of medial tibial stress syndrome. Sports Med 3:436–446, 1986.

5. Detmer DE, Sharpe K, Sutel RF, Girde FM: Chronic compartment syndrome, diagnosis, management outcome. Am J Sports Med 13:162–170, 1985.
6. Dina EM, Mehlman CT: Rhabdomyolysis. A primer for the orthopaedist. Orthop Rev 23:28–32, 1994.
7. Fronek J, Mubarek SJ, Hargens AR, et al: Management of chronic exertional anterior compartment syndrome of the lower extremity. Clin Orthop 220:217–227, 1987.
8. Garth WP, Miller ST: Evaluation of claw toe deformity, weakness of the foot, intrinsic and posteromedial shin pain. Am J Sports Med 19:821–827, 1987.
9. Holder LE, Michael RH: The specific scintigraphic pattern of shin splints of the lower leg. J Nucl Med 25:865–869, 1984.
10. Jackson D: Shin splints, an update. Physician Sportsmed 6:51–61 Oct, 1978.
11. Jackson SW, Bailey D: Shin splints in the young athlete: A nonspecific diagnosis. Physician Sportsmed 3:45–51, 1975.
12. Jones BH, Harris JG, Vish JN, et al: Exercise induced stress fractures and stress reactions of bone. Epidemiology, etiology and classification. Exerc Sports Sci Rev 17:379–422, 1989.
13. Matsen FA, Roobeck LH: Compartment syndrome. Instr Course Lect 38:463–472, 1989.
14. Matsen FA, Wingust RA, Krogmore RD: Diagnosis and management of compartment syndromes. J Bone Joint Surg Am 62:280–291, 1980.
15. McDermott AP, Marbie E, Yabsley RH, et al: Monitoring dynamic anterior compartment pressure during exercise: A new technique using the slit catheter. Am J Sports Med 10:83–89, 1982.
16. Michael RH, Holder LE: The soleus syndrome, a cause of medial tibial stress (shin splints). Am J Sports Med 13:87–94, 1985.
17. Mubarek SJ, Gould RN, Lee YF, et al: The medial tibial syndrome. Am J Sports Med 10:201–205, 1982.
18. Mubarek SJ, Owens CA: Compartment syndrome and its relationship to the crush syndrome. A spectrum of disease. Clin Orthop Rel Res 113:81–89, 1975.
19. Mubarek SJ, Owens CA: Double insicion fasciotomy of the leg for decompression in compartment syndrome. J Bone Joint Surg Am 59:184–187, 1977.
20. Mubarek SJ, Owens CA, Garfin S, et al: Acute exertional superficial posterior compartment syndrome. Am J Sports Med 6:287–290, 1978.
21. Pedowitz RA, Hargens AR, Mubarek SJ: Modified criteria for the objective diagnosis of chronic compartment syndrome at the leg. Am J Sports Med 18:35–40, 1990.
22. Sheehan G: Make '76 the year of the Magic Six. Running wild. Physician Sportsmed 4:29, 1976.
23. Stanitsky CL, McMaster JH, Scanton PE: On the nature of stress fractures. Am J Sports Med 6:391–396, 1978.
24. Styf JR: Intramuscular pressure measurements during exercise. Operat Tech Sports Med 3:244, 1995.
25. Styf JR, Suukula D, Korner LM: Intramuscular pressure and muscle-blood flow during exercise in chronic compartment syndrome. J Bone Joint Surg Br 69:301–305, 1987.
26. Sullivan D, Warren RF, Pauolu H, et al: Stress fractures in 51 runners. Clin Orthop Rel Res 187:188–195, 1987.
27. Turnipseed W, Detmer O, Girdle F: Chronic compartment syndrome, an unusual case for claudication. Am Surg 250:557–562, 1989.
28. Whitelow GP, Wetzler M, Levy AS, et al: A pneumatic leg brace for the treatment of tibial stress fractures. Clin Orthop Rel Res 270:301–309, 1991.
29. Zwas ST, Frank G: The role of scintigraphy in stress and overuse injuries. Nucl Med Annu 109–141, 1989.

JUDITH F. BAUMHAUER ■ MICHAEL J. SHEREFF ■ JOHN S. GOULD

━━━━━ *CHAPTER ELEVEN*

Ankle Pain in Runners

An estimated 50 million sports injuries occur each year in the United States.[66, 195] Eighty to 90% of these injuries include sprains, strains, and contusions.[99, 100, 106] The most common of all athletic injuries are ankle injuries,[99, 106, 123] ranging from 17% to 20% in most sports.[78, 79, 100, 106, 168] Ankle injuries constitute 20% to 25% of total time lost to injury in every running or jumping sport.[167] The estimated rates of ankle injury in runners range from 15% to 30%.[107, 173, 269, 275]

Although ankle injuries are quite common, the complex etiologic factors leading to these injuries are unknown. Diverse components considered to be potential risk factors of injury have been divided into extrinsic and intrinsic variables.[166] Extrinsic factors include the type of sport, playing time, level of competition, equipment, and environmental conditions. Intrinsic factors consist of physical characteristics such as age, sex, fitness level, previous injury, strength, range of motion, joint laxity, and joint stability. The suspected multifactorial deficiencies related to ankle injury have remained elusive.

The impact of loading on the foot and ankle and the effects of ground reactive forces have been extensively studied.[40, 41, 93, 190, 204, 205, 244, 263] These forces are altered by many factors including footwear (barefoot versus shod) and velocity (walking, sprinting). The repetitive transmission of these forces to the foot and ankle have been linked with specific injuries.[88, 158, 204, 222, 223, 239, 274]

The nonspecific symptom of ankle pain has an extensive differential diagnosis (Table 11–1). The differential diagnosis of ankle injuries includes intraarticular pathology, as well as acute fractures and stress fractures, musculotendinous strains, retinacular tears, and nerve injuries. A thorough understanding of the ankle joint and its surrounding soft tissue envelope and bone stability is necessary to obtain the correct diagnosis.

ANKLE JOINT ANATOMY

The ankle joint is composed of an intricate relationship between bony and ligamentous support. The ankle joint is maintained by the cone-shaped talus and its sculptured fit between the tibia and fibula.[122] In a neutral position, the ankle has strong osseous constraints. With increasing plantar flexion, the osseous constraints are removed and the soft tissues and ligaments maintain joint stability. It is in this position that the ligamentous tissues are most susceptible to injury.[22, 30, 101, 160, 207]

The soft tissue structure of the ankle is maintained by three groups of ligaments functioning as static stabilizers: the lateral ligaments, the deltoid ligament, and the syndesmosis complex.

The dynamic stabilizers of the ankle joint consist of the muscles of the anterior, lateral, and posterior compartments of the leg. Muscle weakness and muscle imbalances have

TABLE 11–1 Differential Diagnosis of Ankle Pain

Soft Tissue	Cartilage/Bone
Ligament injury	Osteochondral lesions of the talus
1. Ankle sprain	
2. Syndesmosis injury	Stress fractures
3. Sinus tarsi syndrome	Acute fractures
4. Bassett ligament	Fracture non-unions
5. Anterior tibiotalar impingement syndrome	Osteoarthritis
	Tumors
Tendon injury	
1. Achilles tendon	
2. Peroneal tendon	
3. Posterior tibial tendon	
4. Flexor hallucis longus	
Nerve entrapment syndromes	
Accessory musculature anomalies	

TABLE 11-2 Major Cutaneous Nerve Supply to the Foot

Tibial nerve	Deep peroneal nerve
Saphenous nerve	Sural nerve
Superficial peroneal nerve	

been implicated in persistent ankle pain and recurrent ankle sprains.[12, 13, 27, 136, 261, 273]

Five cutaneous nerves cross the ankle joint to supply the foot (Table 11–2). Nerve entrapment syndromes have been implicated in the causes of chronic ankle pain in runners.[14, 196]

A carefully taken history of the injury is imperative (Table 11–3). The history guides the physician in the physical examination and potentially elucidates an etiologic factor for the injury, such as training error, a rapid increase in mileage, or new running shoes.

GENERAL PHYSICAL EXAMINATION

A systematic approach to palpation of the foot and ankle is important to identify the injured structures. Examination of the foot and proximal fibula rules out other possible injuries occurring concomitantly and masquerading as ankle pain. The areas of maximal tenderness are localized and recorded. Pain over the anatomic locations of the lateral

TABLE 11-3 Components of History Taking

Injury History

Previous ankle injury
Instability symptoms
Taping or bracing practices
Mechanism of injury
Audible pop or snap at the time of injury
Ambulation status initially and currently
Initial treatment received
Time delay in seeking care or follow-up
Duration of symptoms

Sports History

Level of competition
Training methods
Mileage
Timing surface
Footwear/inserts
Weather changes

Medical History

Generalized ligamentous laxity
Limb alignment
Personality traits
Recent illnesses
Other musculoskeletal injuries

or medial ligaments of the ankle is diagnostic of injury. An exception to this rule is pain posterior to the lateral malleolus in a congruous ankle joint. This may represent injury to the peroneal tendon complex rather than the posterior talofibular ligament. Pain in the anterior aspect of the ankle between the tibiofibular articulation may represent a syndesmosis ligament injury. This ligamentous complex can be further assessed by manual compression proximally from the fibula to the tibia, the squeeze test. Pain in the region of the distal tibiofibular articulation suggests a syndesmotic ligament injury.[121]

Routine range-of-motion and manual strength testing of the ankle should be performed to assess the degree of injury and may be used as a baseline during follow-up examinations.

SPECIFIC INJURIES

ACUTE ANKLE SPRAIN

Ligamentous injury to the ankle can involve the lateral, medial, or syndesmosis ligamentous complex. Clear elucidation of the mechanism of injury aids in making the proper diagnosis. Eversion injuries can lead to deltoid ligament tears and, when associated with external rotation of the foot, syndesmosis injuries.[72, 149, 240, 285] Plantar flexion and inversion ankle injuries can lead to rupture of the lateral ligamentous complex of the ankle.[7, 8, 28, 30, 33] The most extensive clinical studies of ankle ligament injuries have been conducted by Brostrom and colleagues.[30–33] They found isolated ruptures of the anterior talofibular ligament (ATFL) in 65% of inversion ankle sprains. A combination injury involving the ATFL and calcaneofibular ligament (CFL) occurred in 20%. A complete rupture of the ligaments resulted in a tear of the joint capsule. The CFL was never ruptured alone. The remainder of their patients had anterior inferior tibiofibular ligament (10%) or deltoid ligament (3%) injuries. The posterior talofibular ligament was rarely injured.[30] Through ankle ligament sectioning[129, 169, 224] and strain pattern studies,[56, 226] the ATFL has been shown to be the primary restraint to inversion injury when the foot is in plantar flexion, whereas the CFL is the main lateral stabilizer in a neutral ankle position.

The classification of ankle sprains is based

on the mechanism of injury.[7, 28, 30, 33, 72, 149, 160, 207] Excessive inversion motion of the tibiotalar joint in various degrees of plantar flexion or dorsiflexion results in an inversion or lateral ankle sprain. Excessive eversion motion of the ankle joint results in an injury to the medial aspect of the ankle and the deltoid ligament, an eversion ankle sprain. An ankle sprain is further stratified into grade I, II, or III based on the severity of the injury.[18, 114] This is evaluated by the patient's symptoms and physical examination findings. Various investigators have further defined the grading system based on histopathologic features of the injured ligaments.[7, 8, 42, 71, 148] Grade I injuries involve a ligament stretch without macroscopic tearing, minimal swelling or tenderness, minimal functional loss, and no mechanical joint instability. A grade II injury is a partial macroscopic ligament tear with moderate pain, swelling, and tenderness over the involved structures. Some loss of joint motion and mild to moderate joint instability are noted. A grade III injury is a complete ligament rupture with marked swelling, hemorrhage, and tenderness. Loss of function and severe joint instability occur.

Mechanical stability of the lateral ankle ligaments can be assessed clinically by the anterior drawer[20, 26, 38, 60, 124, 128, 133, 139, 144, 150, 245] and talar tilt test.[18, 44, 61, 94, 139, 151, 159, 232, 243, 245] Functional instability or the feeling of giving way, a subjective evaluation by the patient, was first described by Freeman[94] and further investigated by Tropp.[272] Tropp defined functional instability as mobility beyond voluntary control. Some researchers report a positive correlation between functional instability and recurrent ankle sprains.[95, 103, 272] The objective evaluation of proprioceptive response time is a research tool currently used to investigate functional instability.[96, 103, 272]

The diagnosis of an acute ankle sprain is based on a thorough history; complete physical examination including observation, palpation, range-of-motion, strength, and provocative stability testing; and radiographic evaluation.

The history should include the mechanism of injury, which allows a practitioner to focus on the anatomic structures likely to be involved. The patient's perceived area of pain may help localize the structures injured. The time interval between the injury and presentation allows one to assess the degree of injury, because edema and ecchymosis are time related. Initial treatment using rest, ice, compression, and elevation (RICE) may also alter the appearance on presentation, as may dependent positioning and continued running or activity. A history of prior ankle injury has been found to correlate with an increased risk of subsequent ankle injury.[78] The use of an ankle brace or tape may suggest functional ankle instability.[72] A popping or snapping sound at the time of injury may represent ligament rupture. The initial and current weight-bearing ability of the patient may aid in assessing the patient's perceived ankle stability.

Initial visualization of the ankle may reveal swelling and ecchymosis on the lateral or medial aspect of the ankle. General physical examination with anatomic localization of the maximal areas of tenderness suggests the diagnosis. Provocative testing such as the anterior drawer and talar tilt tests should be performed to assess the stability of the ligament structures of the ankle.

The anterior drawer test, first described by Landeros and colleagues,[144] evaluates the integrity of the ATFL. It is performed by stabilizing the distal tibia and applying an anteriorly directed force to the heel. The amount of anterior displacement of the talus relative to the tibia is recorded. The amount of anterior displacement in the pathologic ankle is dependent on the magnitude and duration of the stress load, degree of muscle relaxation, type of anesthesia, foot position, and measurement techniques.[163, 216] Research has found that the maximal amount of anterior displacement is produced with the ankle in 10 degrees of plantar flexion.[225] An anterolateral dimple over the area of the ATFL implies a positive result with a compromised ATFL. There is controversy in the literature about an absolute value that depicts a positive result.[20, 60, 128, 133, 144, 150, 151, 216, 232, 245] Various factors can influence the relative amount of physiologic laxity of the ankle, including previous trauma, age less than 15 years, geometric orientation of the lateral collateral ligaments, congenital abnormalities, and genetic conditions including connective tissue disorders.[216] The majority of investigators agree that comparisons with the uninjured ankle are helpful. Lindstrand and Mortensson,[163] using a radiographic anterior drawer stress test and local anesthesia, identified a positive result in those individuals with a calculated displacement difference of greater than 3 mm. These individuals underwent surgical confirmation of the intact or disrupted ATFL.

Ninety percent of ATFL disruptions were identified using this criterion and local anesthesia. Without local anesthesia, only 33% were identified. The traditional subjective grading as mild (minimal displacement), moderate (some displacement), and severe (marked displacement with an anterolateral dimple in the area of the ATFL) is still used in practice today.[42, 72, 227, 234] In an attempt to clarify this issue of millimeters of displacement and specific ligamentous disruption, cadaveric radiographic studies were performed.[5, 109, 280] These used stress view radiographs with and without anterior stress on the heel and before and after cadaveric ligament sectioning of only the ATFL and of the ATFL and CFL. A spectrum of normal values was obtained from 0 to 6 mm of anterior displacement.[109] Depending on the ligament sectioned, the values ranged from 4 to 18.2 mm of total displacement or greater than 2 mm of displacement relative to the contralateral side for the ATFL only. For the ATFL and CFL sectioning studies, the total range was 5 to 22.5 mm of displacement. Until an objective measuring device can be developed with a high intrarater and interrater reliability plus documented validity correlated with surgical confirmation of ligamentous disruption, the subjective grading scale will remain.

The talar tilt test evaluates the integrity of the CFL. With the ankle joint in neutral position and the distal tibia stabilized, an inversion stress is placed on the heel and the tilt deformity of the hindfoot relative to the distal tibia is assessed. Again, the subjective clinical measure of mild (minimal angulation), moderate (some angulation), and severe (marked angulation) is used. The literature lists a great range of normal values for the talar tilt angle assessed by stress radiographs.[25, 61, 105, 151, 159, 216, 245] The talar tilt angle is measured by the angle formed between a line drawn on the distal tibial articular surface and the talar dome. The normal range is 0 to 27 degrees. Local anesthesia may assist with pain control in evaluating talar tilt in an acute ankle injury. Comparison with the contralateral, uninjured ankle is recommended.

Radiographic evaluation begins with the standard views of the ankle: anteroposterior, lateral, and 15 degrees of internal tibial rotation or mortise view. These initial views are examined for potential fracture of the distal tibia, talar processes, talar dome (osteochondral lesions), medial malleolus, lateral malleolus, and anterior process of the calcaneus.

Stress radiographs during clinical provocative testing (anterior drawer and talar tilt tests) may aid in assessing ligament disruption. However, with a wide variation of normal and pathologic values listed in the literature, interpretation of the results is difficult. The position of the foot in dorsiflexion, neutral, or plantar flexion, in association with the amount of displacement or angulation identified on radiographs, has not been well outlined. Comparison views of the uninjured ankle are the most reliable indicator.

The treatment of acute ankle sprains has been extensively studied.[32, 51, 85, 95, 112, 141, 142, 191, 203, 220, 257] The operative and nonoperative options are excellently presented by Kannus and Renstrom.[132] Based on this review, the recommended treatment of acute ankle sprains is physical therapy. This would include active assistive range of motion of the ankle and foot, proprioceptive training, and peroneal muscle strengthening.

Chronic recurrent ankle sprains, whether mechanically or functionally unstable, have been treated with either anatomic lateral ankle ligament repairs[4, 31, 108, 134, 135] or lateral ankle ligament reconstructions.[39, 44, 81, 84, 236, 255, 258, 276] Comparisons between reconstructive techniques have found the Chrisman-Snook procedure to be superior to all other reconstructive techniques. However, the Gould modification of the Brostrom anatomic repair[108] has equal if not better results and is technically easier without weakening the primary evertor of the ankle, the peroneal brevis tendon. Snook commented that the Chrisman-Snook procedure should be considered a salvage procedure for chronic ankle instability.[253]

OSTEOCHONDRAL LESIONS OF THE TALUS

Misdiagnosis or delayed diagnosis of osteochondral lesions of the talus occurs in up 81% of cases of chronic ankle pain.[90] The symptoms of ankle pain, recurrent swelling, ankle instability, or the feeling of catching or locking of the ankle lead a clinician to the diagnosis. These lesions have been classically described as lateral or medial based on the cause,[19, 37, 209, 229] mechanism of injury,[19, 64, 161, 171] and propensity for healing.[37, 229] Lateral lesions account for 43% of osteochondral lesions and are wafer shaped, located in the anterior portion of the talar dome, and caused by a traumatic event such as an inversion ankle injury. Medial lesions (57%) are cup shaped and posterior in location. The suspected cause is osteochondrosis with associated degenerative cysts. Both computed tomography (CT) and magnetic resonance imaging (MRI) have been recommended for delineating these lesions more clearly.

Berndt and Harly described four stages of osteochondral lesions and related these stages to treatment options (Table 11–4). Ferkel and Sgaglione described a CT staging system for these lesions.[90]

The current recommended treatment for Canale and Belding[37] stages I, II, and medial stage III is a short leg non–weight-bearing cast for 6 weeks. If symptoms persist after this treatment, ankle arthroscopy is indicated, with excision, curettage, and drilling of small lesions. Larger lesions may be stabilized with bioabsorbable or buried pins or screws. Lateral stage III lesions and all stage IV lesions are initially treated with excision of the small fragments, curettage, and drilling. Larger lesions, defined as more than one third of the articular surface, require pinning or screw fixation for stabilization.[67]

SYNDESMOSIS INJURIES

The tibiofibular syndesmosis comprises the anterior inferior and posterior inferior tibiofibular ligaments, the transverse ligament, and the interosseous membrane.[116, 262] It maintains the relationship between the tibia and fibula and provides a lateral constraint to the talus within the ankle mortise. The inferior aspect of the syndesmosis also has a pivotal role in maintaining the distal tibiofibular joint. The fibula rotates 3 degrees laterally with dorsiflexion and 3 degrees medially with plantar flexion.[167] With the ankle in plantar flexion and during the push-off phase of running, the fibula migrates distally in response to the contraction of the leg and foot musculature.[242] This distal descent deepens the ankle mortise, tightens the interosseous membrane, and therefore adds to the stability of the ankle.

Syndesmosis ruptures are commonly associated with deltoid ligament injuries[118, 262] and with fractures.[157, 211] Fifty percent of Weber B ankle fractures (fibula fracture occurring at the level of the tibial plafond) have corresponding syndesmosis disruptions.[216, 262] Weber C ankle fractures (fibula fracture occurring above the level of the tibial plafond) often have a corresponding syndesmosis injury.[262]

The mechanism of injury for syndesmosis disruption is a plantar flexion external rotation injury.[97] Fritschy reported an incidence of 12 cases of isolated syndesmosis injuries in 400 ankle ligament ruptures. The athletes participated in various sports including soccer, skiing, and skating.[97]

Athletes with syndesmosis injuries complain of anterior lateral ankle pain in the region of the syndesmosis. The degree of swelling and pain associated with the injury can be significant. Patients have difficulty bearing weight on the injured ankle. Palpation over the syndesmotic ligaments anteriorly causes pain, as does passive external rotation of the foot. Posterior palpation in the corresponding region of the syndesmosis causes less discomfort.[97] Provocative tests, in addition to passive external rotation of the foot, include the squeeze[121] and cotton tests.[262] The squeeze test is performed by compressing the fibula and tibia together at the midcalf. A positive result is pain at the distal tibiofibular articulation. The cotton test is a lateral displacement assessment performed by grasping the heel and talus in one hand and the distal tibia in the other. The maneuver consists of attempting to move the talus laterally in the ankle mortise. Greater than 3 mm of lateral displacement is considered a positive finding of instability.[262] Comparison with the uninjured side is recommended.

After an adequate ankle series (anteroposterior, lateral, and mortise), a stress radiograph in plantar flexion and external rotation may demonstrate lateral diastasis.[97] Greater than 5 mm of clear space medially indicates a syndesmosis disruption.[262] Various additional studies such as an MRI, CT scan, and a bone

TABLE 11–4 Staging System for Osteochondral Fractures of the Talus

Stage	Description
I	Compression of subchondral bone without break in cartilage
II	Partial detached osteochondral fragment
III	Totally detached osteochondral fragment remaining in crater
IV	Displaced osteochondral ligament loose in joint

From Canale ST, Belding RH: Osteochondral lesions of the talus. J Bone Joint Surg Am 62:97–102, 1980.

scan have been advocated in the establishment of the diagnosis.[68, 97, 162, 175]

The treatment of a complete rupture with loss of ankle joint congruity requires surgical intervention with stabilization of the syndesmosis. This can be accomplished through the use of syndesmotic screws, cerclage wires, or Kirshner wires.[36, 97] Failure to maintain a congruous ankle joint can result in tibiotalar arthrosis.[116, 157, 262] A partial syndesmosis injury or strain can be treated with immobilization for a short period in the acute phase of injury to aid in pain control (7 to 10 days).[227] Functional treatment similar to that for an acute ankle sprain is begun. The important difference is in the recovery time, with an acute ankle sprain ranging from 3 to 6 weeks for return to activity and syndesmotic injuries taking an average of 3 months.

ACHILLES TENDON INJURIES

Injury to the Achilles tendon is a common complaint among injured runners.[46, 48, 53, 126, 153, 250] The prevalence of Achilles tendon injury ranges from 6% to 11% in the injured runner population.[53, 126] One study found that 16% of runners with Achilles tendinitis were unable to continue running secondary to pain and recurrence.[53] Diverse factors have been found to incite overuse Achilles tendon injuries, such as hard running surfaces, excessive mileage, change in running technique, shoe design, and the intensity of training.[46, 52, 126, 154, 278, 282] Poor running shoe support design and hyperpronation running gait are considered major factors in these overuse injuries.[11, 52, 126, 164, 201, 251] Cavus foot structure has also been implicated as increasing the risk for Achilles tendon rupture secondary to an inflexible foot with poor shock absorption.[11, 126, 265] Immobilization has been shown to decrease the surface area and diameter of collagen fibers in the Achilles tendon in rats after 5 weeks.[199] This suggests that immobilization has a detrimental effect on tendon strength. Training does not appear to increase collagen fiber size or strength.[267]

The biomechanic strength and the tensile load of the Achilles tendon have shed some light on why this tendon is vulnerable to overuse injury with running. After initial heel strike, the tibia externally rotates, unlocking the transverse tarsal joint, allowing midfoot pronation, and creating a supple midfoot and hindfoot complex to accommodate to the ground. Through this pronation mechanism, the Achilles tendon is subject to a slight rotational force, with a higher tensile load found on medial aspect of the tendon.[52, 126, 165, 200] The tensile strength of the Achilles tendon has been calculated to be approximately 4000 to 5000 N, with the tendon elongating approximately 1 to 2 cm with rupture.[2, 80] Temperature variations may alter these values.[45] Through the use of a cadavaric model, the force applied to the Achilles during running is estimated at six to eight times body weight.[241] This would approach the ultimate tensile strength during each stride. In vivo studies collaborating these findings have not been performed.

Classification of chronic Achilles tendon pain ranges from retrocalcaneal bursitis to peritendinitis, tendinosis, tendinitis, partial rupture, and complete rupture.[2, 218, 221] The previous classification represents a gradual transition of progressive injury from microtrauma secondary to excessive mechanical load to disruption of the collagen bundles, resulting in partial or complete rupture.[2, 218, 221]

The blood supply to the Achilles tendon has been extensively studied.[145] The anatomic finding of a watershed zone approximately 4 to 5 cm proximal to the Achilles tendon insertion is another factor in the vulnerability of this tendon to repeated injury. Peacock[214] and Halstad and coworkers[113] reported that the blood vessels supplying the Achilles tendon decreased in size and number with aging.

Athletes may complain of localized pain at the Achilles tendon insertion, anterior to the tendon (retrocalcaneal bursitis), or in the proximal watershed zone of the tendon (peritendinitis, tendinosis, tendinitis, partial or complete rupture). The duration of symptoms, the initial inciting event leading to the symptoms, and the symptom severity should be elicited.[218] Nelan and associates[200] found pain associated with sprinting to be highly correlated with surgical findings of tendinosis or partial rupture.

Clinically establishing the diagnosis of peritendinosis versus tendinitis is difficult.[218] Fusiform swelling with or without warmth may be evident along the Achilles tendon. Crepitation may also be present with motion. A prominent posterolateral calcaneal tuberosity may cause irritation, erythema, swelling, or warmth at the Achilles tendon insertion secondary to heel counter irritation (pump bump). Footwear modifications with padding or a Silapos pad over the irritated area, with a soft heel counter, are indicated.

The painful arc test may aid in determining if fusiform swelling is within the peritenon or the tendon.[282] As the foot is ranged through full dorsiflexion to full plantar flexion and the swelling moves proximal and distal with reference to the medial and lateral malleoli, tendinitis or tendinosis is suggested. If the swelling remains fixed in reference to the malleoli during the full ankle range of motion, the swelling is contained within the peritenon (peritendinitis).

The Thompson squeeze test and the needle test are used to determine if a complete Achilles tendon rupture is present.[270]

Radiographic studies include initial plain radiographs of the foot. A prominent superior angle of the calcaneal tuberosity (Haglund deformity) on the lateral foot film may cause impingement of the retrocalcaneal bursa against the Achilles tendon, inciting irritation and initiating retrocalcaneal bursitis. Calcific tendinitis may also be evident on plain radiographs. MRI is advocated for suspected cases of tendinitis or tendinosis resistant to conservative measures. MRI can elucidate partial ruptures and degenerative tendon from peritendinitis with excellent specificity and sensitivity.[277] The routine use of MRI in patients with posterior heel pain is not recommended because the majority of patients respond to initial conservative management.[47]

Initial nonoperative treatment consists of modification of activity, patient education, antiinflammatory modalities, heel lift, and gentle stretching. Once the athlete is nontender to palpation and has restored his or her flexibility, slow progressive return to activities is allowed. Faulty body mechanics leading to this injury and any training errors are corrected. Four to 6 months of conservative treatment is recommended before operative intervention.[47, 48, 69, 143, 152, 217, 238, 248, 252]

Surgical treatment is based on the MRI findings obtained after a trial of conservative management. With peritendinitis, the inflammatory peritenon is excised. In tendinosis, the degenerative tendon is excised. In the highly motivated athletic population undergoing surgical treatment for failed conservative management, 70% and 90% had good to excellent results.[152, 175]

The role of cortisone injection is limited.[137] It has been suggested in cases of peritendinitis to decrease inflammation.[137, 156] However, iatrogenic Achilles tendon rupture secondary to inadvertent intratendinous injection has been reported.[43, 184]

PERONEAL TENDON INJURY

Complete rupture of either of the peroneal tendons is extremely rare; the majority occur with an inversion ankle injury.[1, 65, 86, 188] The more common problem of peroneal tendinosis has been reported as a cause of chronic ankle pain in runners.[10, 50] The largest series of longitudinal ruptures of the peroneal tendon in athletes was a retrospective study reported by Bassett and Speer.[10] Eight athletes were found surgically to have longitudinal tears of one of the peroneal tendons after a plantar flexion and inversion ankle injury. The athletes complained of persistent lateral ankle swelling, popping, and retrofibular pain after the initial injury. The ankles were stable on physical examination. Swelling was evident along the retrofibular area of the ankle. Active ankle circumduction revealed retrofibular popping. Passive motion did not recreate this finding. The peroneal tendons did not subluxate or dislocate with this maneuver. Results of all plain radiographs of the ankle were normal. Peroneal tenograms were performed and found to be 100% sensitive but not specific for the degree of tendon disruption. Neither MRI nor CT was performed. Tenograms can demonstrate peroneal entrapment, adhesions, rupture, or tenosynovitis; however, they are an invasive examination with possible complications. Each athlete completed his or her season with taping while wrapping and underwent surgical intervention at the conclusion of the season.

Under local anesthesia, the retrofibular area was explored. The superior peroneal retinaculum was intact in all cases. The peroneus longus tendon was injured in five patients and the peroneus brevis in three. The longitudinal tears ranged from 1 to 3 cm in length. With active circumduction of the ankle, the snapping appeared to be caused by one tendon's moving over another with or without involvement of the longitudinal rent. The longitudinal defect was excised, as was any fusiform swelling, and the tendon was repaired longitudinally. Histologically, the excised specimen demonstrated synovitis and focal myxoid degeneration with or without inflammatory cell invasion. The athletes made a full recovery, with a gradual return to athletic activities after 3 to 4 weeks of immobilization.

Through a cadavaric study,[10] Bassett and Speer found that with an inversion ankle injury and plantar flexion of less than 15 degrees, the peroneal retinaculum would be injured with resulting instability to the peroneal tendons. With plantar flexion in the range of 15 to 25 degrees, both peroneal tendons are perched along the distal fibula. With subsequent inversion motion, tendon damage results. With plantar flexion greater than 25 degrees, the peroneal tendons are well seated behind the fibula, protecting them from injury.

Peroneal tendon dislocation has been reported to account for approximately 0.9% of lower extremity injuries in skiers.[155] This does occur to a lesser extent in other sport activities.[3, 17, 35, 65, 74, 76, 83, 172, 182, 187, 192, 197] The etiology of this particular injury has initiated cadavaric studies examining the anatomic variations of the fibula and retrofibular sulcus. Edwards[76] examined 178 fibulas and found that 82% had a definite sulcus involving the posterior aspect of the lateral malleolus and 18% had either a flat groove or convex surface, which would suggest a possible anatomic cause of this problem. An inversion ankle sprain mechanism and related peroneal tendon dislocation have also been linked, although the most common mechanism is forced dorsiflexion with contraction of the peroneal tendons.[35] The classification of peroneal tendon dislocations has been described by Eckert and Davis. They classify the pathologic findings into three groups: grade I retinacular separation of the anterior lip, grade II peroneal retinacular tear, and grade III avulsion of the lateral malleolus.[75]

The diagnosis of a peroneal dislocation is based on a patient's history and the characteristic swelling and tenderness occurring posterior and superior to the lateral malleolus. Patients with a peroneal dislocation usually report a snapping sensation accompanied by pain in the posterolateral aspect of the ankle. Circumduction of the ankle with palpation over the peroneal tendons may elicit a dislocation or subluxation of the peroneal tendons.

Treatment of this injury is controversial. Escalas and colleagues[83] conservatively treated 38 patients with acute peroneal dislocation injuries with tendon reduction and compressive dressing. Twenty-eight patients later suffered recurrent dislocations. Eckert

and Davis[75] treated seven acute injuries conservatively, and six patients had persistent pain and recurrent dislocation. Of 73 patients with acute injuries treated with acute surgical repair, Eckert and Davis found 76% had excellent results. Stover and Bryan[264] report on 17 acute peroneal dislocations. Seven were treated with non–weight-bearing casts for 4 weeks. Six of these patients had excellent results. Eight patients eventually had conservative management with ankle strapping; seven patients were unsuccessful with this treatment protocol. These seven patients underwent surgical intervention. It is unclear whether these treatment failures were a result of unrecognized ankle instability concurrent with peroneal tendon dislocation, or peroneal tendinosis with longitudinal tears causing persistent pain, or due to recurrent dislocation.

Chronic dislocations of the peroneal tendons are primarily treated surgically.[3, 6, 172, 187, 256] A number of procedures are described as having variable success rates and follow-ups. The treatment options include periosteal reattachment procedures, groove-deepening procedures, tenoplasty procedures, and bone block procedures.

POSTERIOR TIBIAL TENDON INJURY

Acute injuries isolated to the posterior tibial tendon are rare; however, chronic overuse injuries resulting in tenosynovitis, peritendinitis, and tendinosis have been recognized with increasing frequency during the past few years.[98, 120, 130, 131] The mechanism of this injury is thought to be repeated hyperpronation with increasing force generated during running.[15]

Acute injuries such as dislocation of the posterior tibial tendon have been reported with inversion ankle injuries.[73, 147] Another mechanism of injury for a dislocation includes forced eversion with an associated syndesmotic ligament injury.[170, 227, 271] Acute rupture can occur with an associated open laceration injury or avulsion of the accessory navicular.[111, 271]

The breadth of the literature on posterior tibial tendon pathology is based on the progression of tenosynovitis to tendon dysfunction secondary to degeneration.[57, 131] This most commonly occurs in middle-aged or older individuals and is rare in athletes.[57, 98, 120, 130, 131] It may be associated with excessive overuse such as hyperpronation with running.[15] A large spectrum of clinical findings accompanies posterior tibial tendon dysfunction. This ranges from isolated medial ankle pain symptoms without any objective findings to tenderness along the posterior tibial tendon, swelling, inversion weakness with the ankle in plantar flexion, loss of the longitudinal arch, hindfoot valgus, and a positive single limb heel rise test. The single limb heel rise test result is positive when the heel does not invert as the athlete raises onto his or her toes or is unable to rise onto the toes.

Plain radiographs of the ankle and foot may delineate an avulsion injury of the accessory navicular with retraction of the bony fragments. Other additional findings with progressive degeneration of the tendon demonstrate an abnormal talo–first metatarsal angle on both the weight-bearing anteroposterior and lateral foot radiographs.[130, 215] MRI demonstrates posterior tibial tendon abnormalities, such as peritendinitis and fluid within the tendon sheath or degeneration of the posterior tibial tendon with longitudinal tears or rupture.[57, 58, 231]

Initial treatment of an athlete with an intact posterior tibial tendon, a negative result of a single limb heel rise test, and preservation of the longitudinal arch is rest, oral antiinflammatory agents, and a medial heel and sole wedge to decrease pronation forces.[127, 130, 131] A longitudinal arch support can also be used. Conservative treatment should be continued until the pain is resolved. Preexercise and postexercise stretching of the Achilles tendon and a gentle warm-up of the posterior tibial tendon are helpful when the athlete is pain free. Mechanical realignment of hyperpronation is essential to decrease the recurrence of this injury. Changes in running shoes every 400 miles are suggested to maintain midfoot cushioning and arch support and decrease pronation stress.[49, 206]

For those individuals with incompetence of the posterior tibial tendon demonstrated by loss of longitudinal arch, hindfoot valgus, forefoot abduction with varus, a positive result of a single limb heel rise test, and an MRI scan demonstrating degeneration of the posterior tibial tendon, surgical intervention is warranted. The choice of the surgical procedure is controversial. Surgical treatment options include flexor digitorum longus tendon transfer to the posterior tibial tendon with excision of the degenerative posterior tibial tendon with or without distraction arthro-desis of the calcaneal cuboid joint or a varus calcaneal osteotomy.[130, 131, 170, 198, 215, 235] The nonoperative options in this group would include a short articulated ankle-foot orthosis to maintain foot alignment. This brace would function as a static support for the arch and would need to be worn indefinitely. Fixed deformities of the foot associated with posterior tibial tendon dysfunction related to arthritic symptoms and joint degeneration may be treated with arthrodesis of the affected joint.[130, 131, 215] This is rare in the athletic population.

Acute dislocations of the posterior tibial tendon are treated surgically. Conservative treatment has been universally unsuccessful.[73] Relocation of the posterior tibial tendon and surgical repair of the flexor retinaculum with a pants-over-vest type of repair with or without deepening of the retromalleolar groove has been suggested.[73] A bony slide procedure as described by Sharon and colleagues has also been used.[246] A proposed reconstructive procedure recommended for cases with deficient retinaculum uses a portion of the superficial deltoid ligament as well as the flexor digitorum longus tendon sheath to recreate a restraint for the posterior tibial tendon.[73]

POSTERIOR COMPARTMENT FRACTURES

Persistent posterior or posterolateral pain in runners who previously sustained ankle injury may represent a posterior compartment fracture of the ankle. The fracture in 12 of 20 patients with this history and symptoms was an acute os trigonum fracture of the posterolateral tubercle of the talus.[213] An asymptomatic os trigonum fracture is found in 5% of the population and in 14% of the athletic population.[103, 180, 210, 213] A separate case report described a hyperpronation injury with the ankle in plantar flexion, fracturing the posteromedial tubercle of the talus of a runner.[87]

Clinical examination reveals tenderness in the region of the posterior ankle. Motion of the great toe may cause pain because of the close proximity of the flexor hallucis longus tendon between the posterolateral and posteromedial tubercles of the talus.[115]

Initial plain radiographs of the ankle may demonstrate arthrosis of the posterior ankle joint.[213] The talar process fracture may or may not be seen. A special 30-degree subtalar oblique view can sometimes help to distinguish the fracture.[186] Increased uptake of radionuclide in the region of the fractured posterior process or non-union is evident on bone scan.

Initial treatment of a posterior compartment fracture is 6 weeks of cast immobilization. Patients who present late with chronic injuries are initially treated with physical therapy (stretching and strengthening of the ankle) and antiinflammatory modalities for 6 to 8 weeks. In one series of conservatively treated patients, one third responded to physical therapy with progressive return to activity and only occasional symptoms; one patient responded to cortisone injections and cast immobilization; the remainder underwent surgical excision of the fragment with good results.[213]

ANTERIOR TIBIOTALAR IMPINGEMENT SYNDROME

Anterior tibiotalar impingement syndrome represents a group of pathologic conditions causing pain with ankle dorsiflexion secondary to bone or soft tissue interposition. This was first described by Morris in soccer players with anterior ankle pain.[194] The pain is brought on by dorsiflexion of the ankle. McMurray coined the phrase *footballer's ankle,* noting its occurrence in soccer players.[183] Anterior tibial osteophytes and corresponding bone formation in the region of the talar neck causing dorsiflexion impingement at the tibiotalar joint were believed to be the pathology. It was hypothesized that forced plantar flexion of the ankle resulted in anterior capsular injury, leading to the laying down of bone in response to this trauma. O'Donoghue later called the dorsal osteophytes *impingement exostoses.*[208] He and others believed that these exostoses formed in any sport requiring rapid accelerations and decelerations at the extremes of ankle range of motion.[24, 117, 138, 140, 202, 212, 259]

The symptoms consistent with impingement exostoses include pain at the extremes of motion, limited range of motion, and swelling. Objective findings include limited range of motion, particularly in dorsiflexion, and occasional palpable bony irregularities corresponding to the areas of pain. Radiographs demonstrate bony formation and the squaring of the anterior tibial lip. Bone is noted to fill in the area of the talar neck

sulcus. Weight-bearing films in full dorsiflexion may demonstrate osteophyte contact anteriorly and posterior tibial talar joint widening.

Conservative treatment consists of a heel lift, activity modification with limitation of dorsiflexion, rest, and antiinflammatory modalities. Bracing or taping directed toward limiting ankle dorsiflexion may be helpful; however, this may provide only symptomatic relief, with the impending return of pain on discontinuance.[227] Surgical ostectomy can be performed either arthroscopically[117, 125, 174] or through an open procedure[140, 208] and is indicated when conservative management fails to relieve the symptoms or when pain recurs.

Soft tissue lesions leading to tibiotalar impingement include Bassett's ligament[9] and meniscoid lesions.[179, 181, 283] Bassett and colleagues, in 1990, reported on a prominent distal fascicle of the inferior ATFL as a cause of chronic ankle pain after an inversion ankle sprain.[9] They reported on a cadaveric study examining the inferior ATFL and found that the distal fascicle contacted the talar dome in an average of 12 degrees of dorsiflexion. A parallel clinical study confirmed these results. The symptoms produced included anterolateral ankle pain, swelling, and ankle discomfort. They hypothesized that loss of ATFL integrity (after an inversion ankle injury) allowed the talus to subluxate anteriorly and subsequently to make contact with the distal fascicle of the anterior inferior talofibular ligament, leading to tibial talar impingement. Five of seven clinical patients required chondroplasty of the anterolateral talar dome at the time of injury secondary to chondral abrasion from ligament irritation. Arthroscopic debridement of the distal fascicle of the inferior ATFL resulted in excellent long-term follow-up in five of seven patients and a good result in two of seven in one study. No instability was identified on resection.

Meniscoid lesions defined as cartilaginous transformations of a ruptured ATFL were first described by Wolin and associates in 1950.[283] They described the hyalinization of the ATFL in nine patients with chronic ankle pain and functional instability after an inversion ankle sprain. Surgical exploration of these ankles identified the meniscoid lesions at the anterolateral aspect of the ankle, causing irritation in the lateral gutter of the ankle joint.

McGinty and coworkers believed that the meniscoid lesions became interposed between the talus and the lateral malleolus, leading to pain, instability, swelling, and synovitis.[181] They advocated arthroscopic removal of the lesion with resolution of the symptoms and signs. McCarroll and associates similarly recommended surgical removal of the lesions with good results and return to prior level of activity.[179]

One study disputed the hyalinized ligament theory resulting in the ankle joint symptoms and conjectured that generalized synovitis led to the ligament alterations.[174] The recommendations were to perform a complete synovectomy to relieve the symptoms. This resulted in a 75% excellent long-term outcome with a 20% complication rate secondary to synovectomy consisting of sensory paresthesias, superficial infections, and a deep infection.

STRESS FRACTURES

Stress fractures are an injury commonly encountered at sports medicine clinics. Stress fractures account for approximately 10% of all sports injuries[177] and range between 4.7% and 15.6% of injuries to runners.[34, 53, 178]

The first description of a stress fracture was in a soldier,[29] and many of the epidemiology and etiology studies have investigated military recruits.[63, 104, 110, 189, 193, 284] In a population of 320 athletes sustaining stress fractures, runners accounted for 221 of the total number of patients with stress fractures.[176] The most common bone affected was the tibia (49.1%), followed by the tarsals (25.3%), metatarsals (8.8%), femur (7.2%), and fibula (6.6%). There was no significant difference in weekly running mileage and the affected sites. Isolated cases of medial malleolar[247] and lateral process fractures of the talus[21] have also been reported in runners.

Many studies have identified predisposing factors causing bone to be more susceptible to insufficiency fractures (Table 11–5). Stress or fatigue fractures are by definition fractures occurring when normal bone is subject to excessive stress.[228] Etiologic factors resulting in stress fractures include running errors, anatomic variations such as cavus (rigid) or pronated feet, poor footwear, and temporary inactivity.[59, 91, 266]

Primarily two theories have been suggested to explain the etiology of stress fractures in athletes. The first identified progressive muscle weakness as the body fails to absorb stress and transfers that stress to the bone.[54, 92] Skinner and Cook reported on stress fractures of the femoral neck in runners and calculated the load to failure of this bone.[249] The load to failure was found to be higher than that which could be generated with normal running. They therefore concluded that muscle fatigue allowed transfer of stress to the bone during long runs, leading to fatigue fractures. The second theory implicated the force of the muscle pull as an etiologic factor leading to stress fractures.[70, 260] The support of this theory is the occurrence of stress fractures in non–weight-bearing bones such as the humerus in baseball players. Whatever the cause, many researchers agree that a physiologic disturbance occurs in osteoclastic and osteoblastic activities, resulting in a stress fracture.

The symptoms include localized point tenderness over the affected bone, mild to moderate swelling, and pain with activity. The time of onset of the pain can be variable, and often no inciting event can be elicited.

Initial plain radiographs should be obtained; however, bony changes consistent with stress fractures are evident in only 30% to 70% of cases.[55, 110, 185, 230, 233, 237, 268] In addition, the period from the onset of pain to positive radiographic evidence of a stress fracture can vary from 2 weeks to 3 months, depending on the specific bone injured.[82, 219, 266]

A technetium bone scan is an extremely sensitive tool for the diagnosis of stress fractures. The pattern of uptake of the technetium in athletic injuries has been extensively studied.[55, 281] Unlike plain radiographs, results of bone scans are positive within 6 to 72 hours of the onset of pain. The accuracy of bone scan for this entity is very good.

The treatment for stress fractures consists of a two-phase protocol described by Clement.[54] Phase one concentrates on pain control, anti-inflammatory modalities, and activity modifications (swimming, low-resistance cycling, and water running). During this phase, stretching and flexibility are emphasized as

TABLE 11–5 Predisposing Factors Leading to Insufficiency Fractures

Menstrual irregularity	Alcohol intake
	Hypothyroidism
Osteoporosis	Anorexia nervosa
Diabetic or idiopathic neuropathy	Paget disease
	Rheumatoid arthritis
Smoking	

well as local muscle strengthening and re-training.

Phase two is begun when the athlete has been pain free for 10 to 14 days. While continuing the phase one treatment, the athlete is slowly allowed to return to running. Initial alternate running days are encouraged. It has been shown that a rest period decreases the rate of stress fractures from 4.6% to 1.6% in military recruits. Attention to running surface, shoes, and gait is also integrated into the phase two protocol, and orthotics and footwear modifications are used. The majority, greater than 90%, improve with this treatment.[176]

NERVE ENTRAPMENT SYNDROMES

Heel and foot pain are common complaints among runners.[16, 23, 62, 196] Although tarsal tunnel compression of the tibial nerve is a well-recognized nerve entrapment syndrome causing paresthesias in the plantar aspect of the foot, other lesser known peripheral nerve impingements occur, causing ankle pain in runners. In a review examining nerve entrapments of the foot and ankle in runners, 2 of 21 operative cases presented with dorsal ankle pain secondary to compression of the deep peroneal nerve at the superior talus.[196] Palpation of the maximal area of tenderness caused radiating paresthesias into the first web space of the foot. At surgery, a dorsal spur was found on the distal aspect of the talus, causing the deep peroneal nerve compression. Other areas of deep peroneal nerve entrapment, also called *anterior tarsal tunnel syndrome,* include the distal aspect of the inferior extensor retinaculum with or without associated compression of the extensor hallucis longus tendon.[196] Conservative treatment includes immobilization, local injections with lidocaine and cortisone, and nonsteroidal antiinflammatory drugs.[23, 62, 77, 119, 146, 254] With resistant cases, surgical intervention consisting of release of the nerve compression is successful. Preoperative nerve conduction studies or electromyograms are not believed to be necessary. The sensitivity and specificity of electrical diagnostic studies are poor.[16] Postoperative immobilization of the foot and ankle for 2 to 4 weeks is recommended. Mild jogging is begun at 8 weeks, and full training is resumed at 12 weeks.[16, 119, 196]

SUMMARY

Chronic ankle pain in runners can be due to multiple causes. A thorough review of the patient's history with a physical examination concentrating on anatomic structures surrounding the ankle is imperative. The addition of provocative testing and radiographic examinations can aid in elucidating the pathology. After treatment of the injury, attention to training technique, running shoes, and individual gait is integrated into global patient education to decrease the incidence of injury recurrence.

REFERENCES

1. Abraham E, Stirnaman JF: Neglected rupture of the peroneal tendons causing recurrent sprains of the ankle. J Bone Joint Surg Am 61:1247–1248, 1979.
2. Allenmark C: Partial Achilles tendon tears. Clin Sports Med 11:759–769, 1992.
3. Alm A, Lamke LO, Liljedahl SO: Surgical treatment of dislocation of peroneal tendons. Injury 7:14–19, 1975.
4. Althoff B, Peterson L, Renstrom P: Simple plastic surgery of invertebrate ligament damage in the ankle joint. Lakartidningen 78:2857–2861, 1981.
5. Arms SW, Renstrom P, Incavo S, et al: A-P laxity of the human ankle and the effect of AFTC resection. Proceedings of the 64th Annual Meeting of the Orthopaedic Research Society, Atlanta, GA, Feb. 1–4, 1988.
6. Arrowsmith SR, Fleming LL, Allman FL: Traumatic dislocations of peroneal tendons. Am J Sports Med 11:142, 1983.
7. Baldvini FC, Tetzlaff J: Historical perspectives on injuries of the ligaments of the ankle. Clin Sports Med 1:3–12, 1982.
8. Baldvini FC, Vegso JT, Torg JT, Torg E: Management and rehabilitation of ligamentous injuries to the ankle. Sports Med 4:364–380, 1987.
9. Bassett FH, Gates HS, Billys JB, et al: Talar impingement by the anteroinferior tibiofibular ligament. A cause of chronic pain in the ankle after inversion sprain. J Bone Joint Surg Am 72:55–59, 1990.
10. Bassett FH, Speer KP: Longitudinal rupture of the peroneal tendons. Am J Sports Med 21:354–357, 1993.
11. Bates BT, Osternig LR, Mason B, et al: Foot orthotic devices to modify selected aspects of lower extremity mechanics. Am J Sports Med 7:338–342, 1979.
12. Baumhauer JF: A Comparison Study of Ankle Inversion and Eversion Strength in Healthy and Inversion Ankle Sprained Individuals as Assessed by the Cybex II & Dynamometer. Masters Thesis, Middlebury College, Middlebury, VT, 1985.
13. Baumhauer JF, Alosa DM, Renstrom PAFH, et al: A prospective study of ankle injury risk factors. Am J Sports Med 23:564–570, 1995.
14. Baxter DE: Functional nerve disorders in the athletic foot, ankle and leg. Instr Course Lect 42:185–194, 1993.
15. Baxter DE: The foot in running. In Mann RA,

Coughlin MJ (eds): Surgery of the Foot and Ankle, vol 2, 6th ed. St. Louis, Mosby-Year Book, 1993, pp 1225–1235.

16. Baxler DE, Thigpen CM: Heel pain—operative results. J Am Orthop Foot Ankle Soc 5:15–25, 1984.

17. Beck E: Operative treatment of recurrent dislocation of the peroneal tendons. Arch Orthop Trauma Surg 98:247–250, 1981.

18. Bergfeld J, Halpern B: Sports Medicine: Functional Management of Ankle Injuries. American Academy of Family Physicians Syllabus. Kansas City, Gardiner-Caldwell Syner Med, 1991.

19. Berndt AL, Hardy M: Transchondral fractures (osteochondritis dessicans) of the talus. J Bone Joint Surg Am 41:988–1020, 1959.

20. Black HM, Brand RL, Eichelberger MR: An improved technique for the evaluation of ligamentous injury in severe ankle sprains. Am J Sports Med 6:276–282, 1978.

21. Black KP, Ehlert KJ: A stress fracture of the lateral process of the talus in a runner. J Bone Joint Surg Am 76:441–443, 1994.

22. Bland RL, Black HM, Cox JS: The natural history of inadequately treated ankle sprains. Am J Sports Med 5:248–249, 1977.

23. Blockey MJ: Painful heel: Controlled trial of value of hydrocortisone. Br Med J 1:1277–1298, 1956.

24. Boardman KP: Tibiotalar impingement exostoses causing osteochondrometrosis of the ankle. Injury 11:43–44, 1979.

25. Bonnin JGF: The hypermobile ankle. Proc R Soc Med 37:282–286, 1944.

26. Boruta PM, Bishop JO, Braly WG, et al: Acute lateral ankle ligament injuries: A literature review. Foot Ankle 11:107–113, 1990.

27. Bosien WR, Staples OS, Russell SW: Residual disability following acute ankle sprains. J Bone Joint Surg Am 26:95–135, 1955.

28. Brand RL, Collins MDF: Operative management of ligamentous injuries to the ankle. Clinic Sports Med 1:117–130, 1982.

29. Breithaupt MD: Zur Pathologie des Menschlichen Fussen. Medizin Zeitung 24:169–177, 1855.

30. Brostrom C: Sprained ankles I: Anatomic lesions in recent sprains. Acta Chir Scand 128:483–495, 1964.

31. Brostrom L: Sprained ankles IV: Surgical treatment of "chronic" ligament ruptures. Acta Chir Scand 132:551–564, 1966.

32. Brostrom L: Sprained ankles V: Treatment and prognosis in recent ligament ruptures. Acta Chir Scand 132:537–550, 1966.

33. Brostrom L, Liljedahl SO, Lindvall N: Sprained ankles II: Arthrographic diagnosis of recent ligament ruptures. Acta Chir Scand 129:485–499, 1965.

34. Brubaker CE, James SC: Injuries to runners. J Sports Med 2:189–198, 1974.

35. Burman M: Stenosis tenovaginitis of the foot and ankle. Arch Surg 67:686–698, 1953.

36. Canale ST: Ankle injuries. In Crenshaw AH (ed): Campbell's Operative Orthopaedics, vol 3, 7th ed. St. Louis, CV Mosby, 1987, pp 2265–2281.

37. Canale ST, Belding RH: Osteochondral lesions of the talus. J Bone Joint Surg Am 62:97–102, 1980.

38. Cass JR, Morrey BF, Chao EYS: Three-dimensional kinematics of ankle instability following serial sectioning of lateral collateral ligaments. Foot Ankle 5:142–149, 1984.

39. Cass JR, Morrey BF, Katoh Y, Chao EYS: Ankle instability: Comparison of primary repair and delayed reconstruction after long term follow-up study. Clin Orthop 198:110–117, 1985.

40. Cavanagh PR: The biomechanics of running shoe problems. In Segesser B, and Pforringer W (eds): The Shoe in Sport, Chicago, Year Book Medical Publishers, 1989, pp 3–15.

41. Cavanagh PR, Lafortune MA: Grand reaction forces in distance running. J Biomech 13:397–406, 1980.

42. Chapman MW: Sprains of the ankle. Instr Course Lect 24:294–308, 1975.

43. Checknick A, Amit Y, Israeli A, et al: Recurrent rupture of the Achilles tendon induced by corticosteroid injection. Br J Sports Med 16:89–90, 1982.

44. Chrisman OD, Snook GA: Reconstruction of lateral ligament tears of the ankle. J Bone Joint Surg Am 51:904–912, 1969.

45. Ciullo JV, Zarins B: Biomechanics of the musculotendinous unit: Relation to athletic performance and injury. Clin Sports Med 2:71–86, 1983.

46. Clancy WG: Runners injuries. Am J Sports Med 8:287–289, 1980.

47. Clancy WG: Tendinitis and plantar fasciitis in runners. In D'Ambrosia R, Drez D (eds): Prevention and Treatment of Running Injuries. Thorofare, NJ, Slack, 1982, pp 77–87.

48. Clancy WG, Neidhard D, Brand RL: Achilles tendinitis in runners. A report of five cases. Am J Sports Med 4:46–57, 1976.

49. Clanton TO: Etiology of injury to the foot and ankle. In DeLee JC, Drez D Jr. (eds): Orthopaedic Sports Medicine, vol 2. Philadelphia, WB Saunders, 1994, pp 1642–1704.

50. Clanton TO, Schon LC: Athletic injuries to the soft tissues of the foot and ankle. In Mann RA, Coughlin MJ (eds): Surgery of the Foot and Ankle. St. Louis, Mosby-Year Book, 1993, pp 1095–1224.

51. Clark BL, Derby AC, Power GRI: Injuries of the lateral ligament of the ankle. Conservative vs. operative repair. Can J Surg 8:358–363, 1965.

52. Clement DB, Tauton JE, Smart GW: Achilles tendinitis and peritendinitis: Etiology and treatment. Am J Sports Med 12:179–184, 1984.

53. Clement DB, Taunton JE, Smart GW, et al: A survey of overuse running injuries. Physician Sports Med 9:47–58, 1981.

54. Clement DB: Tibial stress syndrome in athletes. J Sports Med 2:81–85, 1974.

55. Collier BD, Johnson RP, Carrera GF, et al: Scintigraphic diagnosis of stress induced incomplete fractures of the proximal tibia. J Trauma 24:156–160, 1984.

56. Colville MR, Marder RA, Boyle JJ, Zarins B: Strain measurement in lateral ankle ligaments. Am J Sports Med 18:196–200, 1990.

57. Conti SF: Posterior tibial tendon problems in athletes. Orthop Clin North Am 25:109–121, 1994.

58. Conti SF, Michelson J, Jahss MH: Clinical significance of magnetic resonance imaging in preoperative planning of posterior tibial tendon ruptures. Foot Ankle 13:208–214, 1992.

59. Cornwall G: Sports Medicine and the pes cavus foot. B C Med J 26:573–574, 1984.

60. Cox JS: Surgical and non-surgical treatment of acute ankle sprains. Clin Orthop Rel Res 198:118–126, 1985.

61. Cox JS, Hewes TF: "Normal" talar tilt angle. Clin Orthop Rel Res 140:37–41, 1979.

62. Cozen L: Bursitis of the heel. Am J Orthop 3:372, 1961.
63. Darby RE: Stress fractures of the os calcic. JAMA 200:131–132, 1967.
64. Davidson AM, Steele AD, MacKensie DA, et al: A review of twenty-one cases of transchondral fractures of the talus. J Trauma 7:378–415, 1967.
65. Davies JA: Peroneal compartment syndrome secondary to rupture of the peroneus longus. J Bone Joint Surg Am 61:783–784, 1979.
66. Dean CH, Hoerner EF: Injury rates in team sports and individual recreation. In Vinger PF, Hoerner EF (eds): Sports Injuries. Boston, John Wright PSG, 1982.
67. DeLee JC: Fractures and dislocations of the foot. In Mann RA (ed): Surgery of the Foot, 5th ed. St. Louis, CV Mosby, 1986, pp 656–715.
68. Denhartog B, Cardone BW, Johnson JE, et al: The role of magnetic resonance imaging in evaluating chronic ankle pain after sprain. American Orthopaedic Foot and Ankle Society Meeting, Boston, July 25–28, 1991.
69. Denstad TF, Roaas A: Surgical treatment of partial Achilles tendon ruptures. Am J Sports Med 7:15–17, 1979.
70. Devas MB: Stress fractures in athletes. J R Coll Gen Pract 19:34–38, 1970.
71. Diamond JA: Rehabilitation of ankle sprains. Clin Sports Med 8:877–891, 1989.
72. Drez DJ, Karchey MF: Ankle ligament injuries: Practical guidelines for examination and treatment. J Musculoskel Med 6:21–36, 1989.
73. Duzounian TJ, Myerson MS: Dislocation of the posterior tibial tendon. Foot Ankle 13:215–219, 1992.
74. Earle AS, Moritz JR, Tapper EM: Dislocation of the peroneal tendons at the ankle: An analysis of 25 ski injuries. Northwest Med 71:108–110, 1972.
75. Eckert WR, Davis EA: Acute rupture of the peroneal retinaculum. J Bone Joint Surg Am 58:670, 1976.
76. Edwards ME: The relations of the peroneal tendons to the fibula, calcaneus and cuboideum. Am J Anat 42:213–253, 1928.
77. Eggers GW: Shoe pad for treatment of calcaneal spur. J Bone Joint Surg Am 39:219–220, 1957.
78. Ekstrand J, Gillquist J: Soccer injuries and their mechanisms: A prospective study. Med Sci Sports Exerc 15:267–270, 1983.
79. Ekstrand J, Tropp H: The incidence of ankle sprains in soccer. Foot Ankle 2:41–44, 1990.
80. Elliott DH: Structure and function of mammalian tendon. Biol Rev Camb Philos Soc 40:392–421, 1965.
81. Elmslie RC: Recurrent subluxation of the ankle joint. Ann Surg 100:364–367, 1934.
82. Engher W: Stress fractures of the medial tibial plateau. J Bone Joint Surg Am 59:767–769, 1977.
83. Escalas F, Figueras JM, Merino JA: Dislocation of the peroneal tendons. Long term results of surgical treatment. J Bone Joint Surg Am 62:451–453, 1980.
84. Evans DL: Recurrent instability of the ankle—a method of surgical treatment. Proc R Soc Med 46:343–344, 1953.
85. Evans GA, Hardcastle P, Frenyo AD: Acute rupture of the lateral ligament of the ankle. To suture or not to suture. J Bone Joint Surg Br 66:209–212, 1984.
86. Evans JD: Subcutaneous ruptures of the tendon of peroneus longus. J Bone Joint Surg Br 48:507–509, 1966.
87. Fabrikant JM, Hlavac HF: Fracture of the posterior process of the talus in runners. A case report. J Am Podiatry Assoc 69:5:329–332, 1979.
88. Falsetti HL, Burke ER, Feld RD, et al: Hematological variations after endurance running with hard- and soft-soled running shoes. Physician Sportsmed 11:118–127, 1983.
89. Ferkel RD, Fasulo GJ: Arthroscopic treatment of ankle injuries. Orthop Clin North Am 25:1:17–32, 1994.
90. Ferkel RD, Sgaglione NA: Arthroscopic treatment of osteochondral lesions of the talus: Long term results. Proceedings of the Annual Meeting of the American Academy of Orthopaedic Surgeons, San Francisco, February 18–23, 1993.
91. Fitch KD: Stress fractures of the lower limbs in runners. Aust Fam Physician 13:511–515, 1984.
92. Frankel VH: Editorial comment. Am J Sports Med 6:396, 1978.
93. Frederick EC (ed): Sports Shoes and Playing Surfaces. Biomechanical Properties. Champaign, IL, Human Kinetics, 1984.
94. Freeman MAR: Instability of the foot after injuries to the lateral ligament of the ankle. J Bone Joint Surg Br 47:669–677, 1965.
95. Freeman MAR: Treatment of ruptures of the lateral ligament of the ankle. J Bone Joint Surg Br 47:661–668, 1965.
96. Freeman MAR, Dean MRE, Hanham IWF: The etiology and prevention of functional instability of the foot. J Bone Joint Surg Br 47:679–685, 1965.
97. Fritschy D: An unusual ankle injury in top skiers. Am J Sports Med 17:282–286, 1989.
98. Funk DA, Cass JR, Johnson KA: Acquired adult flat foot deformity secondary to posterior tibial tendon pathology. J Bone Joint Surg Am 68:95–102, 1986.
99. Garrett WE: Strains and sprains in athletics. Postgrad Med 73:200–209, 1983.
100. Garrick JG, Requa RK: The epidemiology of foot and ankle injuries in sports. Clin Sports Med 7:29–36, 1988.
101. Garrick JG, Requa RK: Role of external support in the prevention of ankle sprains. Med Sci Sports 5:200–203, 1973.
102. Gauffin H, Tropp H, Odenrick P: Effect of ankle disc training on postural control in patients with functional instability of the ankle joint. Int J Sports Med 9:141–144, 1988.
103. Geist ES: Supernumerary bones of the foot—Rontgen study of the feet of one hundred normal individuals. Am J Orthop Surg 12:403–414, 1914.
104. Gilbert RS, Johnson HA: Stress fractures in military recruits—a review of twelve years' experience. Milit Med 131:716–721, 1966.
105. Goldstein LA: Tear of the lateral ligament of the ankle. N Y State J Med 48:199, 1948.
106. Gorrick JG: The frequency of injury, mechanism of injury and epidemiology of ankle sprains. Am J Sports Med 5:241–242, 1977.
107. Gottlieb G, White JR: Responses of recreational runners to their injuries. Physician Sportsmed 8:145–149, 1980.
108. Gould N, Seligson D, Gassman J: Early and late repair of lateral ligament of the ankle. Foot Ankle 1:84–89, 1980.
109. Grace DL: Lateral ankle ligament injuries inversion and anterior stress radiography. Clin Orthop 183:153–156, 1989.
110. Greaney RB, Gerber FH, Laughlin RL, et al: Distri-

bution and natural history of stress fractures in U.S. Marine recruits. Radiology 146:339–346, 1983.

111. Grogan DP, Gasser SI, Ogden JA: The painful accessory navicular: A clinical and histopathological study. Foot Ankle 10:164–169, 1989.

112. Gronmark T, Johnsen O, Kogstad O: Rupture of the lateral ligaments of the ankle. A controlled clinical trial. Injury 11:215–218, 1980.

113. Halstad K, Larsson LC, Lindholm A: Clearance of radiosodium after local deposit in the Achilles tendon. Acta Chir Scand 116:251–256, 1976.

114. Hamilton WG: Sprained ankles in ballet dancers. Foot Ankle 3:99–102, 1982.

115. Hamilton WG: Stenosing tenosynovitis of the flexor hallucis longus tendon and posterior impingement upon the os trigonum in ballet dancers. Foot Ankle 3:74–80, 1982.

116. Hamilton WG: Traumatic Disorders of the Ankle. New York, Springer-Verlag, 1984, pp 1–293.

117. Hardaker WT Jr: Foot and ankle injuries in classical ballet dancers. Orthop Clin North Am 20:621–627, 1989.

118. Harper MC: The deltoid ligament. An evaluation of need for surgical repair. Clin Orthop 226:156–168, 1988.

119. Henneson AS, Westin ND: Chronic calcaneal pain in athletes. Entrapment of the calcaneal nerve? Am J Sports Med 12:152–154, 1984.

120. Holmes GB, Mann RA: Possible epidemiological factors associated with rupture of the posterior tibia tendon. Foot Ankle 13:70–79, 1992.

121. Hopkinson WJ, St. Pierre P, Ryan JB, Wheeler JH: Syndesmosis sprains of the ankle. Foot Ankle 10:325–330, 1990.

122. Inman VT: The Joints of the Ankle. Baltimore, Williams & Wilkins, 1976, pp 30–31, 70–71.

123. Jackson DW: Injury prevention in the young athlete: A preliminary report. Am J Sports Med 6:6–14, 1978.

124. Jackson JP, Hutson MA: Cast brace treatment of ankle sprains. Injury 17:251–255, 1986.

125. Jaivin JS, Ferkel RD: Arthroscopy of the foot and ankle. Clin Sports Med 13:761–783, 1994.

126. James SL, Bates BT, Osternig LR: Injuries to runners. Am J Sports Med 6:40–50, 1978.

127. Janisse DJ: Indications and prescriptions for orthoses in sports. Orthop Clin North Am 25:95–107, 1994.

128. Johannsen A: Radiological diagnosis of lateral ligament lesions of the ankle. Acta Orthop Scand 49:295–301, 1978.

129. Johnson EE, Markolf KL: The contributions of the anterior talofibular ligament to ankle laxity. J Bone Joint Surg Am 65:81–88, 1983.

130. Johnson KA: Tibialis posterior tendon rupture. Clin Orthop Rel Res 177:140–147, 1983.

131. Johnson KA, Strom DE: Tibialis posterior tendon dysfunction. Clin Orthop Rel Res 239:196–206, 1989.

132. Kannus P, Renstrom P: Treatment for acute tears of the lateral ligaments of the ankle. Surgery, cast or early control mobilization? J Bone Joint Surg Am 73:305–312, 1991.

133. Karlsson J: Chronic Lateral Instability of the Ankle (thesis). Gothenburg, Sweden, Gothenburg University, Vasastadens Bokbinder, 1989.

134. Karlsson J, Bergsten T, Lasinger O, Peterson L: Reconstruction of the lateral ligaments of the ankle for chronic lateral instability. J Bone Joint Surg Am 70:581–588, 1988.

135. Karlsson J, Bergsten T, Lasinger O, Peterson L: Surgical treatment of chronic lateral instability of the ankle joint. Am J Sports Med 17:268–274, 1989.

136. Kaumeyer A, Malone T: Ankle injuries: Anatomic and biomechanical considerations for the development of an injury prevention program. J Orthop Sports Phys Ther 1:171–177, 1980.

137. Keck SW, Kelly PJ: Bursitis of the posterior part of the heel: Evaluation of surgical treatment of 18 patients. J Bone Joint Surg Am 47:267–273, 1965.

138. Kelikian H, Kelikian AS: Disorders of the Ankle. Philadelphia, WB Saunders, 1985.

139. Kjaersgaard-Anderson P, Frich LH, Madsen F, et al: Instability of the hindfoot after lesions of the lateral ankle ligaments. Clin Orthop Rel Res 266:170–179, 1991.

140. Kleiger B: Anterior tibiotalar impingement syndromes in dancers. Foot Ankle 3:69–73, 1982.

141. Klein J, Schreckenberger C, Roddecker K, Tiling T: Operative or conservative treatment of recent rupture of the fibular ligament of the ankle. A randomized clinical trial. Unfallchirurgie 91:154–160, 1988.

142. Korkala O, Rusanen M, Jokipii P, et al: A prospective study of the treatment of severe tears of the lateral ligament of the ankle. Int Orthop 11:13–17, 1987.

143. Kvist H, Kvist M: The operative treatment of chronic calcaneal paratendonitis. J Bone Joint Surg Br 62:353–357, 1980.

144. Landeros O, Frost HM, Higgins CC: Post traumatic anterior ankle instability. Clin Orthop 56:169–178, 1968.

145. Langergen C, Lindholm A: Vascular distribution in Achilles tendon—an angiographic and microangiographic study. Acta Chir Scand 116:491–495, 1958.

146. Lapidus RW, Guidotti FP: Painful heel: Report of 323 patients with 364 painful heels. Clin Orthop 39:178–186, 1965.

147. Larsen E, Lauridsen F: Dislocation of the tibialis posterior tendon in two athletes. Am J Sports Med 12:429–430, 1984.

148. Lassiter TE Jr, Malone TR, Garrett WE: Injury to the lateral ligaments of the ankle. Orthop Clin North Am 20:629–640, 1989.

149. Lauge-Hansen N: Fractures of the ankle II. Combined experimental surgical and experimental roentgenologic investigations. Arch Surg 60:957–985, 1950.

150. Laurin C, Mathieu J: Sagittal mobility of the normal ankle. Clin Orthop 108:99–104, 1975.

151. Laurin CA, Ouellet R, St. Jacques R: Talar and subtalar tilt: An experimental investigation. Can J Surg 11:270–279, 1968.

152. Leach RE: Achilles tendon ruptures. In Mack RP (ed): Symposium on the Foot and Leg in Running Sports. St. Louis, Mosby-Year Book, 1982, pp 99–105.

153. Leach RE, Dilorio E, Harney RA: Pathologic hindfoot conditions in the athlete. Clin Orthop 117:116–121, 1983.

154. Leach RE, Janes S, Wasilewski S: Achilles tendinitis. Am J Sports Med 9:92–98, 1981.

155. Leach RE, Lower G: Ankle injuries in skiing. Clin Orthop Rel Res 198:127, 1985.

156. Leach RE, Schepsis AA, Hiroaki T: Achilles tendinitis. Don't let it be an athlete's downfall. Physician Sportsmed 19:87–92, 1991.

157. Leeds HC, Ehrlich MG: Instability of the distal tibio-

fibular syndesmosis after bimalleolar and trimalleolar ankle fractures. J Bone Joint Surg Am 66:490–503, 1984.

158. Light LH, McLellan GE, Klenerman L: Skeletal transients on heel strike in normal walking with different footwear. J Biomech 13:477–480, 1980.

159. Lightowler CDR: Injuries to the lateral ligament of the ankle. Br Med J 289:1247, 1984.

160. Lindenfeld TN: The differentiation and treatment of ankle sprains. Orthopedics 11:203–206, 1988.

161. Lindholm TS, Osterman K, Vankka E: Osteochondritis of the elbow, ankle and hip. Clin Orthop 148:245–253, 1980.

162. Lindsjo U, Hemmirzsson A, Sahlstedt B, Danchwardt-Lillestrom G: Computer tomography of the ankle. Acta Orthop Scand 50:797–801, 1979.

163. Lindstrand A, Mortensson W: Anterior instability of the ankle joint following acute ligament sprain. Acta Radiol Diagn 18:529–539, 1977.

164. Lowdon A, Bader D, Mowat A: The effect of heel pads on the treatment of Achilles tendinitis. A double blind trial. Am J Sports Med 12:431–435, 1984.

165. Lundberg A, Goldi I, Kalin B, et al: Kinematics of the ankle foot complex. Foot Ankle 3:235–238, 1976.

166. Lysens R, Steverlynck A, Vanden Auweele Y, et al: The predictability of sports injuries. Sports Med 1:6–10, 1984.

167. Mack RP: Ankle injuries in athletics. Clin Sports Med 1:71–84, 1982.

168. Maehlum S, Dahlord OA: Acute sports injuries in Oslo: A one year study. Br J Sports Med 18:181–185, 1984.

169. Makhani JS: Lacerations of the lateral ligament of the ankle. An experimental appraisal. J Int Coll Surg 38:454–466, 1962.

170. Mann RA, Thompson FM: Rupture of the posterior tibial tendon causing flat foot. Surgical treatment. J Bone Joint Surg Am 67:556–561, 1985.

171. Marks KL: Flake fracture of the talus progressing to osteochondritis dissecans. J Bone Joint Surg Br 34:90–92, 1952.

172. Martens MA, Noyez JF, Mulier JC: Recurrent dislocation of the peroneal tendons. Results of rerouting the tendons under the calcaneofibular ligaments. Am J Sports Med 14:148–150, 1986.

173. Marti B, Vader JP, Minder CE, et al: On the epidemiology of running injuries: The Bern Grand-Prix Study. Am J Sports Med 16:285–294, 1988.

174. Martin DF, Curl WW, Baker CL: Arthroscopic treatment of chronic synovitis of the ankle. Arthroscopy 5:110–114, 1989.

175. Marymont JV, Lynch MA, Henning CE: Acute ligamentous diastasis of the ankle without fracture evaluation by radionuclide imaging. Am J Sports Med 14:407–409, 1986.

176. Matheson GO, Clement DB, McKenzie DC, et al: Stress fractures in athletes. A study of 320 cases. Am J Sports Med 15:46–58, 1987.

177. McBryde AM: Stress fractures in athletes. J Sports Med 3:212–217, 1975.

178. McBryde AM: In D'Ambrosia R, Dres D (eds): Prevention and Treatment of Running Injuries. Thorofare, NJ, Slack, 1982, pp 21–42.

179. McCarroll JR, Schrader JW, Shelburne KD, et al: Meniscoid lesions of the ankle in soccer players. Am J Sports Med 15:255–257, 1987.

180. McDougall A: The os trigonum. J Bone Joint Surg Br 37:257–265, 1955.

181. McGinty JB, Andrews JR, Diez DJ, et al: Symposium: Arthroscopy of joints other than the knee. Contemp Orthop 9:71–101, 1984.

182. McLennan JG: Treatment of acute and chronic luxations of the peroneal tendons. Am J Sports Med 8:432–436, 1980.

183. McMurray TP: Footballer's ankle. J Bone Joint Surg Br 32:68–69, 1950.

184. Melmed EP: Spontaneous bilateral rupture of the calcaneal tendon during steroid therapy. J Bone Joint Surg Br 47:104, 1965.

185. Merman KO: Less common stress fractures in the foot. Br J Radiol 54:1–7, 1981.

186. Merrill V: Atlas of Roentgenographic Positions and Standard Radiologic Procedures, vol 1, 4th ed. St. Louis, CV Mosby, 1975, p 83.

187. Micheli LJ, Waters PM, Sanders DP: Sliding fibular graft repair for chronic dislocations of the peroneal tendons. Am J Sports Med 17:68–71, 1989.

188. Milgrann JE: Muscle ruptures and avulsions with particular reference to the lower extremities. Instr Course Lect 10:233–243, 1953.

189. Milgrom C, Giladi M, Stein M, et al: Stress fractures in military recruits: A prospective study showing an unusually high incidence. J Bone Joint Surg Br 67:732–735, 1985.

190. Miller DI: Grand reactive forces in distance running. In Cavanaugh PR (ed): Biomechanics of Distance Running. Champaign, IL, Human Kinetics, 1990, pp 203–224.

191. Moller-Larsen F, Wethelung JO, Jurik AG, et al: Comparison of three different treatments for ruptured lateral ankle ligaments. Acta Orthop Scand 59:564–566, 1988.

192. Moritz JR: Ski injuries. Am J Surg 98:493–505, 1959.

193. Morris JM, Blickenstaff LD: Fatigue Fractures: A Clinical Study. Springfield, IL, Charles C Thomas, 1967.

194. Morris LH: Report of cases of athlete's ankle. J Bone Joint Surg 25:220, 1943.

195. Mueller FO, Blyth CS: Fatalities from head and cervical spine injuries occurring in tackle football: 40 years' experience. Clin Sports Med 6(1):185–196, 1987.

196. Murphy PC, Baxter DE: Nerve entrapment of the foot and ankle in runners. Clin Sports Med 4:753–763, 1985.

197. Murr S: Dislocation of the peroneal tendons with marginal fracture of the lateral malleolus. J Bone Joint Surg Br 43:563–565, 1961.

198. Myerson MS, Corrigan J, Schon L, Thompson FM: Tendon transfer combined with calcaneal osteotomy for the treatment of posterior tibial tendon insufficiency: A radiographic investigation. International Foot and Ankle 16(11):712–718, 1995.

199. Nakagawa Y, Totsuka M, Sato T, et al: Effect of disuse on the ultrastructure of the Achilles tendon in rats. Eur J Appl Physiol 59:239–242, 1989.

200. Nelan G, Martens M, Burssens A: Surgical treatment of chronic Achilles tendinitis. Am J Sports Med 17:754–759, 1989.

201. Nichols A: Achilles tendinitis in running athletes. J Am Board Fam Pract 2:196–203, 1989.

202. Nichols JA: Ankle injuries in athletes. Orthop Clin North Am 5:153–175, 1974.

203. Niedermann B, Andersen A, Andersen SB, et al: Rupture of the lateral ligaments of the ankle. Operation or plaster cast? A prospective study. Acta Orthop Scand 52:579–587, 1981.

204. Nigg BM: Biomechanics, load analysis and sports injuries in the lower extremities. Sports Med 2:367–379, 1985.

205. Nigg BM (ed.): Biomechanics of Running Shoes. Champaign, IL, Human Kinetics, 1986.

206. Nigg BM, Bahlsen AH, Denoth J, et al: Factors influencing kinetic and kinematic variables in running. In Nigg BM (ed): Biomechanics of Running Shoes. Champaign, IL, Human Kinetics, 1986, pp 139–159.

207. O'Donoghue D: Treatment of Injuries to Athletes, 3rd ed. Philadelphia, WB Saunders, 1976.

208. O'Donoghue DH: Impingement exostoses of the talus and tibia. J Bone Joint Surg Am 39:835–852, 1957.

209. O'Donoghue DH: Chondral and osteochondral fractures. J Trauma 6:469–481, 1966.

210. O'Rahilly R: A survey of carpal and tarsal anomalies. J Bone Joint Surg Am 35:626–642, 1953.

211. Pankovich AM: Maisonneuve fracture of the fibula. J Bone Joint Surg Am 56:337–347, 1976.

212. Parkes JC II, Hamilton WG, Patterson AH, Rawles JG Jr: The anterior impingement syndrome of the ankle. J Trauma 20:895–898, 1980.

213. Paulos LE, Johnson CL, Noyes FR: Posterior compartment fractures of the ankle—a commonly missed athletic injury. Am J Sports Med 11:439–443, 1983.

214. Peacock EE: Wound Repair, 3rd ed. Philadelphia, WB Saunders, 1984, pp 263–331.

215. Pedowitz WJ, Kavatis P: Flatfoot in the adult. J Am Acad Orthop Surg 3:293–302, 1995.

216. Perlman M, Leveille D, DeLeonibus J, et al: Inversion lateral ankle trauma: Differential diagnosis, review of the literature and prospective study. J Foot Surg 26:95–135, 1989.

217. Plattner P, Mann R: Disorders of tendons. In Mann RA, Coughlin MJ (eds): Surgery of the Foot and Ankle, vol 2, 6th ed. St. Louis, Mosby-Year Book, 1993, pp 805–835.

218. Plattner PF, Johnson KA: Tendons and bursae. In Helal B, Wilson D (eds): The Foot. New York, Churchill Livingstone, 1988, pp 581–613.

219. Prather JL, Nusynitz ML, Snawdy HA, et al: Scintigraphic findings in stress fractures. J Bone Joint Surg Am 59:869–874, 1977.

220. Prins JG: Diagnosis and treatment of injury to the lateral ligament of the ankle. A comparative clinical study. Acta Chir Scand Suppl 486:1–149, 1978.

221. Puddu G, Ippolito E, Postacclini F: A classification of Achilles tendon disease. Am J Sports Med 4:145–150, 1976.

222. Radin EL, Eyre D, Kelman JL, Schiller AL: Effect of prolonged walking on concrete on the joints of sheep. Arthritis Rheum 22:649, 1980.

223. Radin EL, Orr RB, Kelman JL, et al: Effect of prolonged walking on concrete on the knees of sheep. J Biomech 15:487–492, 1982.

224. Rasmussen O: Stability of the ankle joint. Analysis of the function and traumatology of the ankle ligaments. Acta Orthop Scand Suppl 211:1–75, 1985.

225. Renstrom P, Theis M: Biomechanics and function of ankle ligaments: Experimental results and clinical application. J Gen Orthop Trauma 7:29–35, 1993.

226. Renstrom P, Wertz M, Incavo S, et al: Strain in the lateral ligaments of the ankle. Foot Ankle 9:59–63, 1988.

227. Renstrom PAFH, Kannus P: Injuries to the foot and ankle. In DeLee JC, Drez D Jr. (eds): Orthopaedics

228. Richardson EG: Injuries to the hallucal sesamoids in the athlete. Foot Ankle 7:229–244, 1987.

229. Roden S, Tillegard P, Unander-Scharin L: Osteochondritis dissecans and similar lesions of the talus: A report of fifty-five cases with special reference to etiology and treatment. Acta Orthop Scand 23:51–66, 1954.

230. Rosen PR, Micheli LJ, Treres S: Early scintigraphic diagnosis of bone stress and fractures in athletic adolescents. Pediatrics 70:11–15, 1982.

231. Rosenberg S, Cheung Y, Jahss J, et al: Rupture of the posterior tibial tendon. CT and MRI imaging with surgical correlation. Radiology 169:229–235, 1988.

232. Rubin G, Witten M: The talar-tilt ankle and the fibular collateral ligaments: A method for the determination of talar-tilt. J Bone Joint Surg 42:311–326, 1960.

233. Rupani HD, Holder LW, Espinola DA, et al: Three phase radionuclide bone imaging in sports medicine. Radiology 156:187–196, 1985.

234. Ryan JB, Hopkinson WJ, Wheeler JH, et al: Office management of the acute ankle sprain. Clin Sports Med 8:477–495, 1989.

235. Sands A, Grujic L, Sangeorzan B, Hansen JT: Lateral column lengthening through the calcaneocuboid joint. An alternative to triple arthrodesis for correction of flatfoot. Proceedings of the 25th Annual Meeting of the American Orthopaedic Society Foot and Ankle Day, Orlando, FL, February 19, 1995.

236. Sammarco GJ, Diraimondo CV: Surgical treatment of lateral ankle instability syndrome. Am J Sports Med 16:501–511, 1988.

237. Saunders AJ, El Sayed TF, Hilsen AJ, et al: Stress lesions of the lower leg and foot. Clin Radiol 30:649–651, 1979.

238. Schepsis AA, Leach RE: Surgical management of Achilles tendinitis. Am J Sports Med 15:308–315, 1987.

239. Schwellnus MP, Jordaan G, Naokes JD: Prevention of common overuse injuries by the use of shock absorbing insoles. A prospective study. Am J Sports Med 18:636–641, 1990.

240. Sclafani SJA: Ligamentous injury to the lower tibiotalar syndesmosis: Radiographic evidence. Radiology 156:21–27, 1985.

241. Scott S, Winter D: Internal forces at chronic running injury sites. Med Sci Sports Exec 22:357–69, 1990.

242. Scranton PE, McMaster JH, Kelly E: Dynamic fibular function. Clin Orthop 118:76–81, 1976.

243. Sedlin ED: A device for stress inversion or eversion roentgenograms of the ankle. J Bone Joint Surg Am 42:1184, 1960.

244. Segesser B, Pforringer W: The Shoe In Sport. Chicago, Year Book, 1989.

245. Seligson D, Gassman J, Pope M: Ankle instability: Evaluation of the lateral ligaments. Am J Sports Med 8:39–42, 1980.

246. Sharon SM, Knudsen HA, Gastwirth CM: Post traumatic recurrent subluxation of the tibialis posterior tendon. J Am Podiatry Assoc 68:500–502, 1978.

247. Shelbourne KD, Fisher DA, Retting AC, McCarroll JR: Stress fractures of the medial malleolus. Am J Sports Med 16:60–63, 1988.

248. Skech DV: Spontaneous partial subcutaneous ruptures of the tendo Achilles: Review of the literature

Sports Medicine, vol 2. Philadelphia, WB Saunders, 1994, pp 1705–1767.

and evaluation of 16 involved tendons. Am J Sports Med 9:20–22, 1981.

249. Skinner HB, Cook SD: Fatigue failure stress of the femoral neck. A case report. Am J Sports Med 10:245–247, 1982.

250. Slocum DB, James SL: Biomechanics of running. JAMA 205:721–728, 1968.

251. Smart GW, Tauton JE, Clement DB: Achilles tendon disorders in runners—a review. Med Sci Sports Exerc 12:231–243, 1980.

252. Snook GA: Achilles tendon tenosynovitis in long distance runners. Med Sci Sports Exec 4:155–158, 1972.

253. Snook GA: Open forum discussion. Proceedings of the Trans-Pacific Meeting American Orthopaedic Society of Sports Medicine–Japanese Orthopaedic Society of Sports Medicine, Maui, HI, March 20–25, 1993.

254. Snook GA, Chrisman OD: The management of sub-calcaneal pain. Clin Orthop 82:163–168, 1972.

255. Snook GA, Chrisman OD, Wilson TC: Long term results of the Chrisman-Snook operation for reconstruction of the lateral ligaments of the ankle. J Bone Joint Surg Am 67:1–7, 1985.

256. Sobel M, Warren RF, Brourman S: Lateral ankle instability associated with dislocation of the peroneal tendons treated by the Chrisman-Snook procedure. Am J Sports Med 18:539, 1990.

257. Sommer HM, Arza D: Functional treatment of recent ruptures of the fibular ligament of the ankle. Int Orthop 13:157–160, 1989.

258. St. Pierre R, Allman F Jr, Bassett FH, et al: A review of lateral ankle ligamentous reconstruction. Foot Ankle 3:114–123, 1982.

259. St. Pierre RK, Velazco A, Fleming LL: Impingement exostoses of the talus and fibula secondary to an inversion ankle sprain. A case report. Foot Ankle 3:282–285, 1983.

260. Stanitski CL, McMaster JH, Stanton PE: On the nature of stress fractures. Am J Sports Med 6:391–396, 1978.

261. Staples OS: Result study of ruptures of lateral ligaments of the ankle. Clin Orthop 85:50–58, 1972.

262. Stiehl JB: Complex ankle fracture dislocations with syndesmosis diastasis. Orthop Rev 14:499–507, 1990.

263. Stott JRR, Autton WC, Stokes IAF: Forces under the foot. J Bone Joint Surg Br 55:335–344, 1973.

264. Stover CN, Bryan D: Traumatic dislocation of the peroneal tendons. Am J Surg 103:180, 1962.

265. Subotnick S, Sisney P: Treatment of Achilles tendinopathy in the athlete. J Am Podiatry Med Assoc 76:552–557, 1986.

266. Sullivan D, Warren RF, Pavlor H, et al: Stress frac-tures in 51 runners. Clin Orthop 187:188–192, 1984.

267. Suominen H, Kiiskinen A, Heikkinen E: Effects of physical training on metabolism of connective tissues in young mice. Acta Physiol Scand 108:17–22, 1980.

268. Tauton JE, Clement DB, Webber D: Lower extremity stress fractures in athletes. Physician Sportsmed 9:77–86, 1981.

269. Temple C: Hazards of jogging and marathon running. Br J Hosp Med 29:237–239, 1983.

270. Thompson TC, Doherty JH: Spontaneous rupture of tendon of Achilles: A new clinical diagnosis test. J Trauma 2:126–129, 1962.

271. Trevino S, Baumhauer JF: Tendon injuries of the foot and ankle. Clin Sports Med 11:727–739, 1992.

272. Tropp H: Functional instability of the ankle joint (medical dissertation no. 202). Linkoping, Linkoping University, VTT-Grafiska, 1985, pp 1–92.

273. Tropp H: Pronator muscle weakness in functional instability of the ankle joint. Int J Sports Med 7:291–294, 1986.

274. Voloshin A, Wosk J, Brull M: Force wave transmission through the human locomotion system. J Biomech Eng 103:48–50, 1981.

275. Walter SD, Hart LE, McIntosh JM, et al: The Ontario cohort study of running related injuries. Arch Intern Med 149:2561–2564, 1989.

276. Watson-Jones R: Recurrent forward dislocation of the ankle joint. J Bone Joint Surg Br 34:519, 1952.

277. Weistabl R, Stisical M, Newhold A, et al: Classifying calcaneal tendon injury according to MRI findings. J Bone Joint Surg Br 73:683–685, 1991.

278. Welsh RP, Clodman J: Clinical survey of Achilles tendinitis in athletes. Can Med Assoc J 122:193–195, 1980.

279. Werner CO: Lateral elbow pain and posterior interosseous nerve entrapment. Acta Orthop Scand Suppl 174, 1979.

280. White AA III, Johnson D, Griswold DM: Chronic ankle pain associated with the peroneus accessorius. Clin Orthop 103:53–55, 1974.

281. Wilcox JR, Moniot AL, Green JP: Bone scanning in the evaluation of exercise induced stress injuries. Radiology 123:699–703, 1977.

282. Williams JG: Achilles tendon lesions in sports. Sports Med 3:114–135, 1986.

283. Wolin I, Glassman F, Sideman F, et al: Internal derangement of the talofibular component of the ankle. Surg Gynecol Obstet 91:193, 1950.

284. Yale J: A statistical analysis of 3,657 consecutive fatigue fractures of the distal lower extremities. J Am Podiatr Assoc 66:739–748, 1976.

285. Yale J: The Lauge-Hansen classification of malleolar fractures. Acta Orthop Scand 51:181–192, 1980.

THOMAS A. PIETROCARLO

CHAPTER TWELVE

Foot Pain in Runners

The feet are one of the most common areas of injury among runners. This is predictable when one considers the myriad factors affecting a runner's feet. These include biomechanical variations, body weight, running surface, running shoes, cumulative mileage, training errors, and impact factors. However, during the past 25 years, several developments have resulted in a reduction in running injuries of the feet.

Better running shoes have enhanced shock absorption and diminished the risk of overuse and impact-related injuries. Running shoes also tend to have improved stability in the heels because of the use of deeper extended heel counters and dual-density midsoles. This design has created greater stability for pronation-prone runners, thus reducing the incidence of biomechanical-related injuries. We also do not encounter as many extremely long-distance runners as we used to. Knowledge of the benefits of cross-training has resulted in a philosophy of quality miles, not quantity. Runners thus have been able to extend their running careers while suffering fewer lower extremity injuries.

FOOT BIOMECHANICS IN RUNNING

Running is a complex series of interactions involving the feet and lower extremities, with contributions from the trunk and upper body as well. A detailed understanding of the linked biomechanical components of running allows for successful diagnosis and treatment of running-related injuries and, ideally, prevention of problems before they occur.[21]

The gait cycle begins with heel strike and ends with heel strike of the same foot. The stride thus consists of two steps. The gait cycle is further divided into a stance phase and a swing phase. As the speed of gait increases (running), the stance phase decreases and swing phase increases. As the speed of gait continues to increase, both feet are simultaneously off the ground at a point called the nonsupport or float phase. As the speed of running increases, the stance phase decreases, swing phase increases, and float phase increases (Fig. 12–1).[3]

At foot strike, initial contact is made with the lateral aspect of the heel. Heel contact occurs mainly in distance runners. Short-distance runners such as sprinters often contact the ground at midfoot or forefoot.

At heel contact, the foot should be in a supinated position (foot in plantar flexion, adduction, and inversion), with the tibia externally rotated. At the midstance phase of gait, the tibia rotates internally, resulting in

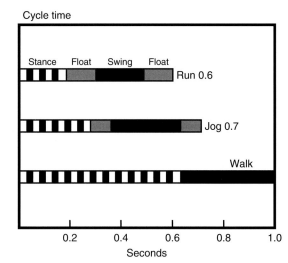

Figure 12–1

As the speed of gait increases, there is a period of time in which both feet are off the ground. This phase is known as the float phase. (From Bateman JE, Trott A: The Foot and Ankle. New York, Thieme-Stratton, 1980.)

eversion of the heel, pronation of the subtalar joint, and unlocking of the midtarsal joint. Pronation (foot in dorsiflexion, eversion, and abduction) is essential for adaption to surface terrain and for shock absorption. An analysis of ground reactive forces in running as com- pared with walking demonstrates the increase in ground reaction force in running. The magnitude of the vertical force in walking rarely exceeds 115% to 120% of body weight, whereas during running and jogging it approaches 275% of body weight (Fig. 12–2).[3]

Figure 12–2

Vertical forces in walking, jogging, and running. (From Mann R, Baxter DE, Lutter LD: Running symposium. Foot Ankle 1(4): 193, 1981.)

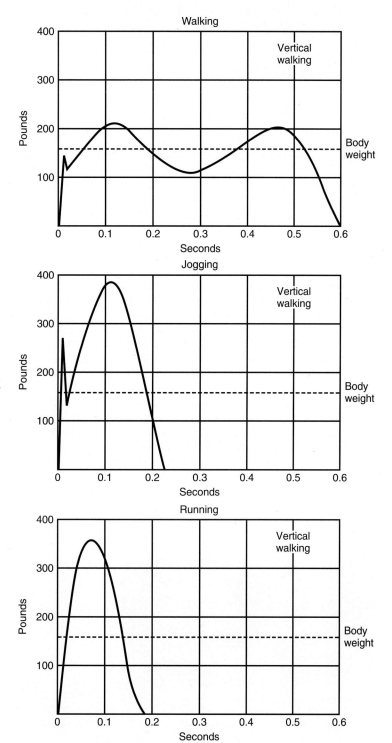

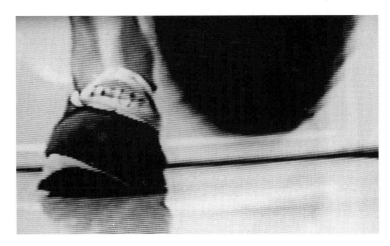

Figure 12–3

Pronation during the midstance phase of the gait.

Pronation continues for approximately 70% of the weight-bearing phase, with maximum pronation at about 40% of the support phase of gait. It is important to realize that pronation is a natural and necessary component in gait. The problem arises with excessive or prolonged pronation during the stance phase, resulting in increased forces being applied to the supporting structures of the foot and leg by requiring additional effort of the intrinsic and extrinsic muscles in an attempt to stabilize the foot during push-off (Figs. 12–3 and 12–4).[13]

Resupination of the foot occurs next as the tibia externally rotates, resulting in stabilization and locking of the midtarsal joint. The plantar aponeurosis also contributes to stability of the forefoot at toe-off. The plantar aponeurosis, which arises from the tubercle of the calcaneus, passes forward and inserts into the base of the proximal phalanges. As the toes are dorsiflexed during the latter part of the stance phase, the aponeurosis is wrapped around the metatarsal heads in a way that not only stabilizes the metatarsophalangeal

(MTP) joints but also helps to elevate the longitudinal arch (Fig. 12–5). The net result is a stable first ray for push-off.[3]

Running biomechanics can be affected by both intrinsic and extrinsic factors. Intrinsic factors stem from a runner's structure and biomechanics. Extrinsic factors negatively affecting foot biomechanics include improper footwear, training errors, an unfavorable running surface, and so on. An appreciation of these factors can help in the diagnosis of running-related injuries. For example, hyperpronation of the feet often predisposes to injury patterns that affect the medial aspect of the feet, ankles, and legs. These include posterior tibial tendinitis, plantar fasciitis, tibial stress syndrome, functional hallux limitus, and so on. Runners with cavus feet have a tendency toward shock-related injuries such as stress fractures, bursitis, and so on.[21]

Another major factor in running injuries is the repetitive stress that accompanies running. An average 150-pound individual who is walking with a step length of 2 1/2 feet for a mile, taking approximately 2210 steps, absorbs at initial ground contact (considering an impact of 80% of the body weight) a total of 253,440 pounds (127 tons), or 63 1/2 tons per foot. If the same individual were running a mile with a step length of 4 1/2 feet, taking approximately 1175 steps, he or she would absorb an initial ground contact (considering an impact of 250% of body weight) a total of 440,625 pounds (220 tons), or 110 tons per foot.[3]

No discussion of foot biomechanics in running would be complete without some discourse about orthotics and their role in the prevention and treatment of running injuries. The purpose of functional orthotics is to com-

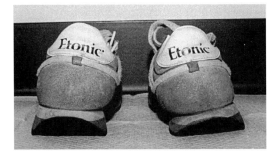

Figure 12–4

Running shoes reflecting abnormal pronation.

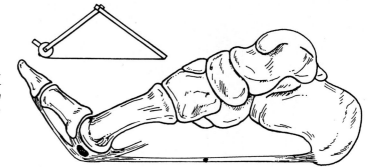

Figure 12–5

Windlass mechanism of plantar aponeurosis. (From Sgarlato TE: A Compendium of Podiatric Biomechanics. San Francisco, College of Podiatric Medicine, 1971.)

pensate for abnormal intrinsic biomechanical factors of the feet by placing the subtalar joint in a neutral position (Fig. 12–6). The neutral position allows the feet to function in a normal manner with a reduced incidence of injury. Orthotics can also be used for myriad other indications, including enhanced shock absorption, accommodation for painful lesions, leg length control, and so on.

Gross and colleagues reported that 75.5% of runners being treated for various running-related injuries including patellofemoral disorders, plantar fasciitis, Achilles tendinitis, shin splints, and miscellaneous problems attained significant improvement with the use of orthotics. Apparent satisfaction was noted, in that 90% of runners continued to use the orthotic devices even after their symptoms

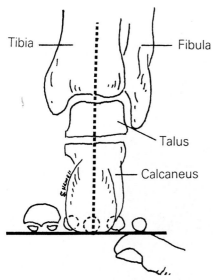

Figure 12–6

Neutral position of the subtalar joint. (From Sgarlato TE: A Compendium of Podiatric Biomechanics, San Francisco, College of Podiatric Medicine, 1971.)

resolved (Fig. 12–7).[10] The use of an appropriate orthotic with a structurally stable shoe can often minimize the risk of injury in a biomechanically compromised runner.

Orthotic devices used in our sports medicine clinic vary from rigid to semirigid to soft or accommodative types. The type of orthotic is determined by analyzing the history and chief complaint; in gait analysis; during both walking and running on a treadmill, with possible video camera analysis when indicated; in evaluation of running shoes and shoe wear pattern; in physical examination; and in biomechanical evaluation.

Rigid or semirigid orthotics are typically used for the treatment of hyperpronation-related injuries. The orthotics are inserted in a manner that positions the subtalar joint in a neutral position based on biomechanical evaluation of the lower extremities.

Orthotics can be modified with the addition of softer, shock-absorbing top covers. Once an orthotic is fabricated, it should be used in running shoes that enhance the effects of the appliance. Shoes must be constructed with a firm heel counter, adequate cushioning of the heel, and forefoot flexibility. When placing an orthotic in a running shoe, it is advisable to remove the insole of the shoe to allow for a precise fit.

Running shoes with firm heel counters result in a combination of increased shock absorption due to heel pad confinement and enhanced hindfoot stability. The latter decreases the possibility of subtalar joint mobility.[14]

Soft or accommodative orthotics are usually indicated when greater shock absorption is needed, as well as in patients with painful plantar lesions. These orthotics are usually made up of a composite of materials including leather, cork, Plastizote and Sorbothane. These orthotics allow for minimal biome-

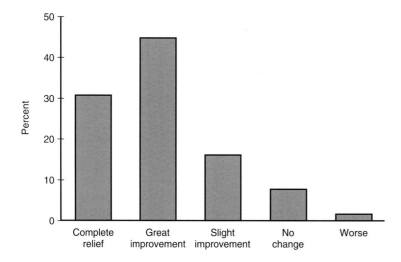

Figure 12–7

The effectiveness of orthotic shoe inserts in long-distance runners (N= 347). (From Gross ML, Davlin LB, Evanski PM: The effectiveness of orthotic shoe inserts in long-distance runners. Am J Sports Med 19:410, 1991.)

chanical correction. They can provide greater support with the addition of firmer reinforcement in the medial longitudinal arch.

DERMATOLOGIC FOOT PROBLEMS

Various skin and nail problems can occur in a runner's foot. These problems are often exacerbated by friction, shoe pressure, and irritation, as well as by heat and moisture retention in running shoes. This section deals with some of the more common disorders.

FRICTION BLISTERS

Friction blisters are a common occurrence in runners. When shearing forces are applied to the skin, a dyshesion occurs intradermally, or between the epidermal and dermal layers, causing an accumulation of fluid or blood (Fig. 12–8)[25] Various factors can contribute to blister development, including improper shoe fit, skin moisture, skin temperature, improperly fitting shoes, bony prominences, and so on.

Prompt treatment of a blister is indicated to avoid pain, inflammation, and possible infec-

Illustration: ©1992. Michael L. Ramsey

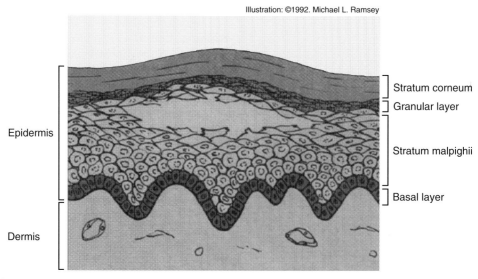

Figure 12–8

Cross section of a characteristic blister formation within the stratum malpighii. (From Ramsey ML: Managing friction blisters of the feet. Physician Sportsmed 20:118, 1992.)

tion. Treatment consists of aspiration or drainage of the fluid content of the blister. The skin should first be cleansed with a topical disinfectant. The actual puncture is made with a sterile needle or scalpel blade. When the blister is drained, the roof should be left intact to form a biologic dressing over the underlying irritated tissue. The blister can then be dressed with a topical antibiotic ointment and covered with a pad, tape, or bandage. Padding can consist of felt pads cut with appropriate apertures to accommodate the underlying blister.

Blisters are prevented by reducing friction on the feet (Table 12–1). Selecting running shoes that fit properly is imperative. Runners should also be aware of any underlying bony prominences such as bunions or hammertoes that need to be accommodated when purchasing shoes. Socks that absorb or wick away moisture are also beneficial. Newer materials such as polypropylene allow the skin to breathe while wicking away moisture. Reducing perspiration when necessary with an astringent agent such as aluminum chloride hexahydrate (Drysol) can be beneficial. Insoles that resist friction (neoprene) can be inserted in shoes. Applying petroleum jelly to friction-prone areas is inexpensive and effective. Finally, padding pressure-prone areas with moleskin or tape can be helpful.

CONTACT DERMATITIS

Contact dermatitis can occur as a result of an allergic reaction to one or more components of running shoes. This condition is quite rare. Potential allergens in shoes include the

TABLE 12–1 Tips on Preventing Blisters

Use a skin spray (Tuf Skin) to toughen the skin.
To protect the toes from excessive friction, apply an adhesive bandage or athletic tape. Be sure to remove the tape between workouts to allow the skin to breathe.
Socks must fit properly (avoid tube socks). Poorly fitting socks may roll up when damp and cause blisters.
To absorb the maximum amount of moisture, socks should contain natural fibers such as cotton and wool.
If you wear two pairs of socks, apply powder between them.
Pad areas of pinching and rubbing with moleskin.
If blisters are recurrent, apply liberal amounts of petroleum jelly to the foot before putting on your socks.
Wear shoes that fit correctly.

toe box material, tanning agents used in leather, dyes, metal eyelets, and so on. The typical eruption usually involves the dorsal aspect of the feet and toes and clinically presents with pruritus and erythema. Hyperhidrosis is a common factor that can cause leaching of the allergic material from the shoe. A shoe screening patch test is available to identify individuals who are susceptible. Treatment consists of avoiding shoes that contain allergic material and symptomatic relief with topical steroid creams.

TINEA PEDIS

Tinea pedis is one of the most common infections affecting runners' feet. A combination of moisture, darkness, and heat, all found in runners' shoes, are contributing factors. Acute tinea pedis occurs in the digital web space; the fourth web space is most commonly affected. Symptoms include pruritus, weeping, oozing, erythema, and skin maceration. Chronic cases of tinea pedis, however, often appear dry, scaly, and erythematous, with involvement of the side of the foot in a moccasin-like distribution.

The most common causative fungal organisms include *Trichophyton rubrum* and *Trichophyton mentagrophytes*. Diagnosis is typically made by examination and a skin scraping of the lesions, which is evaluated microscopically after preparation with potassium hydroxide. The fungal organisms are characterized microscopically by branching hyphae and mycelia.[17]

Treatment consists of drying the feet with a topical astringent, wearing proper socks, changing socks frequently, and applying topical antifungal medications. The most commonly used medications contain miconazole, tolnaftate, haloprogin, or clotrimazole. In persistent infections, an oral antifungal medication may be helpful. If untreated, fungal infections may become secondarily infected with bacteria.

PLANTAR WARTS

Plantar warts are common in both runners and nonrunners. It is commonly thought that excess moisture on the feet may have a contributing role. The causative organism of a wart is a papilloma virus. Although plantar

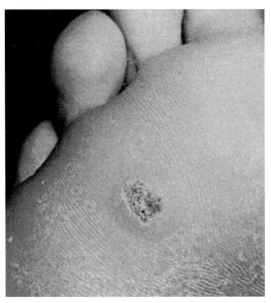

Figure 12–9

Plantar verruca.

warts are among the most common skin maladies, they are also often difficult to treat.

Recurrence is frequent, and although many therapeutic options exist, no single method is effective against all lesions.[24] Warts are sometimes difficult to diagnose because of their similarity to hyperkeratosis (Fig. 12–9). Warts, however, demonstrate small petechial hemorrhages that bleed easily on debridement. Plantar warts usually are characteristically painful when pinched at the margins, whereas a callus is usually tender to direct pressure.

Treatment for warts can vary widely and includes application of keratolytic agents with periodic debridement of the lesions, topical vesicants, antimetabolite injections (bleomycin), drying agents, liquid nitrogen, electrocautery, curettage, and carbon dioxide laser ablation. Physicians should be aware that some individuals may be unable to run because of the invasive nature of some of these treatment options. In our practice, periodic debridement combined with application of topical salicylic acid has worked well, in that athletes are able to continue running with little interruption. If a wart is resistant to treatment, curettage or ablation with a carbon dioxide laser works reasonably well. However, a certain hiatus from running is needed while the area heals. Some studies have shown that oral medications (cimetidine) may show promise in the treatment of plantar verruca.

BLACK TOENAILS

Subungual hematoma is a common finding in runners. The hallux is the most commonly affected toe, although all toes are susceptible. The hematoma is usually caused by repeated pressure and trauma associated with tight-fitting shoes, inadequate height in the toe box, or inadequate shoe length (Fig. 12–10).

The nail apparatus is a complex composition of matrix and nail plate, proximal and underlying soft tissue, cuticle, and nail bed, with underlying phalanx and ligamentous supports between the bone and the bed. The nail bed is composed of vascularized epithelium that is longitudinally ridged in parallel alignment. These ridges provide space for blood or serous fluid to accumulate after trauma. A natural separation exists between the nail plate and the matrix at the lunula, where the nail plate tightly adheres to the underlying nail bed distally.[26]

Subungual hematoma in a runner is typically an insidious problem and is not necessarily acutely painful. In acute cases associated with pain, the nail plate needs to be decompressed, draining the underlying hematoma. Decompression can be performed with a high-speed drill, sterile needle, or electrocautery. Multiple portals may be needed to drain the nail. It is not uncommon for the nail to loosen afterward and to avulse owing to separation from the nail bed. The nail typically regrows, although it may be thicker than normal.

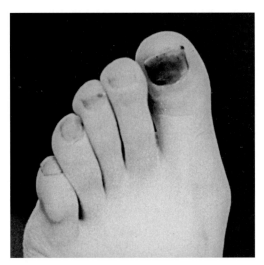

Figure 12–10

Subungual hematoma in the hallux.

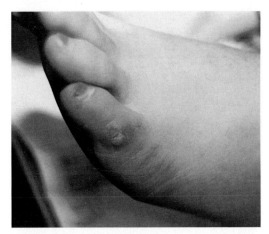

Figure 12–11

Corn (heloma durum) of the fifth toe.

CORNS

A corn is a conical wedge of keratinized tissue with the apex pointing toward the subcutaneous tissue. A corn has a central core that can be very painful (Fig. 12–11).[15]

The two types of corns are hard corns (heloma durum) and soft corns (heloma molle). Hard corns are usually present on the lateral aspect of the proximal interphalangeal (PIP) joint of the fifth toe and on the dorsal aspect of the PIP joints in the second to fourth digits. Corns found over the PIP joints are often associated with hammertoe deformities, whereas those overlying the distal interphalangeal joint or tip of the toe are typically found in mallet toes. Soft corns are most commonly encountered in the fourth web space as a result of the irritation between the head of the proximal phalanx of the fifth toe and the base of the proximal phalanx of the fourth toe. The corn remains soft owing to retained moisture in the web space.

Conservative treatment consists of debridement of the lesion with a number 15 scalpel blade or repeated abrasion with a pumice stone. Padding can be applied using various pads and appliances.

Careful selection of shoes with adequate room in the toe box is important for prevention of lesions. When corns are disabling and unresponsive to conservative measures, an arthroplasty may be indicated.

CALLUSES (HYPERKERATOSIS)

Calluses are thickening of the skin generated by excessive localized pressure either from abnormal anatomic intrinsic factors or from factors such as improperly fitting shoes.

Plantar keratosis may be diffuse (Fig. 12–12) or punctate in appearance. Diffuse lesions are typically caused by shearing forces beneath the metatarsal heads and faulty biomechanics. One of the more menacing callus problems for athletes is the intractable plantar keratosis. The lesion usually is highly painful (Figs. 12–13 and 12–14) and is localized to the area under one or more metatarsal heads.

If untreated, calluses can significantly alter a runner's gait, leading to further injury. The intractable plantar keratosis is typically caused by plantar flexion of the involved metatarsal or a prominent plantar condyle.

Conservative treatment initially consists of debridement of the lesions. In some cases, topical application of salicylic acid for 1 week can soften the lesion and permit adequate resection. Padding consisting of aperture pads, metatarsal pads, and often orthotics with accommodative extensions and pocketing for painful metatarsal heads may be helpful (Figs. 12–15 and 12–16). In resistant cases, surgery may be indicated. This involves plantar condylectomies or elevating metatarsal osteotomies.

FOREFOOT INJURIES

HALLUX VALGUS

Hallux valgus is a complex deformity consisting of lateral deviation of the proximal

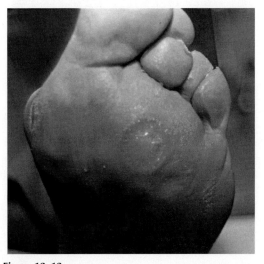

Figure 12–12

Diffuse plantar keratosis.

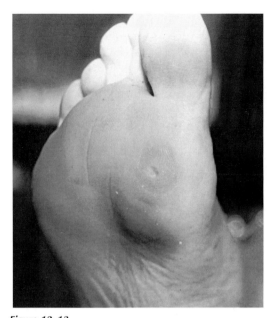

Figure 12–13

Intractable plantar keratosis of the first metatarsal head.

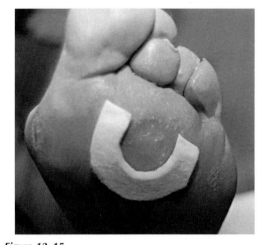

Figure 12–15

Padding for a shearing callus.

phalanx, medial deviation of the first metatarsal, and valgus rotation of the hallux.[8] Also accompanying the deformity is lateral subluxation of the sesamoid and contracture of the extensor and flexor tendons of the hallux (Fig. 12–17). Hallux valgus can be a source of irritation in runners owing to shoe irritation and impaired function of the first MTP joint.

The etiology of hallux valgus can be varied and diverse: hereditary factors, inadequate footwear (high heels, narrow toe box), pronation of the feet, or increased metatarsus primus varus are some of the more common causes.

Assessment of symptomatic hallux valgus in runners should begin with a careful physical examination. In examination of the foot, alignment in weight-bearing, range of motion of the great toe joint, palpation of the sesamoids, alignment of lesser toes, and evidence of neuritic toe pain associated with the bunion should be taken into account. Weight-bearing radiographs should be taken, with

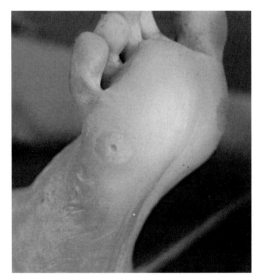

Figure 12–14

Intractable plantar keratosis of the fifth metatarsal head.

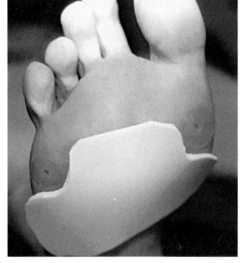

Figure 12–16

Padding for multiple intractable plantar keratoses.

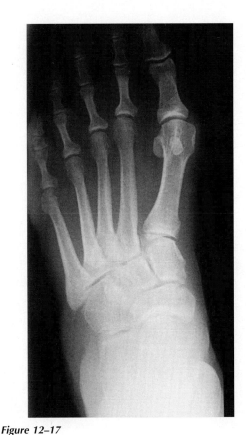

Figure 12–17

Hallux valgus deformity.

measurement and analysis of the intermetatarsal angle, hallux valgus angle, hallux interphalangeus angle, relative metatarsal protrusion, joint congruency, and sesamoid position.

Treatment for symptomatic hallux valgus in runners initially is focused on accommodating the deformity in the running shoes by selecting shoes that are adequately wide and deep in the toe box. With hyperpronation of the feet, an orthosis to balance and align the feet may be particularly effective. If conservative measures should fail to alleviate symptoms, surgery may be an option. The primary goals of bunion surgery are resection of the medial eminence of the metatarsal head, reduction of the intermetatarsal angle, establishment of a congruous joint, and realignment of the sesamoids.

The choice of surgical methods is based on physical examination findings and radiographic evaluation. If the maximal pain is located over the medial eminence and the medial aspect of the metatarsal is enlarged, resection may be all that is necessary.

If the intermetatarsal angle is elevated, but

less than 13 to 14 degrees, a chevron osteotomy is indicated and may be performed in association with a phalangeal osteotomy where indicated (Fig. 12–18). In cases in which the intermetatarsal angle exceeds 14 degrees and the joint is subluxed, a proximal osteotomy with a distal soft tissue procedure is indicated (Figs. 12–19 and 12–20). Proper postoperative rehabilitation is imperative to prevent stiffness of the first MTP joint postoperatively. Cross-training activities can begin as soon as 4 weeks postoperatively, including swimming, biking, and upper body conditioning.

HALLUX RIGIDUS

Hallux rigidus represents degenerative arthritis of the MTP joint of the great toe. It is characterized by limited range of motion of the great toe in both dorsiflexion and plantar flexion. Normal range of motion in the first MTP joint is 30 degrees of plantar flexion and 80 degrees of dorsiflexion.

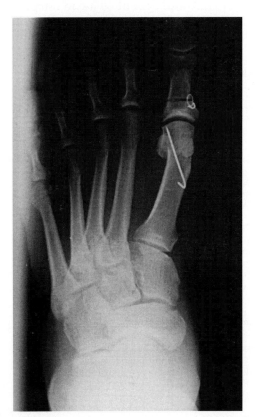

Figure 12–18

Postoperative hallux valgus correction by chevron and proximal phalanx osteotomy.

The cause of hallux rigidus has been the object of much debate. Several theories have been proposed, including an elongated first metatarsal,[5] dorsiflexion of the first metatarsal,[16] osteochondritis dissecans, avascular necrosis, systemic arthritis, trauma, and infection (Table 12–2).

Hallux rigidus presents several problems to a runner. The size of the exostoses can result in shoe rubbing and irritation from the toe box of the shoe. Stiffness of the first MTP joint may result in abnormal biomechanics, and the runner may compensate by running on the lateral border of the foot or abducting the foot to roll over the medial aspect of the hallux.

These forms of compensation may result in proximal leg pain. Initial findings on examination include but are not restricted to painful, limited range of motion of the first MTP joint. It is not uncommon to observe a hyperextension deformity of the hallux interphalangeal joint that develops as a result of compensation for lack of motion in the first MTP joint. Palpable thickening and enlargement of the joint are also present owing to osteophyte formation. Radiographic findings may show joint space narrowing, osteophyte formation,

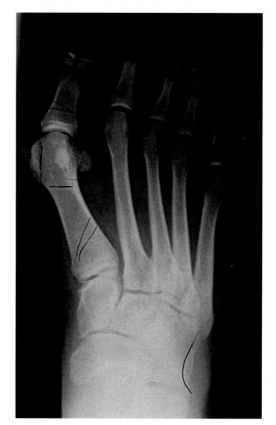

Figure 12–19

Severe hallux valgus deformity.

and loose bodies (Fig. 12–21). Secondary degenerative changes in sesamoids are not uncommon.

Conservative measures in the treatment of hallux rigidus often provide symptomatic relief but generally do not alter the natural course of the disease process. Initial steps are aimed at relieving pressure placed on the enlarged joint by poorly fitting running shoes. This may be accomplished by wearing shoes with soft uppers or shoes with adequate depth and width of the toe box to accommodate the enlarged joint. Shoe modifications include an extended steel shank with a rocker-bottom sole. Oral antiinflammatory medications may lessen symptoms, and intraarticular steroid injections can be used when oral medications are not effective. In the event that conservative measures fail, surgical intervention may be indicated.

Numerous surgical procedures have been described for the treatment of hallux rigidus. Each procedure can be classified according to the specific area of the MTP joint undergoing

TABLE 12–2 Etiology of Hallux Rigidus

Traumatic
  Osteochondral first MTP joint injury
  Intraarticular first MTP joint fracture
  Hallucal sesamoid dysfunction secondary to fracture
    of the sesamoid
  Malunion/nonunion of extraarticular first metatarsal
    fracture
  Epiphyseal injury
Anatomic/structural
  Abnormally long proximal phalanx of the hallux
  Abnormally long first metatarsal
  Elevated first metatarsal
Biomechanical
  Hypermobile first ray
  Excessive hindfoot pronation
Metabolic
  Arthritic conditions affecting the first MTP joint
  Osteochondral defects of the first MTP joint
Neuromuscular
  Extrinsic and/or intrinsic muscle imbalance affecting
    the first ray
Iatrogenic
  Excessive elevation of the first metatarsal
  Excessive lengthening of the first metatarsal
  Excessive fibrosis
  Hallucal sesamoid dysfunction
  Malalignment of the first MTP joint
  Osteochondral injury of the first MTP joint
  Septic arthritis

MTP, metatarsophalangeal.

Cheilectomy procedures are often indicated, with resection of at least one third of the dorsal aspect of the metatarsal head, any osteophytes present at the base of the proximal phalanx, and loose bodies. Implant arthroplasties and fusions should be avoided.

SESAMOID INJURIES

Sesamoid injuries in runners are not uncommon. More than 50% of body weight is transmitted through the great toe complex, including the MTP joint and the tibial and fibular sesamoids.[6] This weight, combined with the repetitive nature and increased ground reaction forces in running, can contribute to sesamoid injuries. Additional predisposing factors leading to sesamoid injuries include cavus feet with a rigid plantar-flexed first ray and hyperpronation of the foot associated with a lateral drift of the sesamoids.

The initial complaints of sesamoid pain may include tenderness and occasionally swelling directly beneath the first metatarsal head. The symptoms are made worse with dorsiflexion of the hallux and direct pressure over the sesamoids. Runners often experience pain with forceful push-off of the great toe and with toe walking.

Radiographic analysis is imperative to diagnose the cause of the sesamoid pain. Radiographs should include weight-bearing anteroposterior, lateral, oblique, and sesamoid axial views. It is not uncommon to see multiple sesamoids on radiographic examination. Ten to 33% of all feet have bipartite or multiple sesamoids.[12] In addition to routine radiographs, bone scans and computed tomography (CT) scans may be necessary to confirm a diagnosis of sesamoid injury.

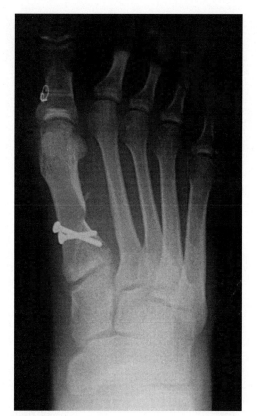

Figure 12–20

Correction of hallux valgus with base wedge osteotomy of the first metatarsal.

operation. Surgery consists of the five following categories: (1) remodeling arthroplasty, (2) resection arthroplasty, (3) arthrodesis, (4) replacement arthroplasty, and (5) periarticular osteotomy.

In runners, the goals of treatment should include increased range of motion, reduction of the size of the joint, maintenance of the length of the toe, and reduction in symptoms.

Figure 12–21

Dorsal osteophyte (arrow) associated with hallux rigidus.

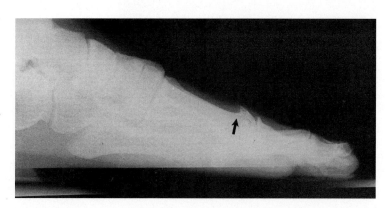

The various types of injuries to the sesamoids in runners are discussed next.

Sesamoiditis

Sesamoiditis can involve chondromalacia of the sesamoids, tendinitis of the flexor hallucis brevis tendon, or synovitis of the MTP joint. Predisposing factors often include cavus foot deformity. Treatment is aimed at reducing inflammation and accommodating the deformity with an orthotic to unweight the sesamoid apparatus.

Stress Fracture

Stress fractures account for 40% of all sesamoid injuries (Fig. 12–22). They must be differentiated from bipartite or multipartite sesamoids. Bone scans or CT scans may be helpful in differentiating the injuries. Treatment includes rest. In the event that non-union occurs, bone grafting or excision may be indicated. After excision, however, an angular deformity of the hallux may occur.

Osteochondritis

Osteochondritis can occur as the primary problem or may follow repetitive stress injury and initial stress fracture with subsequent fragmentation (Fig. 12–23). A component of this is implied avascular necrosis.[1]

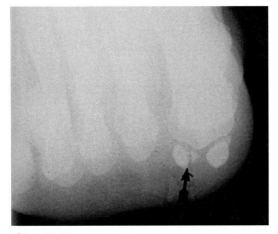

Figure 12–22

Stress fracture (arrow) of a fibular sesamoid.

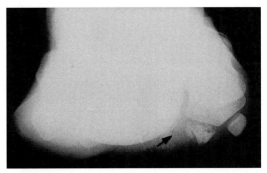

Figure 12–23

Osteochondritis (arrow) of a fibular sesamoid.

METATARSOPHALANGEAL JOINT PAIN

Lesser MTP joint pain is common in runners. Although many of the joints may be affected, the second MTP joint seems to be the most commonly injured. Various causes must be considered, including capsulitis, synovitis, degenerative arthritis, Freiberg's infraction, neuroma, synovial cyst, systemic arthritis, and stress fracture.[27] In our experience, synovitis/capsulitis is the most common condition in the forefoot.

Several factors can contribute to lesser MTP joint synovitis. Biomechanical factors such as a hypermobile first ray and a long second metatarsal result in second MTP synovitis, whereas ankle equinus and anterior ankle impingement may cause diffuse forefoot pain. Other factors may include plantar fat pad atrophy, hammertoe deformity, and plantar flexion of the metatarsal.

Physical findings associated with MTP joint synovitis can include swelling of the joint, toe pain with hyperextension, flexion of the joint, and pain with dorsal plantar manipulation of the MTP joint (drawer sign).[7] In this test, vertical subluxation of the patient's toes places pressure on the plantar capsule, eliciting pain.

Other physical findings may include hammertoe deformity associated with the synovitis, medial or lateral deviation of the toe, and possibly subluxation or dislocation of the joint. Radiographic findings may help confirm this.

Treatment is almost always conservative and generally successful. The treatment is aimed at reducing swelling and pain with ice massage and antiinflammatory medications.

Removing stress from the joint with metatarsal relief padding often incorporated into orthotics can greatly help. If the toe is dorsally subluxed, taping the toe into correct alignment can reduce the buckling effect on the metatarsal head. Shoe modifications including a firm shank with a rocker-bottom sole have been effective in chronic cases. In resistant cases, an intraarticular injection is indicated. This should be used judiciously, however, because repeated injections may be destructive to the ligamentous capsular support of the joint.[18] Surgery, if necessary, may consist of synovectomy and possibly metatarsal osteotomy, although it is rarely indicated.

MORTON'S NEUROMA

A neuroma represents an entrapment of the common digital nerve at the point of bifurcation into the proper digital nerve. The most common site of involvement is the third metatarsal interspace and, to a lesser extent, the second interspace (Fig. 12–24). The nerve becomes entrapped between the adjacent metatarsal heads and the transverse metatarsal ligament. Forefoot loading with intermeta-

tarsal stress leads to chronic inflammation and perineural fibrosis.

An affected runner often experiences symptoms such as pain, burning, paresthesias, and numbness in the adjacent toes. The symptoms are often improved by removing the shoe and massaging the foot. The runner may also notice a clicking in the forefoot when walking and running.

The symptoms of Morton's neuroma can usually be re-created by compressing the forefoot laterally while pressing upward in the involved interspace with the thumb of the opposite hand. This often produces a palpable click with referred pain to the adjacent toes (Mulder's sign) (Fig. 12–25). If the diagnosis of neuroma is in question, blocking the interspace with a local anesthetic and having the patient wear the shoes that exacerbate the symptoms may be revealing.[8] Initial treatment consists of wearing running shoes that are wide enough to avoid compressing the forefoot. An orthosis with metatarsal padding may aid in decompressing the nerves by causing metatarsal splaying.

Injecting the nerve with a mixture of local anesthetic and steroid may afford long-term relief. If conservative measures fail, resection of the neuroma is indicated. Recurrence or

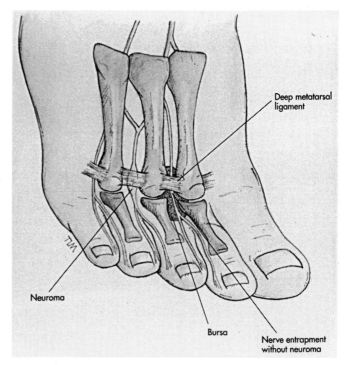

Figure 12–24

Anatomy of intermetatarsal nerve entrapment. (From Baxter DE: The Foot and Ankle in Sport. St. Louis, CV Mosby, 1995.)

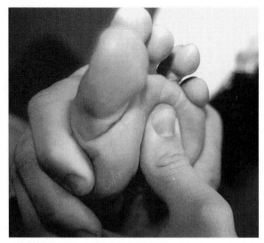

Figure 12–25

Eliciting Mulder's sign.

stump neuroma formation is a possibility, although the success rate is usually quite high.

STRESS FRACTURES

The most common areas for the occurrence of stress fractures in runners are the feet and ankles. A stress fracture is defined as a partial or complete fracture of bone due to its inability to withstand nonvisible stress applied in a rhythmic, repeated, subthreshold manner. Stress fracture remains the appropriate diagnostic term for performance-affecting bone pain secondary to repetitive stress with positive signs on bone imaging of any type.[20] Almost any of the bones in the foot may be subject to stress fractures (Table 12–3).

The original description of the injury is generally attributed to a Prussian military physi-

cian named Breithaupt, who described the clinical signs and symptoms and the time course in development of a stress fracture of a metatarsal. This was commonly known as a march fracture or Deutschlander fracture after radiographs some 40 years later revealed the bony changes.[19]

When considering the pathogenesis of stress fractures, it should be remembered that bone is a heterogeneous, anisotropic, living tissue that requires stress for normal remodeling and function. Bone is continuously remodeling to adapt to the biomechanical environment. When excessive stresses are applied, such as in running, the remodeling process is accelerated to maintain the integrity and function of the osseous system. If the remodeling process lags behind, the disruptive effects of repetitive stress lead to a stress fracture. Thus, stress fractures are a result of a dynamic process, not a single occurrence such as an acute fracture.[22]

The diagnosis of stress fractures includes a detailed history with emphasis on any change in the runner's normal training program related to mileage, shoes, surface terrain, and so on. Physical findings include localized tenderness, swelling, elevation of temperature, and sensitivity to vibratory sensation. Radiographic findings for the first 1 to 2 weeks after the onset of symptoms are often negative. After 2 weeks, stress fractures may demonstrate periosteal new bone formation or an actual cortical break (Fig. 12–26). After 4 weeks, frank callus formation may appear. Stress fractures of cancellous bone such as the calcaneus typically present radiographically as localized areas of increased density. This appearance is due to the combination of trabecular microfractures along lines perpendicular to the offending stress and new bone deposition along fractured trabeculae (Fig. 12–27). These findings may not be present until 2 to 4 weeks after the onset of symptoms.[22]

If clinical findings are suggestive of stress fracture but results of conventional radiographs are negative, bone scanning with the radionuclide technetium 99m diposphonate, either three phase or single phase, can provide diagnosis as early as 2 to 8 days after the onset of symptoms (Figs. 12–28 and 12–29). It is important to remember that bone scanning cannot distinguish fractures from other processes such as infection or neoplasm.

Treatment consists of relative rest. Most stress fractures of the foot heal in 4 to 6

TABLE 12–3 Stress Fractures of the Foot and Ankle in Runners (Percentage)

Metatarsals		55
First	37	
Second	25	
Third	19	
Fourth	2	
Fifth	6	
Lateral malleolus		30
Medial malleolus		9
Os calcis		4
Talus		<1
Navicular		2
Sesamoid		<1

From Grama WA, Kalenak A: Clin Sports Med, p 448, 1991.

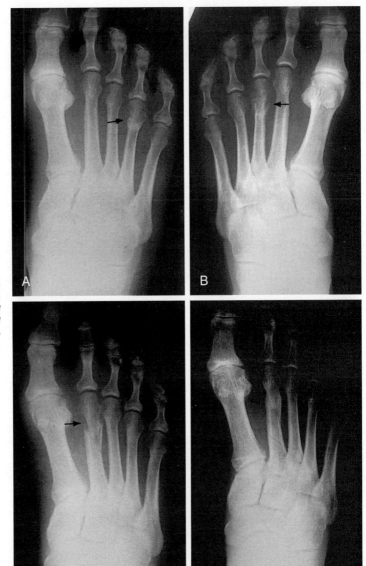

Figure 12–26

Series of repetitive stress fractures involving the second, third, and fourth metatarsals during a 3-year period in a 45-year-old marathon runner. Note the comminuted fracture of the second metatarsal due to running after the stress fracture occurred.

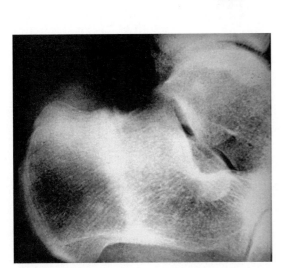

Figure 12–27

Stress fracture of the calcaneus.

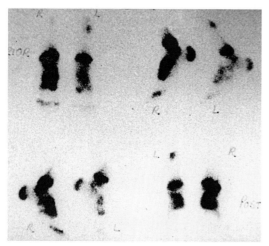

Figure 12–28

Positive bone scan of a navicular stress fracture in a runner.

weeks. During the healing period, it is important to keep the runner involved in some form of low-impact cross-training activities. These can include swimming, running in the deep end of a pool with a wet vest, biking, upper body conditioning, and so on.

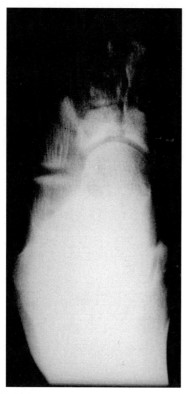

Figure 12–29

Tomogram confirming stress fracture of navicular.

HINDFOOT INJURIES

HEEL PAIN

Inferior heel pain is one of the most common complaints in runners treated at our sports medicine clinic. The multitude of causes includes but is not limited to

- Heel pain syndrome
- Plantar fasciitis
- Fat pad atrophy
- Plantar fascia rupture
- Tarsal tunnel syndrome
- Lateral plantar nerve entrapment
- Stress fracture
- Tumors
- Seronegative arthritis

In order to make an accurate diagnosis, a thorough medical history and examination need to be performed, with particular attention to exact localization of the heel pain (Fig. 12–30).

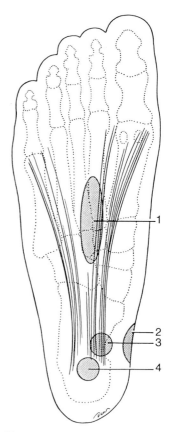

Figure 12–30

Local causes of plantar heel pain. 1, Plantar fasciitis; 2, lateral plantar nerve compression; 3, heel pain syndrome; 4, fat pad atrophy. (From Pfeffer G: Plantar heel pain. In Baxter D [ed]: The Foot and Ankle in Sports. St. Louis, Mosby-Year Book, 1995, p 196.)

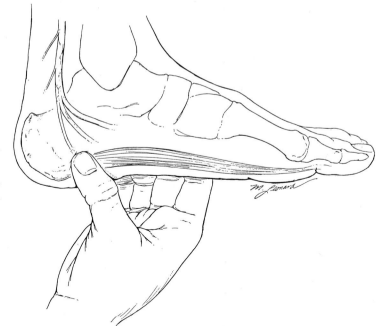

Figure 12–31

Site of maximum tenderness in plantar fasciitis/heel spur syndrome. (From Shor L: Plantar fasciitis. In Myerson M [ed]: Current Therapy in Foot and Ankle Surgery. St. Louis, Mosby-Year Book, 1993, p 178.)

Heel Pain Syndrome

Heel pain syndrome is the most common cause of inferior heel pain in runners. The classic symptoms are pain in the heel on rising in the morning and bearing weight on the heel or after sitting for long periods. The pain and stiffness typically improve with activity, but after prolonged activity the pain returns. The maximum amount of pain is usually present on the medial aspect of the calcaneus at the insertion of the plantar fascia and intrinsic muscles (Fig. 12–31). Radiographic evaluation of the heel may or may not demonstrate a spur. Aside from localized tenderness over the plantar medial aspects of the calcaneus, biomechanical evaluation often shows tightness of the Achilles tendon and either hyperpronated or cavus foot deformity.

Heel pain syndrome is a condition that is to be treated conservatively. Initial treatment consists of reduced running, ice massage, plantar fascia and Achilles stretching, antiinflammatory medication, strapping of the foot, and often some type of biomechanical support of the foot.

This may initially consist of an over-the-counter arch support or, when indicated, a custom-made orthotic. Physical therapy, modalities, and night splints can be helpful; in resistant cases, a steroid injection at the insertion of the fascia may be needed. Conserva-

tive measures are generally successful in 95% of cases and should be used for 6 to 12 months. Surgical intervention is reserved for recalcitrant cases and for when all other possible causes of the heel pain have been investigated and ruled out.

Fat Pad Atrophy

Fat pad atrophy is typically encountered in runners older than 40 years. The result of atrophy is a loss of shock absorption in the heel. The pain is more diffuse and is felt over the central portion of the heel. The plantar tuberosity of the heel is easily palpable. Treatment typically consists of wearing shock-absorbing running shoes with a heel cup or viscoelastic heel pad.

Plantar Fasciitis

Plantar fasciitis typically occurs over the midportion of the plantar fascia and is usually exacerbated by dorsiflexion of the toes and direct pressure over the fascia. This must be differentiated from tendinitis of the flexor hallucis longus tendon. The tendon is typically aggravated with resistance to plantar flexion of the hallux. Differential diagnosis must also include a partially torn plantar fascia, in which a gap in the tendon is often palpable.

Once again, conservative treatment con-

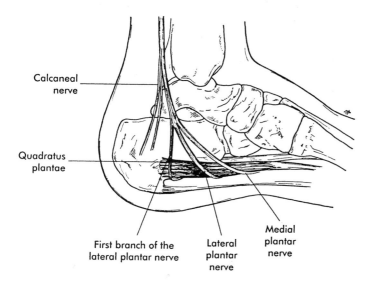

Figure 12–32

Entrapment of the first branch of the lateral plantar nerve of the medial aspect of the heel. (From Pfeffer G: Plantar heel pain. In Baxter D [ed]: The Foot and Ankle in Sports. St. Louis, Mosby-Year Book, 1995, p 196.)

sisting of ice, massage, physical therapy, anti-inflammatory drugs, and so on is indicated. Orthotic treatment is typically indicated for the long term.

Entrapment of the First Branch of the Lateral Plantar Nerve

One of the most commonly overlooked causes of chronic heel pain in athletes is entrapment of the first branch of the lateral plantar nerve (Fig. 12–32).[4] The first branch innervates the periosteum of the medial calcaneal tuberosity, the long plantar ligament, the abductor digiti quinti, and the flexor brevis muscles. The exact site of entrapment usually is between the deep fascia of the abductor hallucis muscle and the medial caudal margin

of the medial head of the quadratus plantae muscle. The usual symptom of entrapment is maximum tenderness at this site.

Treatment consists of rest, oral antiinflammatory medications, ice massage, physical therapy, steroid injections, and orthotics. If conservative treatment fails, surgical release of the entrapped nerve is indicated.

POSTERIOR HEEL PAIN—HAGLUND DEFORMITY

An abnormal prominence of the postero-superior aspect of the heel is referred to as a Haglund deformity. The deformity was originally described by Haglund in 1928 (Figs. 12–33 and 12–34).[11]

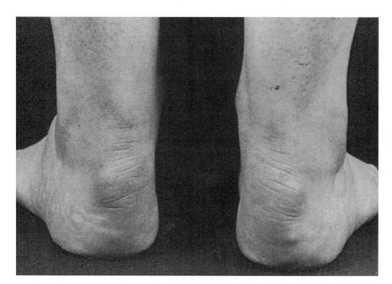

Figure 12–33

Clinical appearance of Haglund's deformity.

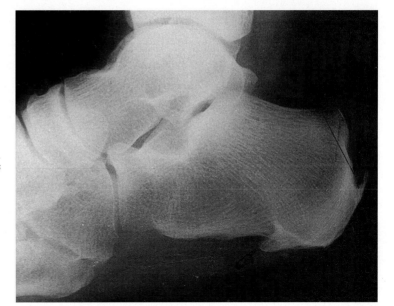

Figure 12–34

Radiographic appearance of Haglund's deformity.

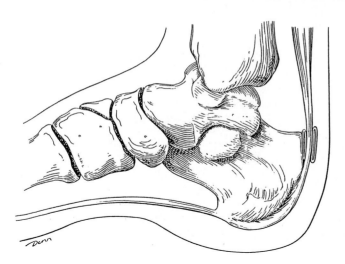

Figure 12–35

Retrocalcaneal and superficial bursae associated with Haglund's deformity. (From Frey C: Surgical management of Haglund's deformity. In Myerson M [ed]: Current Therapy in Foot and Ankle Surgery. St. Louis, Mosby-Year Book, 1993, p 166.)

Figure 12–36

Bone resection in Haglund's deformity. (From Frey C: Surgical management of Haglund's deformity. In Myerson M [ed]: Current Therapy in Foot and Ankle Surgery. St. Louis, Mosby-Year Book, 1993, p 166.)

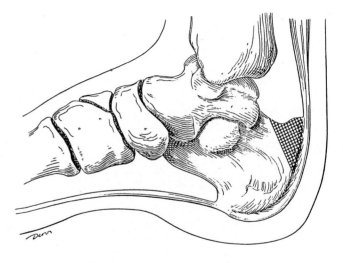

The symptoms of the Haglund deformity are typically brought about by friction and pressure from the heel counter of the running shoe and are exacerbated by medial and lateral shearing due to hypermobility of the heel during the stance phase of running. The hyperconvexity of the heel may cause irritation of the overlying distal Achilles tendon as well as the retrocalcaneal and superficial bursa (Fig. 12–35).

Initial treatment for the Haglund deformity is aimed at reducing the inflammation with ice, antiinflammatory medications, physical therapy, and padding of the heel counter of the shoe. A heel cup or heel lift may alter the pitch of the heel to reduce irritation. Steroid injections where bursitis is present should be avoided owing to proximity of the Achilles tendon. When all conservative measures fail, surgical treatment may be indicated. Surgical treatment consists of resection of the superior portion of the calcaneus, with preservation of the Achilles tendon insertion (Fig. 12–36). Removal of a chronically inflamed or fibrotic bursa can be performed simultaneously.

INSERTIONAL ACHILLES TENDINITIS

Achilles tendinitis with necrosis within the distal Achilles tendon or calcification within the distal Achilles tendon is a common cause of posterior heel pain. Not uncommon is an underlying Haglund deformity exacerbating the symptoms.

The pain associated with this condition is directly over the insertion of the tendon. In cases of insertional calcification, an enlargement of the heel may be present. Conservative treatment consists of Achilles stretching, heel lift, ice massage, and physical therapy. In recalcitrant cases, surgical intervention may be indicated. Surgery consists of splitting the Achilles tendon posteriorly with resection of the underlying calcification and debridement of the necrotic tendon. Resection of a concomitant Haglund deformity can be performed at the same time.

REFERENCES

1. Anderson RB, McBryde AM: Sesamoid foot problems in the athlete. Clin Sports Med 7:51, 1988.
2. Baxter DE: The heel in sports. Clin Sports Med 13:683, 1994.
3. Baxter DE, Mann RA: Running symposium. Foot Ankle 1:191, 1981.
4. Baxter DE, Pfeffer GB: Treatment of chronic heel pain by surgical release of the first branch of the lateral plantar nerve. Clin Orthop 279:229, 1992.
5. Bonney G, McNab I: Hallux valgus and hallux rigidus: A critical survey of operative results. J Bone Joint Surg Br 34:366–385, 1952.
6. Coughlin MJ: Arthrodesis of the first metatarsophalangeal joint as salvage for failed Keller bunionectomy procedure. J Bone Joint Surg Am 69:68–75, 1987.
7. Coughlin MJ: Second metatarsophalangeal joint instability in the athlete. Foot Ankle 14:309–319, 1993.
8. Frymeyer JW (ed): Orthopedic Knowledge Update—4. American Academy of Orthopedic Surgeons, 1993, pp 645–648.
9. Geiringer SR: Biomechanics of the running foot. Biomechanics Nov–Dec:37–40, 1995.
10. Gross ML, Davlin LB, Evanski PM: Effectiveness of the orthotic shoe inserts in the long distance runner. Am J Sports Med 19:409–412, 1991.
11. Haglund P, Beitrag ZW: Klinikder Achillessehre. Aschr Orthop Chir 49:49–58, 1928.
12. Hamilton WG: Surgical anatomy of the foot and ankle. Clin Symp 37(1), 1985.
13. James SL, Jones DC: Biomechanical aspects of distance running. JAMA 221:1014–1016, 1972.
14. Jorgenson U: Body load in heel strike running: the effect of firm heel counter. Am J Sports Med 18:178, 1990.
15. Katchis SD, Hershum EB: Broken nails to blistered heels. Physician Sports Med 21:101, 1993.
16. Kelikian H: Hallux Valgus, Allied Deformities of the Forefoot, and Metatarsalgia. Philadelphia, WB Saunders, 1965.
17. Lillich JS: Dermatologic infections and nail disorders. In Baxter DE (ed): The Foot and Ankle in Sports. St. Louis, CV Mosby, 1995, p 133.
18. Mann RA, Mizel MA: Monoarticular non-traumatic synovitis of the metatarsophalangeal joint: A new diagnosis? Foot Ankle 6:18–21, 1985.
19. Markley KL: Stress fractures. Clin Sports Med 6:405, 1987.
20. McBryde AM: Stress fractures. In Baxter DE (ed): Foot and Ankle in Sports. St. Louis, CV Mosby, 1995.
21. McKenzie DC, Clement DB, Taunton JE: Running shoes, orthotics and injury. Am J Sports Med 2:334, 1985.
22. Myer SA, Saltzman CL, Albright JF: Stress fracture of the foot and leg. Clin Sports Med 12:395, 1993.
23. Omara EF, Rye B: Dermatologic disorders of the foot. Clin Sports Med, 835, 1994.
24. Ramsey ML: Plantar warts. Physician Sportsmed 20:69, 1992.
25. Ramsey ML: Managing friction blisters of the feet. Physician Sportsmed 20:118, 1992.
26. Scioli MN: Managing toenail trauma. Physician Sportsmed 20:108, 1992.
27. Sobel M: Simplifying the approach to metatarsalgia. J Musculoskel Med 10:76, 1993.

CARL FOSTER ■ MANFRED LEHMANN

CHAPTER THIRTEEN

Overtraining Syndrome

Frank Shorter's achievements in the early and middle 1970s represent every runner's secret fantasy: Graduate from prestigious Ivy Leage college as a "promising" runner; train exceptionally hard just at the very end of your collegiate career, and run above expectations at the nationals; move to Florida (later Colorado) as a full-time athlete; train rigorously (reportedly in the range of 200 km per week with the additional stress of living and training in the heat or at high altitude) during the buildup for the 1972 Olympics; become the "top gun"; win a spot on the Olympic team; win gold at the Olympics (not to mention fifth place in the 10 km); repeat 4 years later with silver at the Olympics; "retire" to fame and fortune as an attorney, clothing manufacturer, commentator, celebrity, age group runner, and so on. Hollywood couldn't write a better script.

Frank Shorter blossomed under the rigors of hard training. The story could just as easily have been otherwise, as it was for Frank's competitor Dr. Ron Hill of Great Britian. As well documented by Tim Noakes,[44] Hill was the dominant international long-distance runner of the late 1960s and early 1970s. He was very much the pre-race favorite in Munich. Hill was also famous for his dedication to training. In preparation for major championships, including the 1972 Olympiad, Hill increased his already substantial training into the range of 180 to 200 km per week. Hill was also extraordinarily consistent in his training, reportedly having a streak of approximately 10 years without missing a single day of running. Unfortunately, Hill often failed to live up to expectations in major championships. If one uses Hill's training loads as reported by Noakes and plots race results during the period of nearly a decade in relation to training load, a region of best performance is noted in the range of 150 to 170 km per week (Fig. 13–1), with his third best race after "only" 115 km per week. How is it that one runner can flourish under very hard training while another fails?

The fact is that serious athletic training represents a risk—a risk of pushing a talented body to the furthest limits of its ability to absorb stress in hopes of achieving that last bit of improvement that separates the champion from the also-ran. The margin of victory is very small. An analysis of speed-skating performances at the 1988 Calgary Olympiad (indoor venue with consistent ideal weather and ice conditions)[49] demonstrates that the difference in average velocity between all the gold and all the silver medal performances was 0.3%. The difference in all the gold and all the fourth-place performances was 1.3%. Assuming the mathematic risk of translating these percentage differences from speed skating to marathon running, one might expect 24 seconds between gold and silver and 1:45 between gold and fourth place. These are, in fact, very realistic competitive margins and demonstrate the small margin between success and failure at the highest competitive levels. Is it any wonder that athletes and their coaches feel compelled to risk total failure in an attempt to ensure that they are adequately prepared for major competitions? Many of the chapters of this text describe the various mechanical factors that can affect hips, knees, ankles, and feet subjected to continuing high levels of stress—the orthopedic overuse injuries. This chapter discusses the overtraining syndrome, a less discrete but no less formidable obstacle to success in the athletically motivated, the factor that possibly separated Frank Shorter from Ron Hill.

THE TRAINING RESPONSE

The nature of the training response is defined by the legend of the farm boy who lifted

173

Ron Hill Training Load vs Performance

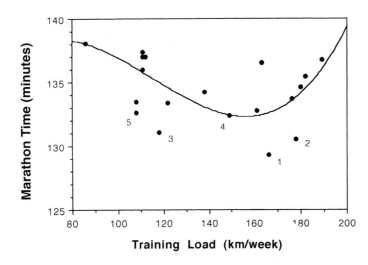

Figure 13–1

Relationship of reported training load (km/week) to marathon racing performance over a period of several years in the British marathon runner Dr. Ron Hill.[42] Note that the best-fit relationship suggests that optimal performance occurs in the range of 160 km/week. The numerals on the figure indicate the first through fifth best performances for Dr. Hill. Of particular interest is the progressively slower performances observed as the training load exceeds 180 km/week. (Adapted by permission from T. Noakes, 1991, Lore of Running, *3rd ed. [Champaign, IL: Human Kinetics Publishers], 298–299.)*

a young calf. The next day he lifted the same (now marginally larger) calf, and the next day, and the next day, and the next day until he was a legendary strongman capable of lifting a fully grown bull. We adapt to stresses. This phenomenon is described in quantitative terms by a model proposed by Banister and colleagues in Canada.[12, 38] At the end of each training session, the momentary performance capacity of an athlete has actually decreased because fatigue accumulated during the session is larger than the momentary gain in fitness. By the time of the next training session (assuming enough time has elapsed to allow full recovery), the performance capacity is slightly greater because the gain in fitness is now larger than the fatigue remaining from the training session. In most contemporary athletes (many of whom are training twice daily), full recovery often does not occur before the next training session. Because full recovery from a heavy training session may require 48 hours or more,[19, 53, 54] it seems reasonable to assume that most serious contemporary athletes are inadequately recovered most of the time. Accordingly, although fitness continues to increase incrementally, performance may remain depressed from pretraining levels if the magnitude of fatigue resulting from training remains above the accrued fitness. Thus, at any given time, the momentary performance capacity of an athlete is the summated product of the athlete's intrinsic performance capacity, modified by the accumulated fitness and fatigue resulting from training.

During ordinary training, coaches and athletes choose a training load that keeps fatigue at only moderate levels, allowing performance to improve slowly as fitness increases. However, it is a widely held belief that occasional periods of very severe training (sufficient to depress performance capacity significantly) may result in larger ultimate levels of performance when the training load is eventually reduced. This practice is referred to as *overreaching* (Fig. 13–2). Overreaching is typically carried out for periods ranging from a few days to a couple of weeks. In fact, most contemporary athletes train using cycles of deliberate overreaching interspersed with regeneration cycles (Fig. 13–3). The steady progression of record performances, and particularly the increased depth of performances at a very high level, testifies to the general effectiveness of this pattern of training, which is usually referred to as *periodization*. However, the limited experimental data that address this issue do not generally support the need for overreaching.[7]

If overreaching is too profound, is continued for too long, or is coupled with too many other stresses, an athlete's performance may fail to recover when the training load is reduced. Even if the regeneration cycle is extended, performance may fail to return to expected levels. Given the time urgency of athletic competition, failure to perform well at the time you expect to perform well can destroy a season. The necessity of performing well on a specified date certainly is stressful, and the instincts of coaches and athletes often

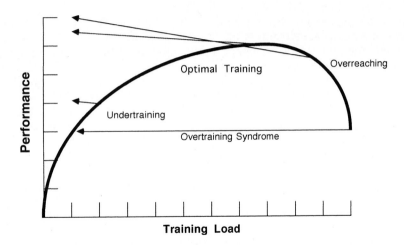

Figure 13–2

Schematic response of performance to changes in training load. In a general sense, performance improves as training load is increased, up to the point of optimal training. At heavier training loads, overreaching, performance may be expected to deteriorate. At any given training load, a small improvement in performance may be expected for a short time after a decrease in training load. The best performances are probably obtained with reduced training after mild overreaching. However, if the magnitude of overreaching is too large or is continued too long, performance fails to improve with reduction in training, overtraining syndrome.

act to make the situation worse. The instinctive response of most coaches and athletes to "competitive incompetence" is to assert that they are "out of shape" and to train harder. Thus, a seriously overreached athlete tends to be given exactly the wrong therapy—more

training. We believe that this inappropriate response to either accidental or deliberate overreaching is central to many, if not most, cases of overtraining syndrome.

If a broad definition of overtraining syndrome is accepted, overtraining syndrome

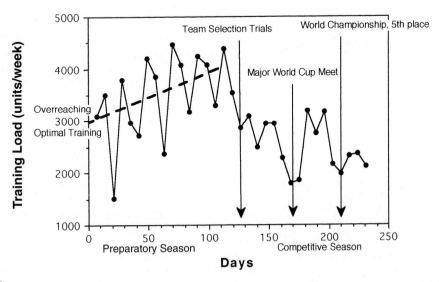

Figure 13–3

Schematic yearlong training periodization scheme in an elite athlete (fifth place in World Championship). Note that during the preparatory season, 2 weeks of overreaching (above the dashed diagonal line, representing the athlete's estimated adaptive ability) are followed by a week of comparatively light training to allow regeneration. Even during the comparatively reduced training during the competitive season, major reductions in the training load occur before major competitions.

may be comparatively common among elite athletes. Studies of elite distance runners suggest that approximately two thirds may experience overtraining syndrome at some time during their careers.[39, 40] Other studies suggest that 20% to 50% of swimmers, basketball players, and soccer players may be overtrained during a competitive season.[21, 23, 28, 29, 31, 55] Thus, overtraining syndrome is neither a trivial nor a rare problem among serious athletes. Its incidence is comparable to discrete injuries relative to its effect on athletic careers.

Various terms have been applied to this unhappy state. At least as long ago as 40 years, the swimming coach J.E. "Doc" Counsilman recognized and wrote about the problem of "staleness."[8] Other early workers, particularly in Europe, also described similiar conditions. [19, 26, 28, 29, 31, 54] As this phenomenon has been more exensively studied, the term *overtraining syndrome* has come to be generally applied.[19, 26, 28, 29] Some authors use the term *overtraining* also to describe the process of heavier than usual training. This has led to much confusion because a given term may be used both as a verb (the athlete is overtraining) and as a noun (the athlete is overtrained). For consistency, we prefer to use the term *overreaching* for the act of engaging in unusually heavy training and to reserve the term *overtraining* for the complex pathophysiologic-behavioral syndrome that results from too severe or too prolonged overreaching.

ELEMENTS OF OVERTRAINING SYNDROME

Overtraining syndrome is an imperfectly described condition. There are few if any good experimental models. Indeed, because overtraining syndrome has such a negative influence on the likelihood of competitive success, few athletes train hard enough to risk overtraining syndrome without a specific competitive goal. Only the studies by Lehmann and colleagues[27, 30, 33] with distance runners and recreational athletes, Fry and associates[16, 17] with Special Forces soldiers, and Snyder and others[24, 50, 51] with cyclists have even minimally satisfied the goal of producing overtraining syndrome experimentally.

Historically, at least two seemingly unrelated conditions appear to be associated with overtraining syndrome. The first is the classic or so-called sympathetic form of overtraining characterized by a state of hyperexcitability. The second is the modern or so-called parasympathetic form of overtraining characterized by a state of phlegmatic behavior. Early studies from Europe refer to these syndroms as *basedowoid* and *addisonoid* forms of overtraining.[19, 26, 28, 29] The former calls to mind a thyroid hyperfunction (morbus Basedow) and the latter an adrenal hypofunction (morbus Addison), although thyroid or adrenal pathophysiology has never been demonstrated in clinical overtraining syndrome. The sympathetic form of overtraining is comparatively less common and seems more likely to occur in explosive types of sports such as sprinting, jumping, and throwing. The parasympathetic form of overtraining is the more common variety and is the usual form in long-distance runners. Although seemingly discrete conditions, these two syndromes are probably sequential presentations of the same pathophysiologic state. Some generally accepted observations from the two varieties of overtraining syndrome are presented in Table 13–1.

HYPOTHESES REGARDING GENESIS OF OVERTRAINING SYNDROME

In addition to being a loosely defined syndrome, overtraining syndrome is also essentially refractory to definitive treatment. The only treatment seems to be a fairly prolonged (~6 months) reduction in the training load, a prescription not likely to be particularly welcomed by coaches and athletes. It seems fair to suggest that overtraining syndrome is a manifestation of the exhaustion stage of the general adaptation syndrome model proposed by Seyle. Support for this suggestion is provided by the observation that other stressors in addition to exercise training (travel, job stress, social stress, frequent competition, inadequate nutrition) seem to predispose an athlete to overtraining syndrome. Indeed, overtraining syndrome is probably a cousin of the burnout syndrome noted in other groups subjected to prolonged periods of stress (students, soldiers, artistic performers, physicians, business executives). Overtraining syndrome has been hypothetically linked to five different causes: neuroendocrine dysfunction, sympathetic/parasympathetic imbalance, catabolic/anabolic imbalance, amino acid imbalance, and carbohydrate deficit.

TABLE 13–1 Pathophysiologic Findings in Classic (Sympathetic) Versus Modern (Parasympathetic) Forms of Overtraining Syndrome

Sympathetic	Parasympathetic
Impaired performance	Impaired performance
Easily fatigued	Easily fatigued
Restlessness, hyperexcitability	Depression, phlegmatic behavior
Disturbed sleep	Sleeps easily
Anorexia, weight loss	Normal appetite, constant weight
Increased resting heart rate	Very low resting heart rate
Slow recovery heart rate after exercise	Quick recovery of heart rate after exercise
Increased resting blood pressure	Hypoglycemia during exercise
Postural hypotension	Decreased submaximal and maximal lactate
Slow return of blood pressure after exercise	Decreased libido (men), amenorrhea (women)
Loss of competitive desire	Loss of competitive desire
Increased incidence of infections	Increased incidence of infections
Decreased maximal lactate	

NEUROENDOCRINE DYSFUNCTION

Barron and colleagues[2] reported reduced cortisol, adrenocorticotropic hormone, growth hormone, and prolactin release after insulin-induced hypoglycemia in overtrained distance runners. Because pituitary luteinizing hormone, thyroid-stimulating hormone, and prolactin release in response to luteinizing hormone–releasing hormone and thyroid-releasing hormone did not differ from that of controls, hypothalamic dysfunction with normal pituitary function was suggested. However, Keizer and associates[25] noted a reduction in pituitary β-endorphin release, suggesting possible pituitary dysfunction. Because lower concentrations of free testosterone are frequently observed in overtrained male athletes,[30] the underlying mechanism may be more complex, involving central (hypothalamic, pituitary) and peripheral (e.g., diminished gonadal blood flow and adrenal overload during prolonged periods of severe training) alterations. In addition, based on quite different already achieved levels of adaptation, different mechanisms may explain contradictory results in well-experienced and adapted athletes[2, 30] as compared with less-experienced athletes during an early stage of their careers.[33]

Further support for the hypothalamic-pituitary dysfunction hypothesis is provided by studies of female athletes who develop amenorrhea with severe exercise training.[37] Impaired ovarian function consequent to severe training is thought to be related to diminished pituitary hormone secretion secondary to alterations in the hypothalamic control of gonadotropin release. In women, exercise-related amenorrhea appears to be similar to that induced by illness, weight loss, and psychologic or environmental stress. Because one common finding in overtrained male athletes is a loss of libido and decreases in serum free testosterone concentration, it seems reasonable to suggest that a generalized failure of reproductive function is an early marker of overtraining syndrome.[9, 22, 37]

SYMPATHETIC/PARASYMPATHETIC IMBALANCE

Lehmann and coworkers[36] have demonstrated a substantial (40% to 70%) decrease in nocturnal urinary catecholamine secretion in overtrained distance runners and in soccer players as a late marker of overtraining syndrome, a finding that has been independently confirmed.[41] This phenomenon was observed only after prolonged periods of severe training or competition and seemed to disappear with prolonged periods of regeneration (Fig. 13–4). It was believed to be attributable to a decrease in intrinsic sympathetic activity. This in turn may be attributable less to fatigue of catecholamine production than to inhibitory effects dependent on an amino acid imbalance with increased brain levels of aromatic amino acids (phenylalanine, tryptophan, tyrosine) and increased hypothalamic dopamine and tryptophan concentrations. Evidence for this hypothesis has been demonstrated in animal models.[45] Although direct experimental evidence is lacking, the importance of other stressors producing sympathetic arousal (lack of sleep; occupational/educational demands; social demands; travel, particularly interna-

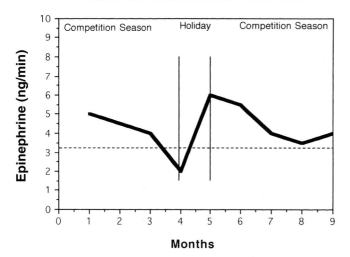

Nocturnal Catecholamine Secretion

Figure 13–4

Schematic demonstration of decreased nocturnal catecholamine secretion in soccer players during a competitive season. Note the decline in catecholamine secretion just before the winter holiday (at which time the athletes were demonstrating evidence of overtraining syndrome) and the recovery after the regeneration period. (Adapted from Lehmann M, Schnee W, Scheu R, et al: Decreased nocturnal catecholamine excretion: Parameter for an overtraining syndrome in athletes. Int J Sports Med 13:236–242, 1992.)

tional travel; competition) in reducing the exercise training load necessary to produce overtraining syndrome argues for an alteration of catecholamine release as a contributor to the reduced urinary catecholamine excretion with overtraining. However, plasma catecholamine responses at submaximal workloads may be elevated, as observed in elite swimmers suspected of having overtraining syndrome[23] or in overtrained distance runners.[30, 33, 36] This difference in basal urinary catecholamine excretion and plasma catecholamine response clearly remains an area for further inquiry.

CATABOLIC/ANABOLIC IMBALANCE

Because of the great training loads endured by contemporary athletes (particularly long-distance runners), these athletes may have significant difficulty maintaining adequate nutritional intake. In studies including a large increase in the volume of training,[30] decreases in the serum concentration of various nutritional markers (serum albumin, summed serum amino acids, glucose) were observed.

Adlercreutz and colleagues[1] have suggested that the typical directional changes in free testosterone (decrease) and cortisol (increase) during heavy training are consistent with a catabolic milieu. This unfavorable change in free testosterone/cortisol has also been noted by others in various groups of athletes during periods of severe training.[18, 22, 52–54] However, in one of the few experimental models of overtraining syndrome,[30] no clear change in

the free testosterone/cortisol ratio was noted despite convincing clinical evidence of overtraining syndrome. Additionally, in a parallel study that used higher-intensity exercise as the increased training stress (and in which no clinical evidence of overtraining syndrome was noted), a significant decrease in serum free testosterone was observed.[30]

AMINO ACID IMBALANCE

Newsholme and associates[43] have noted that the increased uptake of branched-chain amino acids by muscle tissue during severe sustained exercise (often associated with glycogen depletion and hyper–fatty acidemia) may lead to an increase in the ratio of aromatic (e.g., free tryptophan/branched-chain amino acids). This in turn may lead to an increased uptake of tryptophan in the brain and an increased synthesis of the neurotransmitter 5-hydroxytryptamine (5-HT). Given that evidence shows that tiredness and sleepiness may be partially dependent on the brain concentration of 5-HT, the researchers hypothesized that the relative imbalance of aromatic/branched-chain amino acids may be associated with the central fatigue of overtraining syndrome.[56] Many data support this as a central point in the generation of overtraining syndrome. 5-HT–containing cells are located in clusters in both the pons and upper medulla (rapheal nuclei). These areas have connections to most areas of the brain, particularly to areas associated with motor, neuroendocrine, and emotional function (all areas of disturbance with overtraining syndrome). Given the connections of 5-HT–containing cells to the hypothalamus and the importance of hypothalamic function as a central regulator, other neuroendocrine abnormalities could be induced by 5-HT–mediated hypothalamic dysfunction.

The ratio of branched-chain amino acids/tryptophan is depressed after severe acute exercise.[3, 32] In animal models, this was associated with accumulation of 5-HT in the brain of exhausted animals.[46] In severe acute exercise in humans (ultradistance triathlon), a generalized decrease in several serum amino acids was combined with an increase in several others including free tryptophan.[32] Experimental supplementation with dietary branched-chain amino acids or with tryptophan has not, however, been demonstrated to improve endurance in cyclists during a single acute bout of exhaustive exercise.[35] In an experimental model of increased training volume and intensity in runners, Lehmann and colleagues[30] noted unfavorable changes in the ratio of branched-chain amino acids/free tryptophan in a group demonstrating clinical evidence of overtraining syndrome (increased

training volume) and in a group demonstrating no evidence of overtraining syndrome (increased training intensity). Thus, at present, experimental evidence supporting the conceptually attractive imbalanced amino acid hypothesis remains unconvincing.

CARBOHYDRATE DEFICIT

The peripheral fatigue that is common in athletes during strenuous training is at least partially related to a chronic depression of muscle glycogen concentration and phosphocreatine, which in turn leads to an increase in the level of nerve stimulation required for a given muscle action. Costill and associates[5, 6] have suggested that at least part of the overtraining phenomenon is related to chronic muscle glycogen depletion. Evidence supporting the importance of muscle glycogen depletion during acute fatigue is evident in the pattern of suppressed blood lactate accumulation during exercise in muscle glycogen–depleted athletes[15] and in a decrease in the ratio of blood lactate to ratings of perceived exertion (Fig. 13–5).[50]

Figure 13–5

Schematic representation of the relationship between the rating of perceived exertion (RPE) and blood lactate during incremental exercise testing. During severe training, primarily as a result of muscle glycogen depletion, the RPE increases and the blood lactate concentration decreases at any given workload. Blood lactate vs. RPE values in the lightly shaded region imply fairly normal recovery from training. Values in the darkly shaded region suggest either inadequate recovery or inadequate carbohydrate intake.

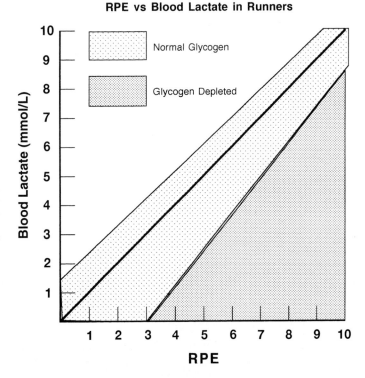

Studies by Snyder and coworkers[51] using a severe training model with maintenance of muscle glycogen demonstrated the development of overtraining syndrome despite normal levels of resting muscle glycogen. Interestingly, despite normal resting muscle glycogen concentrations, the blood lactate/rating of perceived exertion ratio was decreased (0.82 vs. 0.64 at the power output associated with a blood lactate level of 4.0 $mmol^{-1} \cdot L^{-1}$ before intervention). Considering the frequency of severe muscle glycogen depletion in athletes, these data make it unlikely that muscle glycogen depletion per se is the primary cause of overtraining syndrome. However, given the potential cascade phenomenon of muscle glycogen depletion–hyper–fatty acidemia–amino acid imbalance–central fatigue, frequent periods of muscle glycogen depletion may have a role in causing overtraining syndrome.

OTHER ABNORMALITIES WITH OVERTRAINING SYNDROME

Two other features that seem to be comparatively common in overtraining syndrome are changes in mood state and relative immunologic incompetence. As a part of the accumulation of hypothalamic 5-HT, an overall disturbance in mood state is a potential. Athletes typically use terms such as "washed out," "lacking in energy," "need a vacation," "grumpy," "poor concentration," "forgetful," and "trouble sleeping," all of which describe conditions consistent with either classic or modern overtraining syndrome.[19, 21, 39, 40] Lehmann and associates[30] have demonstrated a regular relationship between a "trivial" four-point symptom index based primarily on muscle soreness and general fatigue. We have used a rather more specialized questionnaire (Table 13–2) and have demonstrated a regular

TABLE 13–2 Psychophysical Complaint Index

Complaint Index
How do you feel today? Put a slash through the index at the point that best represents how you feel about each of the complaints that athletes often have. The words-expressions are intended to serve as guides.

No complaints					Moderate complaints				Severe complaints	
0	1	2	3	4	5	6	7	8	9	10

Feel great					Feel OK				Feel horrible	
0	1	2	3	4	5	6	7	8	9	10

Fresh					Tired				Exhausted	
0	1	2	3	4	5	6	7	8	9	10

Good morning!					Is it morning already?				Oh s---!	
0	1	2	3	4	5	6	7	8	9	10

Perky					OK				Lethargic	
0	1	2	3	4	5	6	7	8	9	10

Dynamic					Sluggish				Toast	
0	1	2	3	4	5	6	7	8	9	10

Muscles feel good					A little sore				Muscles ache	
0	1	2	3	4	5	6	7	8	9	10

Total score _____ / 7 = average score _____

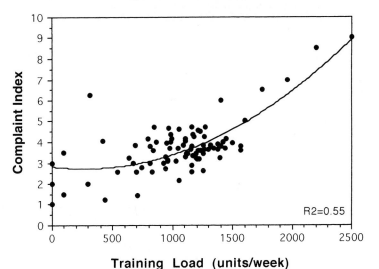

Training Load vs Complaint Index

Figure 13–6

Relationship of training load (computed as the summated [weekly] product of training duration × rating of perceived exertion for each training session[14]) to an index of psychophysical complaints.

relationship between the mean complaint index and the weekly training load (Fig. 13–6).

A common finding among heavily training athletes is an apparent increased susceptibility to infectious disease. This observation apparently was made as early as 1928 after the St. Moritz Winter Olympics. This is paradoxic, in that mild to moderate exercise is thought to enhance immune function, primarily by an increased lymphocyte response to mitogenic stimulation and by a generalized increase in the number of natural killer cells. Hard training without evidence of maladaptation does not result in abnormal immune cell function.[20, 42] It is generally to be expected that among seriously training athletes, minor illnesses (e.g., colds) will cause more days of lost training than injuries. Newsholme and others[43, 45, 46] have suggested that intense/long-duration exercise may cause a marked decrease in the plasma glutamine level. Because adequate levels of plasma glutamine are thought to be essential for lymphocyte proliferation and the function of macrophages and because skeletal muscle is probably the largest source of plasma glutamine, an exertion-related net inward transport of glutamine may lead to reductions in plasma glutamine and, accordingly, may have a negative effect on immune function. This hypothesis is supported by decreases in plasma glutamine in overtrained athletes.[43] These decreases persist well into the recovery period, even after performance has begun to normalize. Although not statistically significant, the direc-

tional changes in plasma glutamine levels in overtrained runners (decrease) and nonovertrained runners (increase) observed by Lehmann and colleagues[34] provide some support for the glutamine hypothesis.

At present, no data demonstrate whether nutritional supplementation with glutamine could act to prevent the immunosuppression that occurs with heavy training. Net transport of glutamine from the gut to the blood is thought to be a comparatively inefficient process. Additionally, although convincing evidence supports the value of ascorbate on immune function after severe acute exercise,[47] it is unclear whether this operates via a glutamine-mediated mechanism or via a negative interaction of free radicals and leukocyte function.[10]

TRAINING CONSIDERATIONS

The development of overtraining syndrome is clearly related to an imbalance in the training/recovery relationship. However, because exercise is usually defined in terms of its intensity, frequency, and duration, a single variable has not been identified to describe the magnitude of the input to the system provided by exercise. Banister and others[12, 38] have suggested that the summated product of heart rate and time can provide a single number representation of the training load. Edwards[11] has discussed the concept of heart rate–based training zones and time in zone

TABLE 13–3   Modified Rating of Perceived Exertion Scale

Approximately 30 minutes after the completion of a training session, ask the athlete to describe the overall effort put into the training session:

Rating	Verbal Description
0	Rest
1	Very easy
2	Easy
3	Moderate
4	Somewhat hard
5	Hard
6	
7	Very hard
8	
9	Very, very hard
10	Maximal

as an approach to quantitating training load. Because of concerns about the practicality of using a heart rate–based system, the problem of accounting for very high-intensity exercise (which might produce a higher than maximal heart rate, were that possible), and concerns about integrating resistance training into the system, we have developed a system that uses a modification of the Rating of Perceived Exertion (RPE) Scale developed by Borg (Table 13–3) to rate the overall intensity of an entire training session. When this training intensity score is multiplied by the duration of that session, a single-number representation of that training session is produced. This number relates well to the average heart rate during steady-state exercise[14] and to the relative time in heart rate–blood lactate–defined training

zones.[13] Integrated over convenient time intervals (weekly), an index of the total training load (intensity × duration) may be generated (Table 13–4).

We have demonstrated that training load during the 6 weeks preceding a cycle time trial is related to the performance capacity of the athlete (Fig. 13–7). The nature of this relationship follows the negatively accelerating function of any dose-response relationship. The total training load is also related to an athlete's complaints during training (Fig. 13–6).

Bruin and coworkers,[4] using racehorses as an experimental model, have demonstrated that the constancy of the training load may be just as important in the generation of overtraining syndrome as the total training load. During heavy training, horses develop a syndrome (poor performance, nervousness, anorexia) that is in many ways similar to the so-called classic or sympathetic form of overtraining syndrome. Bruin's group noted that the horses tolerated progressive increases in the total training load (hard days progressively more severe) as long as the training on intervening regeneration days was kept very light. However, as soon as the training load was increased by making the regeneration days more difficult, the horses developed overtraining syndrome. This observation fits both practical models of training athletes (hard day–easy day) and expectations related to sympathetic-parasympathetic imbalance, imbalanced amino acid, and glycogen deple-

TABLE 13–4   Evaluation of the Load, Monotony, and Strain Associated with a Training Program

Day	Training Session	Duration (min)	Rating of Perceived Exertion	Load
Sunday	Run 30 km, hilly	135	5	675
Monday	Jog 5 km, easy	25	2	50
Tuesday	Jog 5 km, 6 × 1000 m/400 m			
	At anaerobic threshold, jog 5 km	80	5	400
Wednesday	Run 15 km	65	4	260
Thursday	Jog 5 km, 10 × hill loop			
	Fartlek, jog 5 km	80	6	480
Friday	Jog 5 km, easy	25	2	50
Saturday	Jog 3 km, easy	15	2	30
	Race 15 km	52	9.5	494
	Jog 2 km, easy	10	2	20

Daily mean load	351.2
Daily standard deviation of load	241.8
Monotony (daily mean/daily standard deviation)	1.45
Weekly load (daily mean load × 7)	2459
Strain (total load × monotony)	3573

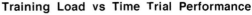

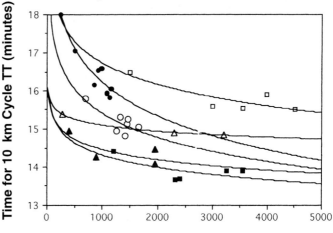

Figure 13–7

Relationship of training load to performance in a 10-km cycle time trial in several athletes during a 1-year period. Training load is computed as the weekly average over the 6 weeks preceding the time trial.

tion models of the genesis of overtraining syndrome. It suggests that training monotony in conjunction with the total training load provides the stress that can lead to overtraining syndrome. It also fits with the experiences of Ron Hill, our introductory example, in that he was apparently unwilling to take true recovery days during periods of training before major competitions.

As a test of the training monotony hypothesis, we have monitored several athletes during fairly prolonged periods of training and competition. Training load was calculated using our RPE × duration method (see Table 13–4). Training monotony was calculated on a weekly basis as the weekly summated load multiplied by the mean daily load divided by the standard deviation of load (see Table 13–4). Because monotonous training at low total loads is unlikely to produce overtraining syndrome, we use the load × monotony as an index of training strain.

Figure 13–8 depicts plots of training load, monotony, and strain in an elite athlete during 2 years of training. Note that in addition to lower total training loads during the second year, the training monotony (x/sd) is also lower, leading to a lower calculated training strain during the second year. When you appreciate that 2 hours of daily training with a perceived exertion of "hard" (5) equals 4200 units of training load, you can note that the athlete trains very hard, often in excess of 5000 units per week. During the first year, this athlete had complained of nonspecific malaise early during the preparation year (~day 100) and performed very poorly at the

major selection trials (day 235). The next year, with a reduced total training load, a decrease in training monotony, and consequently a very reduced training strain, the athlete trained comfortably through the year and recorded personal best performances at the time of the major selection trials. Additionally, it may be seen that during the first year, many weeks had no regeneration days (20 minutes or less of easy intensity exercise), whereas in the second year every week had at least one (and often more) true regeneration day. It should be noted, however, that on days when serious training was conducted, the load was as high or higher during the second as in the first year.

Figure 13–9 shows plots of the occurrence of illnesses as a function of training strain in several athletes. Although individual levels of strain required to produce illness are rather different between athletes, each athlete seems to have a clearly identifiable personal threshold. On this basis, we have been able to account for 84% of the episodes of illness solely on the basis of exceeding the individual training strain threshold. For reasons that remain unclear, for about 25% of the times in which athletes exceed their threshold, illness does not result. Our impression is that training monotony is relatively more important than total training load relative to the genesis of illnesses. Studies have provided independent confirmation of the association between the relative loading of the training program and the incidence of illness.[48]

Thus, data in animal models, performance-related data, and illness-related data suggest

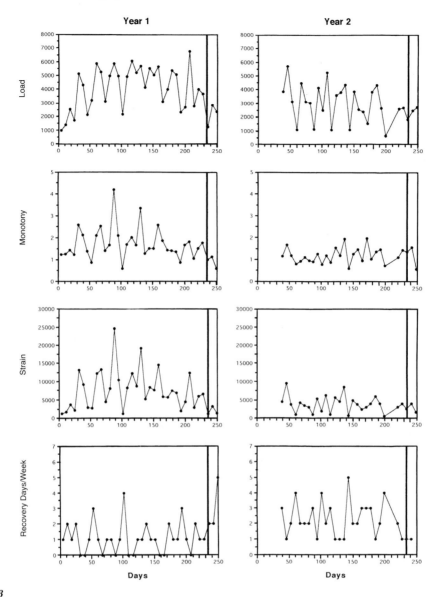

Figure 13–8

Serial trends in training load, monotony, strain, and recovery days/week during 2 years of preparation in an elite athlete. During year 1, the athlete complained of nonspecific malaise and competitive incompetence early in the preparation period (~day 100). Performance at the major competion of the year (~day 235) was very unsatisfactory. Note the high total training load, monotony, and strain and the generally low number of recovery days per week during this year. During year 2, the athlete reduced the total training load, monotony, and strain, primarily by adding more recovery days during each week. The athlete reported doing much better during the training year and recorded personal best performances at the major competition of the year (~day 235).

that not only the training load but indices of training monotony may contribute to the genesis of negative outcomes consistent with overtraining syndrome. Given the interest in training periodization shown by most coaches, it may be that subsequent analyses of training data from athletes presenting with overtraining syndrome will suggest a strategy for preventing the development of this problem.

DIAGNOSIS OF OVERTRAINING SYNDROME

Because overtraining syndrome is probably multifactorial in origin and rather inconsistent in presentation, diagnosis becomes primarily the remaining possibility once other problems have been ruled out. Certainly, in any athlete who presents with a nonspecific decline in performance and any or all of the symptoms listed in Table 13–1, the presence of significant metabolic disease or infection should be ruled out. In its absence, the remaining diagnosis becomes overtraining syndrome.

Simple blood tests are unlikely to be very revealing. Results from experimental studies of overtraining syndrome (long-distance runners) are not particularly specific.[18, 28, 52] Because most athletes do not have control laboratory studies performed during periods of light training, out-of-range individual laboratory values are difficult to interpret. Further, because heavy training is often associated with substantial short-term changes in hydration status, leading to hemoconcentration or hemodilution, depending on the time interval

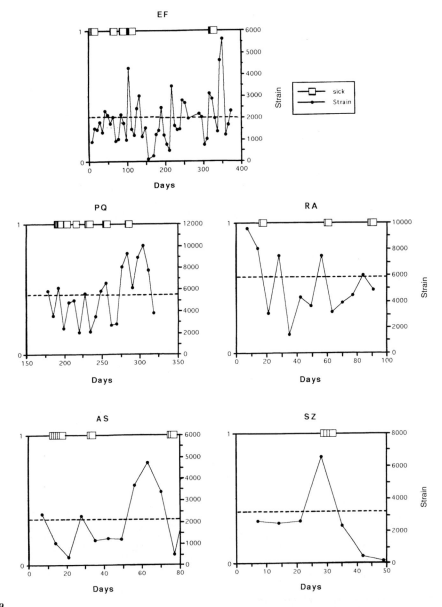

Figure 13–9

Representative plot of training strain (load × monotony) (circles) in relation to illnesses (squares) in several athletes. Each athlete has a fairly clearly identifiable threshold of training strain that seems to be associated with subsequent illnesses.

since the last training session, plasma concentrations of various metabolites may be hard to interpret. In general, in overtrained athletes a generalized decrease in leukocytes, iron, and ferritin is expected. Further, fasting blood glucose level may be rather low, as may be serum levels of albumin, globulins, fatty acids, and ammonia. Finally, serum testosterone level is likely to be low, serum cortisol level high, and basal norepinephrine excretion low in an overtrained athlete. Assuming that the athletic oligomenorrhea affecting heavily training female athletes is part of the same larger dysresponse to training, reproductive hormone levels may be low. None of these observations, however, is definitive for overtraining syndrome.

CONCLUSION

Athletes certainly seek to push the limits of their ability to respond to stress in quest of the less than 0.5% improvement that can separate the champion from the also-ran. Accordingly, overtraining syndrome will continue to be a problem in the athletic community. It seems clear that whatever mechanisms emerge to explain this phenomenon (Fig. 13–10), an imbalance in the training load–recovery relationship is the primary factor contributing to the genesis of overtraining syndrome. New approaches to periodizing the training load, including variation of training load within time periods as small as 1 week, may be of great importance to preventing overtraining syndrome. Additional factors causing stress on an athlete's system, including occupational, educational, social, and nutritional factors, and particularly including multiple time zone travel and frequent competition, may act to increase the likelihood of developing overtraining syndrome at any given level of training stress. It also seems clear that the stresses likely to provoke overtraining syndrome are highly individual and that even athletes with similar performance capabilities may have very different thresh-

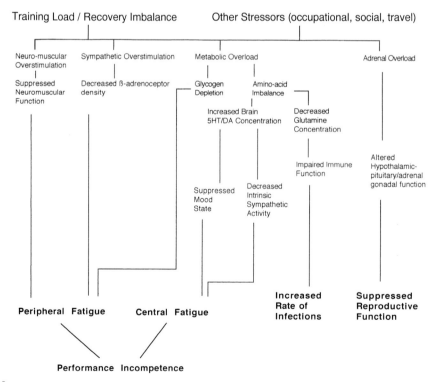

Genesis of Overtraining Syndrome

Figure 13–10

Overall schematic of factors likely to be related to the development of overtraining syndrome.

olds in relation to developing overtraining syndrome.

At the most commonsense level, one must systematically evaluate the performance of athletes to determine whether overtraining syndrome is present or not. No athlete who is progressing (better training sessions or better competitions) has overtraining syndrome. However, in already adapted athletes, failure to progress in training or competition should be viewed as a clear warning of possible overtraining syndrome. Given the degree to which overtraining syndrome is refractory to treatment, early recognition and an aggressive approach to reducing the overall level of stress on the athlete are critical.

Managers, coaches, trainers, and physicians involved in the preparation of athletes must be prepared to remain objective to detect impending overtraining syndrome and be willing to modify planned training schedules quickly to interrupt the cycle of overreaching–reduced performance–emotional panic–increased training–overtraining syndrome. In particular, health professionals (who, unlike coaches/trainers, can stand apart from emotional involvement with the day-to-day training program) need to be prepared to exert their authority to interrupt impending overtraining syndrome. To return to the analogy with which we introduced this chapter, had someone with recognizable credentials (a physician, physiologist, trainer, coach) been able to convince Ron Hill that his insistence on increasing his ordinarily successful training schedule before major competitions and on running every single day regardless of fatigue, illness, or injury only interfered with his recovery from real training sessions, the results of the Munich Olympic marathon might have been very different. Instead of a comparatively easy victory, Frank Shorter might have had competition all the way to the finish line. At the same time, and particularly if they are not themselves experienced with heavy training, health professionals must remember that (1) athletes are capable of tolerating training loads without any sequelae that are beyond the comprehension of most ordinary individuals and that (2) the risk of developing overtraining syndrome (or for that matter any training-related injuries) is a calculated risk that many athletes and coaches are more than willing to take. Put differently, many would prefer to fail gloriously than to feel that they will stand on the starting line less than fully prepared.

REFERENCES

1. Adlercreutz H, Harkonen K, Kuoppasalmi K, et al: Effect of training on plasma anabolic and catabolic steroid hormones and their response during physical exercise. Int J Sports Med 7(Suppl):27–28, 1986.
2. Barron JL, Noakes TD, Levy W, et al: Hypothalamic dysfunction in overtrained athletes. J Clin Endocrinol Metab 60:803–806, 1985.
3. Bloomstrand E, Hassmen P, Ekblom B, Newsholme EA: Administration of branched chain amino acids during sustained exercise—effects on performance and on plasma concentration of some amino acids. Eur J Appl Physiol 63:83–88, 1991.
4. Bruin G, Kuipers H, Heizer HA, Vander Vusse GJ: Adaptation and overtraining in horses subjected to increasing training loads. J Appl Physiol 76:1908–1913, 1994.
5. Costill DL, Bowers R, Branham G, Sparks K: Muscle glycogen utilization during prolonged exercise on successive days. J Appl Physiol 31:834–838, 1971.
6. Costill DL, Flynn MG, Kirwan JP, et al: Effects of repeated days of intensified training on muscle glycogen and swimming performance. Med Sci Sports Exerc 20:249–254, 1988.
7. Costill DL, Thomas R, Robergs RA, et al: Adaptations to swimming training: Influence of training volume. Med Sci Sports Exerc 23:371–377, 1991.
8. Counsilman JE: Fatigue and staleness. Athl J 15:16–20, 1955.
9. Cumming DC, Wheeler GD, McColl EM: The effects of exercise on reproductive function in men. Sports Med 7:1–17, 1989.
10. Duthie GG, Robertson JD, Maughan RJ, Morrice PC: Blood antioxidant status and erythrocyte lipid peroxidation following distance running. Arch Biochem Biophys 282:78–83, 1990.
11. Edwards S: The Heart Rate Monitor Book, Sacramento, CA, Fleet Feet Press, 1990.
12. Fitz-Clarke JR, Morton RH, Banister EW: Optimizing athletic performance by influence curves. J Appl Physiol 71:1151–1158, 1991.
13. Foster C: Exercise session RPE reflects global exercise intensity (abstract). J Cardiopulm Rehabil 14:332, 1994.
14. Foster C, Hector LI, Welsh R, et al: Effects of specific vs cross training on running performance. Eur J Appl Physiol 70:367–372, 1995.
15. Foster C, Snyder AC, Thompson NN, Kuettel K: Normalization of the blood lactate profile in athletes. Int J Sports Med 9:198–200, 1988.
16. Fry AC, Kraemer WJ, van Borselen F, et al: Catecholamine responses to short term high intensity resistance exercise overtraining. J Appl Physiol 77:941–946, 1994.
17. Fry RW, Morton AR, Garcia-Webb P, et al: Biological responses to overload training in endurance sports. Eur J Appl Physiol 64:335–344, 1992.
18. Fry RW, Morton AR, Garcia-Webb P, Keast D: Monitoring exercise stress by changes in metabolic and hormonal responses over a 24-hour period. Eur J Appl Physiol 63:228–234, 1991.
19. Fry RW, Morton AW, Keast D: Overtraining in athletes: An update. Sports Med 12:32–65, 1991.
20. Gabriel H, Urhausen A, Valet G, et al: Diagnostic approach towards recognizing overtraining by lymphocyte immunophenotyping in endurance trained athletes. Int J Sports Med 15:358A, 1994.
21. Gutmann MC, Pollock ML, Foster C, Schmidt DH:

Training stress in Olympic speed skaters: A psychological perspective. Physician Sportsmed 12:45–57, 1984.

22. Hakkinen K, Parkarinen A: Serum hormones in male strength athletes during intensive short term strength training. Eur J Appl Physiol 63:194–199, 1991.

23. Hooper SL, Mackinnon LT, Gordon RD, Bachmann AW: Hormonal responses of elite swimmers to overtraining. Med Sci Sports Exerc 25:741–747, 1993.

24. Jeukendrup AE, Hesselink MKC, Snyder AC, et al: Physiological changes in male competitive cyclists after two weeks of intensified training. Int J Sports Med 13:534–541, 1992.

25. Keizer H, Platen AP, Koppesdraar H: Blunted β endorphin responses to corticotropin releasing hormone and exercise after exhaustive training. Int J Sports Med 12:97A, 1991.

26. Kuipers H, Keizer HA: Overtraining in elite athletes: Review and directions for the future. Sports Med 6:79–92, 1988.

27. Lehmann M, Baumgartl P, Wiesenack C, et al: Training-overtraining: Influence of a defined increase in training volume vs training intensity on performance, catecholamines and some metabolic parameters in experienced middle and long distance runners. Eur J Appl Physiol 64:169–177, 1992.

28. Lehmann M, Foster C, Keul J: Overtraining in endurance athletes: A brief review. Med Sci Sports Exerc 25:854–862, 1993.

29. Lehmann M, Foster C, Keul J: Overtraining in middle and long distance runners. In Fahey TD (ed): Encyclopedia of Sports Medicine and Exercise Physiology. New York, Garland (in press).

30. Lehmann M, Gastmann U, Peterson G, et al: Training-overtraining: Performance and hormone levels after a defined increase in training volume versus intensity in experimental middle and long distance runners. Br J Sports Med 26:233–242, 1992.

31. Lehmann M, Gastmann U, Steinacker JM, et al: Overtraining in endurance sports. Med Sport Boh Slov 4:1–6, 1995.

32. Lehmann M, Huonker M, Dimeo F, et al: Serum amino acid concentrations in nine athletes before and after the 1993 Colmar ultra triathlon. Int J Sports Med 16:155–159, 1995.

33. Lehmann M, Knizia K, Gastmann U, et al: Influence of a 6-week, 6 days per week training on pituitary function in recreational athletes. Br J Sports Med 27:186–192, 1993.

34. Lehmann M, Mann H, Gastmann U, et al: Unaccustomed high mileage vs intensity training related changes in performance and serum amino acids. Int J Sports Med 17:187–192, 1996.

35. Lehmann M, Schiestl G, Schmidt K, et al: BCAA supplementation related performances in cyclists. Eur J Appl Physiol 69(Suppl):36, 1994.

36. Lehmann M, Schnee W, Scheu R, et al: Decreased nocturnal catecholamine excretion: Parameter for an overtraining syndrome in athletes. Int J Sports Med 13:236–242, 1992.

37. Loucks AB: Effect of exercise training on the menstrual cycle: Existence and mechanisms. Med Sci Sports Exerc 22:275–280, 1990.

38. Morton RH, Fitz-Clarke JR, Banister EW: Modeling human-performance in running. J Appl Physiol 69:1171–1177, 1990.

39. Morgan WP, Brown DR, Raglin JS, et al: Psychological monitoring of overtraining and staleness. Br J Sports Med 21:107–114, 1987.

40. Morgan WP, Costill DL, Flynn MG, et al: Mood disturbance following increased training in swimmers. Med Sci Sports Exerc 20:408–414, 1988.

41. Naessens G, Lefevre J, Priessens M: Practical and clinical relevance of urinary basal noradrenaline excretion in the follow up of training processes in semiprofessional soccer players. Clin J Sports Med (in press).

42. Ndon JA, Snyder AC, Foster C, Wehrenberg WB: Effects of chronic intense exercise training on the leukocyte response to acute exercise. Int J Sports Med 13:176–182, 1992.

43. Newsholme EA, Parry-Billings M, McAndrew N, Bugettt R: A biochemical mechanism to explain some characteristics of overtraining. Med Sport Sci 32:79–93, 1991.

44. Noakes TD: Lore of Running. Champaign, IL, Human Kinetics Press, 1991, pp 263–361.

45. Parry-Billings M, Bloomstrand E, McAndrew N, Newsholme EA: A communication link between skeletal muscle, brain and cells of the immune system. Int J Sports Med 11(Suppl 2):122–128, 1990.

46. Parry-Billings M, Budgett R, Koutedekis Y, et al: Plasma amino acid concentration in the overtraining syndrome: Possible effects on the immune system. Med Sci Sports Exerc 24:1353–1358, 1992.

47. Peters EM, Goetzsche B, Grobbelaar B, Noakes TD: Vitamin C supplementation reduced the incidence of postrace symptoms of upper respiratory tract infection in ultramarathon runners. Am J Clin Nutr 57:170–174, 1993.

48. Snouse S, Rundell KF: Injury and illness occurrence for elite short track speed skaters. Proceedings of the 3rd IOC World Congress on Sport Sciences, Atlanta, September 1995.

49. Snyder AC, Foster C: Physiology and nutrition for skating. In Lamb, DR, Knuttgen HG, Murray R, (eds): Perspectives in Exercise Science and Sports Medicine, vol 7. Carmel, IN, Cooper Publishing Group, 1994, pp 181–219.

50. Snyder AC, Jeukendrup AE, Hesselink MKG, et al: A physiological, psychological indicator of overreaching during intensive training. Int J Sports Med 14:29–32, 1993.

51. Snyder AC, Kuipers H, Cheng B, et al: Overtraining following intensified training with normal muscle glycogen. Med Sci Sports Exerc 27:1063–1069, 1995.

52. Urhausen A, Gabriel H, Kindermann W: Blood hormones as markers of training stress and overtraining. Sports Med 20:251–276, 1995.

53. Urhausen A, Kinderman W: Behavior of testosterone, sex hormone binding globulin and cortisol before and after a triathlon competition. Int J Sports Med 8:305–308, 1987.

54. Urhausen A, Kullner T, Kinderman: A 7-week follow up study of the behavior of testosterone and cortisol during the competition period in rowers. Eur J Appl Physiol 56:528–533, 1987.

55. Verma SK, Mahindroo SR, Kansal DK: Effect of four weeks of hard physical training on certain physiological and morphological parameters of basket-ball players. J Sports Med 18:379–384, 1978.

56. Wilson W, Maughan RJ: Evidence for the role of 5-HT in fatigue during prolonged exercise. Int J Sports Med 14:297–300, 1993.

JOHN G. PATY, JR.

━━━ *CHAPTER FOURTEEN*
Arthritis and Running

The benefits of running include positive effects on the cardiovascular system, improved weight control and psychologic well-being, and positive effects on the musculoskeletal system including improved bone density and decreased disability.[29, 30, 34] The risk of osteoarthritis with running has evolved from the high incidence of soft tissue and bone injury in runners;[32, 41, 49, 52] osteoarthritis occurring in other sports-related activities;[38] and reports suggesting occupation-related osteoarthritis.[16, 38] This chapter reviews the clinical and pathologic features of osteoarthritis, as well as data related to running and osteoarthritis. Comments on the likelihood of its occurrence in runners are also included.

DEFINITION OF OSTEOARTHRITIS

Osteoarthritis is characterized by "joint symptoms and signs which are associated with defective integrity of articular cartilage, in addition to related changes in the underlying bone and at the joint margins."[3] A classification for subsets of osteoarthritis has been proposed by Altman and colleagues (Table 14–1).[3] Osteoarthritis may be idiopathic or secondary. Examples of idiopathic osteoarthritis include localized forms affecting the hands, feet, knees, hips, and spine and a generalized form that involves three or more peripheral joint areas and the spine. Secondary forms of osteoarthritis are due to trauma, congenital or developmental diseases such as Legg-Calvé-Perthes disease of the hip, epiphyseal dysplasia, or metabolic diseases such as hemochromatosis. Secondary osteoarthritis may also occur in calcium pyrophosphate deposition disease and follows other forms of arthritis such as rheumatoid arthritis and endocrine diseases such as acromegaly.

PATHOLOGY OF OSTEOARTHRITIS

Osteoarthritis is characterized pathologically by abnormalities in the cartilage and subchondral bone. Articular cartilage is avascular and requires mechanical loading to remain healthy, receiving nutrients from the synovial fluid by diffusion and imbibition. The lower zones of the cartilage receive nutrition via the subchondral bone. The avascular state is crucial to cartilage integrity, and increased vascularization of subchondral bone that penetrates into the cartilage is one of the pathologic features of osteoarthritis. Early in the course of osteoarthritis, water content and ground substance (proteoglycan) that holds together the collagen fibers (type II) that form articular cartilage are increased.

With the progression of degenerative changes, a loss of the ground substance and a change in collagen fiber arrangement and size occur.[8] Histochemical staining of the cartilage with safranin O reveals a loss of metachromasia in the superficial layers of the cartilage, but deeper one may see increased staining around clusters of chondrocytes that are attempting to repair the joint cartilage. These changes are accompanied by fraying, fissures (fibrillations), deep clefts, thinning, and ultimately loss of cartilage. Lysosomal proteases, metalloproteinases, and collagenases released by the chondrocytes may account for much of the cartilage loss.[8] As cartilage thins, underlying bone is exposed.

Remodeling and appositional new bone formation of the subchondral bone as a result of subchondral microfractures are early findings in osteoarthritis and account for the subchondral sclerosis seen on radiographs. Subchondral bone cysts form as a result of synovial fluid penetration into the subchondral bone (Table 14–2).[19] The osteophytes or

TABLE 14–1   Classification for Subsets of Osteoarthritis

I. Idiopathic
  A. Localized
    1. Hands: e.g., Heberden and Bouchard nodes (nodal), erosive interphalangeal arthritis (nonnodal), scaphometacarpal, scaphotrapezial
    2. Feet: e.g., hallux valgus, hallux rigidus, contracted toes (hammer/cock-up toes), talonavicular
    3. Knee
      a. Medial compartment
      b. Lateral compartment
      c. Patellofemoral compartment (e.g., chondromalacia)
    4. Hip
      a. Eccentric (superior)
      b. Concentric (axial, medial)
      c. Diffuse (coxae senilis)
    5. Spine (particularly cervical and lumbar)
      a. Apophyseal
      b. Intervertebral (disc)
      c. Spondylosis (osteophytes)
      d. Ligamentous hyperostosis (Forestier disease, or skeletal diffuse idiopathic hyperostosis [DISH])
    6. Other single sites: e.g., shoulder, temporomandibular, sacroiliac, ankle, wrist, acromioclavicular
  B. Generalized: includes three or more areas listed above
    1. Small (peripheral) and spine
    2. Large (central) and spine
    3. Mixed (peripheral and central) and spine
	II. Secondary
	  A. Posttraumatic
	  B. Congenital or developmental diseases
	    1. Localized
	      a. Hip diseases: e.g., Legg-Calvé-Perthes, congenital hip dislocation, slipped capital femoral epiphysis, shallow acetabulum
	      b. Mechanical and local factors: e.g., obesity (?), unequal lower extremity length, extreme valgus/varus deformity, hypermobility syndromes, scoliosis
	    2. Generalized
	      a. Bone dysplasias: e.g., epiphyseal dysplasia, spondyloapophyseal dysplasia
	      b. Metabolic diseases: e.g., hemochromatosis, ochronosis, Gaucher disease, hemoglobinopathy, Ehlers-Danlos disease
	  C. Calcium deposition disease
	    1. Calcium pyrophosphate deposition disease
	    2. Apatite arthropathy
	    3. Destructive arthropathy (shoulder, knee)
	  D. Other bone and joint disorders: e.g., avascular necrosis, rheumatoid arthritis, gouty arthritis, septic arthritis, Paget disease, osteopetrosis, osteochondritis
	  E. Other diseases
	    1. Endocrine diseases: e.g., diabetes mellitus, acromegaly, hypothyroidism, hyperparathyroidism
	    2. Neuropathic arthropathy (Charcot joints)
	    3. Miscellaneous: e.g., frostbite, Kashin-Beck disease, Caisson disease

Adapted from Altman R, Asch E, Bloch D, et al: Development of criteria for the classification and reporting of osteoarthritis. Arthritis 29:1039–1049, 1986.

osteochondrophytes (spurs) arise in the synovium at the joint margins[1] and are accompanied by neovascularization from the subchondral bone. Vascular engorgement and healed microfractures account for increased stiffness in subchondral bone. During impact, both cartilage and subchondral bone compress as they absorb the forces of weight-bearing. At higher impact, subchondral bone is a more important shock absorber, and increased stiffness there may result in greater forces in the cartilage with subsequent further degenerative changes.[8]

DIAGNOSIS OF OSTEOARTHRITIS

For the diagnosis of osteoarthritis of the knee, clinical findings such as knee pain and radiographic features of joint space narrowing, subchondral sclerosis, and marginal osteophytosis provide a high degree of sensitivity and specificity.[3] However, when Brandt and colleagues arthroscopically examined 92

patients with chronic knee pain and radiographic evidence of mild osteoarthritis by the Kellgren and Lawrence criteria or joint space narrowing,[7] 7 of 17 patients whose radiographic findings were normal by marginal osteophytosis or joint space narrowing had advanced tibiofemoral and patellofemoral compartment changes of cartilage loss. Additionally, 16 patients with radiographic criteria of osteoarthritis had no abnormalities on arthroscopy. The researchers concluded that radiographs are not a reliable tool for evaluating osteoarthritis.[7] This discrepancy between radiographic and anatomic findings underscores one of the problems in making a diagnosis of osteoarthritis. This feature is particularly pertinent because most of the studies published on running and osteoarthritis have used radiologic criteria only.

Clinical diagnosis of osteoarthritis, therefore, is based on a history of joint pain, physical findings of bony enlargement and crepitus or limited motion, and radiographic findings of spurring, joint space narrowing, and subchondral sclerosis. The most commonly used radiologic criteria are based on the Kellgren and Lawrence classification.[23] With a standard anteroposterior view of the hips, knees, and feet and a posteroanterior view of the hands and lateral view of the cervical and lumbar spines, the Kellgren criteria are as follows: grade zero (none); grade one (doubtful)—slight joint space spurring; grade two (minimal)—definite osteophytes and possible joint space narrowing; grade three (moderate)—multiple osteophytes with definite joint space narrowing and subchondral sclerosis; and grade four (severe)—large osteophytes with marked joint space narrowing, subchondral sclerosis, and bony deformity.[7, 23]

Alexander also emphasizes the importance of distinguishing traction spurs where ligaments attach but do not obliterate the joint level and osteophytosis. He notes that failure to distinguish between traction spurs from osteophytosis may lead to overinterpretation of radiographs. He also states that long, continued, vigorous exercise is not a cause of osteoarthritis and notes the high incidence of overuse injuries in musicians, particularly keyboard and string players, but not an increased incidence of osteoarthritis. He also notes two other important clinical features. Although osteophytes do occur early in osteoarthritis and cartilage abnormalities may be present, patients with radiologic evidence of osteophytosis may show no evidence of progression for long periods. Additionally, tibial spines are not traction spurs but are articular surfaces covered with thick cartilage.[1] Altman and coworkers proposed that progression of osteoarthritis in the hips and knees could best be assessed by an anteroposterior radiograph that evaluated the hips for joint space narrowing and cyst formation and the weight-bearing knee view by narrowing, spurs, and subchondral sclerosis.[4]

PATHOGENESIS OF OSTEOARTHRITIS

Osteoarthritis may occur because of one or more predisposing factors, including biomechanical, genetic, biochemical, hormonal, age, and gender.[42] Davis and associates found close correlation of bilateral knee osteoarthritis with obesity and a strong correlation of trauma with unilateral osteoarthritis of the knee.[10] Greater body weight was associated with a more rapid progression of the osteoarthritis. Those with osteoarthritis are three and a half times more likely to be obese at the age of 20, two to three times more likely to have performed heavy work, and five times more likely to have suffered an injury.[10] Leisure activity was not significantly different in 46 severely osteoarthritic patients who had had total knee arthroplasty compared with 46 community controls.[24]

Although 75% of those older than 70 years have radiographic evidence of osteophytosis, age by itself is not a necessary nor a sufficient cause of osteoarthritis. Biochemically, cartilage changes due to aging and to osteoarthritis are quite different. Unlike osteoarthritic cartilage, aging cartilage shows a decrease in water content, an increase in proteoglycans, and normal cartilage proteases.[19, 36]

IMPACT LOADING IN THE PATHOGENESIS OF OSTEOARTHRITIS

Impact loading has been proposed as an important factor in osteoarthritis. Radin and colleagues subjected eight sheep to 4 hours of walking on concrete per day.[46] Four control sheep walked on wood chips. After 9 months,

TABLE 14–2 Radiographic-Pathologic Correlations in Osteoarthritis

Pathologic Abnormalities	Radiographic Abnormalities
Cartilaginous fibrillation and erosion	Localized loss of joint space
Appositional new bone formation on cancellous subchondral bone trabeculae and bony end-plate	Bony eburnation
Fibrous-walled, mucus-containing cysts resulting from synovial fluid intrusion or myxoid degeneration	Subchondral cysts
Revascularization and enchondral ossification in remaining cartilage	Osteophytes
Compression of weakened and deformed trabeculae	Bony collapse
Fragmentation of osteochondral surface; bone and cartilage metaplasia in joint capsule	Intraarticular osseous bodies

Adapted from Hamerman D: The biology of osteoarthritis. N Engl J Med 320:1323, 1989.

the experimental sheep were limping. Radiographs showed calcification of the knee and elbow ligaments, and cartilage fibrillation and decreased cartilage hexosamine levels were noted in the experimental animals.

Impact loading for running is two and a half to three times body weight forces at the tibiofemoral interface and is one time body weight for walking. Strength and flexibility of the hips and knees are key factors in absorbing shock during running. Allen proposes a theoretic concept of load and repetition from no-load repetition with subsequent disuse atrophy to the very highest load and repetition, when bone and joint injury may occur.[2] Almost 25 years ago, Radin and associates proposed that the subchondral bone became stiff in early osteoarthritis as a result of healing microfractures.[47] The subchondral bone loses its shock absorbency, with subsequent increased stress on the cartilage. Osteoarthritis results from repetitive impulse loading. Consistent with the impact load concept as a cause of osteoarthritis, Glyn and coworkers reported a low incidence of osteoarthritis in the hips and knees on the affected side when compared with the unaffected side in patients who had polio at a young age.[17]

In contrast to these reports, Panush and Lane noted that repetitive impulse loading alone in humans (up to one million cycles per year) does not lead to osteoarthritis. Prior injury to the cartilage meniscus or anterior cruciate ligament, however, leads to osteoarthritis of the knee (Fig. 14–1). As many as 50% of those with anterior cruciate ligament injury and 10% of those with meniscectomy develop osteoarthritis, observed in long-term follow-up. These authors and others have also noted that immobilization may hasten articular degeneration.[36, 39] Some animal studies have suggested but not proved a causative role of exercise in osteoarthritis.[39]

OCCUPATION-RELATED OSTEOARTHRITIS

With regard to impact loading, occupational injuries provide some clues. Skeletons from prehistoric times document osteoarthritis in the shoulders of young people, invoking activity as a factor. However, results of studies of occupation-related osteoarthritis are conflicting.[16] Most of the studies have been based solely on osteophyte formation on radiographs, and patients with previous trauma have not been excluded. Because 40% to 70% of patients with radiographic changes of osteophytosis may be symptom free,[1, 31, 39] the correlation between osteophytosis and actual joint deterioration may be poor. Epidemiologic data suggest that mechanical stress alone does not lead to osteoarthritis.[16] Hadler has noted that the literature supporting osteoarthritis in industry is mostly anecdotal.[18] He notes a high incidence of radiologic abnormalities in nonindustrial symptomatic and asymptomatic controls, with poor correlation between radiographic findings and symptoms. Prospective studies were noted to be conspic-

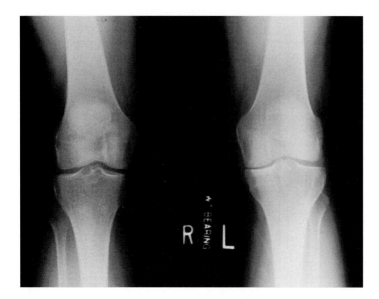

Figure 14–1

Severe left knee medial joint space narrowing and subchondral sclerosis in a 15 miles/week 61-year-old woman who had left knee pain and effusion and who had quit running because of knee pain. She had a history of previous "meniscal tear."

uously absent. There is a similar dearth of prospective studies of running surveys and injury (discussed later).

Osteoarthritis of the knee in the first national Health and Nutrition Examination Survey (HANES I) was associated with knee bending in occupation, body mass index (BMI) (kg/m² >30), and black race.[5] Bone and joint changes in pneumatic drillers were examined by Burke and coworkers.[9] They noted a previous report of osteoarthritis in the elbows and shoulders of pneumatic drillers. However, in a retrospective survey of 34 unselected pneumatic drillers with a mean duration of employment of 10.3 years, they found no evidence of joint space narrowing but did find spurring of the olecranon at the triceps insertion in nine patients, a common finding in miners using pneumatic tools, but found radiologic changes of mild osteoarthritis with joint spurring in only two elbow joints. They concluded that the incidence of osteoarthritis in pneumatic drillers was low. Panush and colleagues commented on previous studies suggesting the role of repetitive use as a predisposing factor in osteoarthritis of the shoulders and elbows of pneumatic drill operators, disc syndromes in dock workers, and hand arthritis in millworkers and seamstresses.[40] They noted that Burke and coworkers suggested that impact without injury was not associated with osteoarthritis and that results of previous studies were misinterpreted.

SPORTS-RELATED OSTEOARTHRITIS

Kujala and associates examined 117 male Finnish world class athletes for osteoarthritis.[27] They looked at former runners, soccer players, weight lifters, and shooters who had competed between 1920 and 1965 in either the Olympic games, world or European games, or intercountry competition. Osteophytosis of either the tibiofemoral or patellofemoral compartment qualified as knee osteophytosis. Radiographic osteoarthritis of the knee was statistically greater in soccer players in the tibiofemoral joint and in weight lifters in the patellofemoral joint. The highest correlation of osteoarthritis, however, was between BMI and previous trauma. Fifty percent of the study group with previous knee injury requiring hospitalization had osteoarthritis. An 11% incidence of osteoarthritis was noted in the lowest-profile BMI (BMI

<21.35) and a 50% incidence in those with BMI in the highest quartile at the age of 20 years (BMI >23.89) (Fig. 14–2).[27] Others have described an increased incidence of osteoarthritis in the lumbar spine, cervical spine, knees, and elbows of wrestlers; the carpometacarpal joints of boxers; the shoulders and elbows of baseball players; and the patellofemoral articulation in cyclists.[40] Panush and Lane noted a 90% prevalence of abnormal knee radiographic findings in American football players at age 23.[39]

CHONDROMALACIA PATELLAE

Before discussing osteoarthritis in running, I would like to comment on chondromalacia patellae and patellofemoral arthralgia. Patellar pain in runners is usually due to patellofemoral arthralgia. Most do not have chondromalacia patellae, an intra-articular softening of the patellar cartilage; nor do they have more advanced osteoarthritis of the patellofemoral compartment. Many runners with patellofemoral pain have biomechanical abnormalities such as rearfoot or forefoot varus, abnormal patellar alignment, or excessive pronation. As with all disorders of the extensor mechanism of the knee, the pain is most notable when a patient squats, gets out of a chair, or climbs or descends stairs. In adolescents, increased patellar pressures may occur as a result of quadriceps inflexibility secondary to overly rapid bone growth. Lateral excursion secondary to a lax medial retinaculum, weak quadriceps, tight lateral stabilizing structures, or a flattened lateral femoral condyle may also contribute to patellofemoral arthralgia. Arthroscopic findings, however, do not reveal patellar cartilage abnormalities. Chondromalacia patellae should be suspected clinically, however, if a patient has excessive grating, popping, catching, locking, or giving way. A positive patellar inhibition sign does not help to distinguish chondromalacia patellae from patellofemoral arthralgia.[11, 41, 44]

RUNNING AND OSTEOARTHRITIS

Naturally occurring or experimental osteoarthritis affects many animals, including horses, sheep, rabbits, dogs, rats, and mice.[51] Reimann produced the partial changes of early osteoarthritis in rabbits 10 weeks after valgus angular osteotomy of the tibia.[48] He

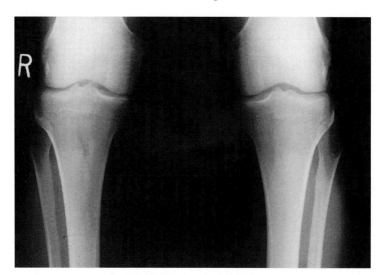

Figure 14–2

Narrowing of the medial compartment of the right knee in a 59-year-old, 6-foot 4-inch 230-lb (BMI = 28 kg/m²) low-mileage runner who presented with right knee pain, bilateral knee crepitance (right greater than left), and right knee effusion. He had had previous symptoms in his left knee and had quit running because of pain in his right knee.

concluded that alteration of the load bearing produced no radiologic or macroscopic changes of osteoarthritis. However, loss of metachromasia (proteoglycan decrease), fibrillation, and clefts with moderate subchondral sclerosis were found.

Subluxation may be the major factor in the development of knee osteoarthritis in dogs who have had rupture of the cranial cruciate ligament. Korvick and coworkers demonstrated subluxation of the knee in cranial cruciate ligament–deficient dogs.[26] Despite the animals' trying to reduce the load on the affected limb by carrying the limb in greater flexion, subluxation occurred in the stance phase. Studies by Videman[53] and by Kaiki and associates[22] address the effects of running on osteoarthritis produced by immobilization in rabbits and chemically induced osteoarthritis in rats. Videman showed that near maximal running in rabbits with immobilization-induced osteoarthritis was associated with no further progression of osteoarthritis than in controls. In the study by Kaiki and colleagues, two injections of 2% hydrogen peroxide produced worse osteoarthritis in running than in nonrunning rats. Nonrunning and saline-injected rats had no histologic evidence of osteoarthritis, compared with 14% of the one-injection running rats and 100% of the running rats who had two hydrogen peroxide injections.[22] The animal data are suggestive but not conclusive that running may have a negative effect on osteoarthritis in the biomechanically impaired or injured foot.

In 1975, Puranen and associates examined the radiographs of 74 former Finnish championship runners whose average age was 55 and who had begun running between the ages of 12 and 25 years.[45] The runners' mileages were not reported. Radiographs of the 74 runners compared with 115 controls revealed an incidence of 4% of radiologic changes of osteoarthritis in the athletes versus 8.7% in the controls. Three of the 60 runners examined did have "true osteoarthritis," with hip pain and radiologic changes. Puranen and associates concluded that repetitive strain does not contribute to the development of osteoarthritis. They concluded that "anatomically and physiologically, it is not strange that the hips of competitive runners should be spared osteoarthritis, for the hip is designed for walking and running, and motion is necessary for the nutrition of the cartilage. By intermittent compression and release, the synovial fluid enters and leaves the cartilage very much in the same way as air enters and leaves the lungs under alternating pressures. On the other hand, both prolonged immobilization and continuous pressure for only 6 days across the living, cartilage-covered joint surfaces produce ulceration and destruction of the cartilage."

In 1981, we reported knee effusions in 46 long-distance runners who had been running 1500 miles or more per year.[6] A positive bulge sign in one or both knees was noted in more than 25% of runners and 9% of the controls. All subjects were asymptomatic. Mileage of those with and those without effusions was not significantly different. A significant association was noted between the effusion and radiographic changes consistent with early osteoarthritis (i.e., prominent tibial spines). The report concluded that runners have transient asymptomatic effusions, which may be indicative of early degenerative disease or joint adaptation to running. Further study, including long-term evaluation of the effects of distance running on weight-bearing joints, will determine whether the observed effusions and radiographic findings are an age- or running-related phenomenon.

In 1983, McDermott and Freyne noted that 6 of 20 runners with knee pain had osteoarthritis.[35] Five of the six subjects with radiologic degenerative changes had clinical findings consistent with osteoarthritis, and all subjects had genu varum. A history of trauma was noted in 4 of the 6 runners, and 3 of the 14 nonosteoarthritic runners reported previous injury. A significant association was noted with genu varum, previous knee injury, and the number of years of running. Although they had no significant difference in their weekly mileage, the affected group ran 61.8 miles per week versus 41.2 miles per week for the unaffected group. Although they had no increased incidence of chondromalacia patellae, three of the six affected runners had patellar osteophytosis in addition to tibiofemoral compartment disease. Interestingly, only two of the six subjects agreed to reduce their mileage. One of the runners was quite instructive. He was a 37-year-old who was running 90 miles per week and had been running for 22 years. He had a history of a torn lateral meniscus of the right knee at age 26 years and had had a meniscectomy. On clinical examination, he was noted to have decreased flexion in his right knee, patellofemoral crepitus, and genu varum. His radiographs showed marked narrowing of the lateral compartment of the right knee and patellar and tibiofemoral osteophytes. Despite these abnormalities, the patient continued to train and compete. The researchers concluded that "the high incidence of trauma and genu varum in the affected group, both of which are recognized as predisposing factors to osteoarthrosis, suggest that running per se was not necessarily the main aetiological factor."

In 1985, Sohn and Micheli reported on a survey of former college varsity athletes, 504 varsity cross-country runners and 287 swimmers.[50] The follow-up was 2 to 55 years, with a mean of 25 years. The age ranged between 23 and 77 years. A similar incidence of severe knee and hip pain was noted in swimmers and runners. Hip pain was defined as none or mild, causing noticeable pain but not interfering with leisure or occupational activity;

and severe, requiring modification of daily living. Fifteen and one-half percent of the runners and 19.5% of the swimmers had mild or severe pain. Two and one-tenth percent of the swimmers and 0.8% of the runners had had surgery for relief of joint pain (four total hips in four runners and seven surgical procedures in six swimmers, including four total hip replacements). The researchers noted a similar degree of pain in all age groups and no differences in average mileage between those runners who complained of pain and those who did not. No significant differences in the years of running were noted between those who complained of pain and those who did not. The investigators concluded that there was no relationship between running and osteoarthritis but cautioned that the average mileage was 25 miles per week and the conclusion may not apply to high-mileage runners. However, because there were no differences between the mileage of the symptomatic versus asymptomatic runners, they stated that high mileage (50 to 140 miles per week) may not necessarily be associated with osteoarthritis.

In 1986, Lane and colleagues reported on 41 long-distance runners 50 to 72 years of age compared with 41 matched controls.[29] The male and female runners had 40% more bone mineral density than the controls. Female runners appeared to have more sclerosis and spur formation on the spine and weight-bearing knee radiographs but not on the hand films. No differences were noted between the groups in joint space narrowing, crepitation, joint stability, or symptomatic osteoarthritis. They concluded that running was not associated with clinical osteoarthritis. They also noted an increase in joint space width in the runners. They observed that 86% of women and 78% of men older than 65 years have radiographic evidence of osteoarthritis. They commented on a high incidence of first metatarsophalangeal asymptomatic osteophytosis in ballet dancers. They also noted the possible selection bias in this study (as in many others). Runners may be more resistant to osteoarthritis, and those with joint disability who had quit running before the study would not have been included.

In 1993, Lane and colleagues reported a 5-year follow-up (they had previously reported a 2-year follow-up in 1989)[28] of 33 of the original 41 runners reported in 1986, compared with 33 of the controls matched for age, years of education, and occupation.[31] The prospective nature of this study is an attempt to correct the study biases noted previously. During the 5-year period, one runner had quit running because of lower extremity joint pain, one had stopped because of a running injury, and two had quit because of illness. Both runners and controls had similar progression of osteoarthritis noted radiographically in their hands. Female runners had statistically significant increases in joint space narrowing on their 1989 versus 1984 knee radiographs. Controls had significantly increased osteophytosis and combined radiologic scores for sclerosis and joint space narrowing and spurs on their 1989 radiographs compared with their 1984 radiographs. The researchers noted that the scores for male runners were significantly changed as a result of spurring but not joint space narrowing. They noted no differences in radiologic progression of osteoarthritis in runners and controls and emphasized that osteophytosis alone without joint space narrowing or clinical evidence of pain or swelling and crepitus is not clinical osteoarthritis. The 1989 radiologic scores were best predicted by the 1984 radiologic scores. Excluding the 1984 radiologic scores, the best predictors for radiologic progression of osteoarthritis in the hands were older age, higher disability, and female sex. Higher 1989 knee scores were associated with older age, faster pace per mile, and greater weight. Older age in 1984 best predicted lumbar spine progression. Those who were older and taller had more knee progression, and male sex was associated with lumbar spine radiologic progression.[31]

Another retrospective study in 1986 by Panush and associates[40] compared 17 male runners (average age of 56 years) who had been running 28 miles per week for 12 years with 18 nonrunning controls. They found no differences in clinical or radiologic changes of osteoarthritis. Although no statistical differences were noted in the physical characteristics of the subjects, the runners were about 10 pounds lighter and 5 years younger than the controls. The researchers concluded that an average of 28 miles per week for longer than 10 years including marathons was not associated with clinical or radiologic osteoarthritis.[40] A preliminary 8-year follow-up of the originally studied runners indicates that 73% of the runners are still running.[39]

In 1990, Konradsen and colleagues[25] reported their results of a retrospective analysis of 27 Danish male runners who were still active and had been running for a median of 40 years, 12 to 24 miles per week. They included all male Danish orienteering runners who had qualified for county teams in the years 1950 through 1955. Thirty-three athletes fulfilled this criterion; three of them could not be located or had died. Three of the remaining original 30 runners were not running because of work or back pain and one as a result of osteoarthritis. The one runner who stopped running because of osteoarthritis had had bilateral hip replacements in 1980 and 1983 and had run until 1978. Six of the 27 runners had pain while running. When compared with 27 nonrunning controls, no differences were found radiologically or clinically. The investigators comment that their study eliminates selection bias because they started with county orienteers in the 1950s.

In contrast to these previous studies finding no association between osteoarthritis with running, Marti and coworkers reported in a retrospective analysis that runners had a significantly higher incidence of osteoarthritis of the hip than controls.[33] They examined 27 former elite long-distance runners and compared them with 9 former bobsled riders and 23 controls. Age and mileage run in 1973 (97 km per week) were predictive of degenerative joint disease of the hip in 1988. Pace rather than mileage alone was considered a significant factor. Runners had a statistically higher incidence of radiologic scores including subchondral sclerosis, osteophyte formation, and joint space narrowing. Four of the five runners with joint space narrowing had hip pain, and two of the four runners had quit running. All four joint space–narrowing abnormalities were in runners versus none in the bobsled riders and controls. Eight of the runners, none of the bobsled riders, and one control had osteophytosis. Runners had a statistically significant increased incidence of hip pain.

Ernst commented on the discrepancy between the Marti study and previous studies.[15] He noted that the patients in the Lane study were lighter and had relatively low mileage (229 minutes per week).[31] The runners in the Panush study were younger and had lower body weight.[40] He also noted in the Finnish study by Puranen's group[45] that the training mileage between 1930 and 1960 was much lower than that of the elite athletes of the 1970s. Marti and colleagues and Ernst conclude that high-mileage running cannot be excluded as a cause of osteoarthritis of the hip.

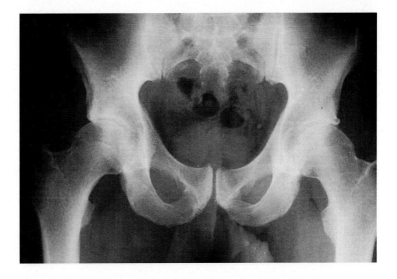

Figure 14–3

Severe joint space narrowing and subchondral sclerosis are present bilaterally, right worse than left, in a 47-year-old high-mileage, fast-paced physician runner who presented with a painful right hip and limited range of motion.

My own bias is that the European researchers may be correct. I attended three high-mileage, long-term runners (>40 miles per week for >10 years) with osteoarthritis of the hip. Severe joint space narrowing with osteophytosis was present in two runners, and osteophytosis with subchondral sclerosis was present in another. Although these runners are highly selected, it is difficult to discount the possibility that their high mileage may have contributed to their hip disease (Figs. 14–3 to 14–5).

SPONDYLOARTHROPATHIES

With the high incidence of injuries in runners, physicians should also be aware of the similarities between lower extremity soft tissue injury and the spondyloarthropathies. Although running is not a cause of these arthritides, they may be exacerbated by running. Ankylosing spondylitis or Reiter syndrome may be confused with running injury, and quiescent spondyloarthropathy may be activated by running activity.[43] I have not infrequently encountered young runners with hip, shin split, or heel pain (which was initially attributed to running) as a result of a spondyloarthropathy. In addition to these historical features, clinical clues may include a history of conjunctivitis, urethritis, or psoriasis; evidence of inflammatory synovitis or a sausage-shaped toe on physical examination; and radiographic evidence of sacroiliitis or osteitis pubis (Table 14–3).[43]

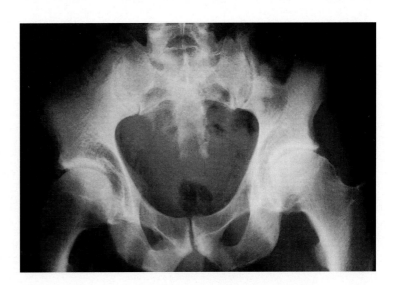

Figure 14–4

Severe joint space narrowing, subchondral sclerosis, and osteophytosis of the left hip in a 56-year-old runner insurance executive who presented with left hip pain, abnormal gait, and markedly restricted motion. The patient had run five marathons and three ultramarathons in the 6 months before friends remarked that he was limping.

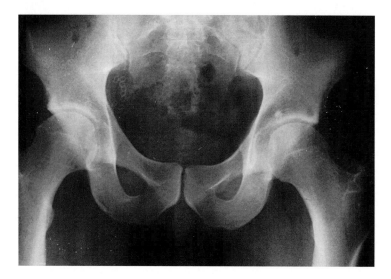

Figure 14–5

Osteophytosis and subchondral sclerosis are present in the right hip of a 32-year-old, 40 mile/week, 6.5 minute/mile training pace stockbroker who had reduced mileage and pace because of right hip pain.

TREATMENT

Treatment of runners with osteoarthritis differs from that of nonrunners with osteoarthritis because runners usually refuse to stop running.[35] To runners, a prescription to give up running to avoid injury is as logical as telling patients with pneumonia to give up breathing to avoid aerolized bacteria or viruses.[41] As with treatment modalities for nonarthritic runners, including high-quality shoes,[12, 37] orthotics when necessary,[20, 41] and warm-up and stretching exercises,[52] physicians must also advise arthritic runners on mileage. Nonsteroidal antiinflammatory drugs may be prescribed as for nonarthritic runners,[54] along with physical therapy directed at strengthening and improving flexibility,[21] but caution must be used in prescribing non-

steroidals for runners because symptoms may be masked[41] and reports describe possible accelerated progression of osteoarthritis in nonrunners who use these drugs.[13] A reduction in mileage below that which produces symptoms either during or after running, along with mild analgesics, is appropriate. I often encourage patients to substitute other aerobic activities such as swimming and exercise biking.[14] However, as noted previously, it is often next to impossible to convince runners to stop running activity completely.

CONCLUSION

Although the case is not closed, moderate running activity (≤25 miles per week) is not associated with osteoarthritis in a previously

TABLE 14–3 The Similarities Between Lower Limb Soft Tissue Injury and the Peripheral Presentation of Spondyloarthritis

	Common Soft Tissue Injuries of the Lower Limbs	Soft Tissue Involvement in Spondyloarthritis
Hip Girdle	Groin strains	Pelvic enthesopathies (adductor especially)
	Adductor, hamstring tendinitis	
	Symphysis instability	Symphysitis
Knee	Johansson-Sinding-Larsen	
	patellar ligament tendinitis	Enthesopathies of tibial tubercle and
	Osgood-Schlatter apophysitis	patellar poles
Hindfoot	Plantar fasciitis	Plantar fasciitis
	Achilles	Achilles
	Paratendinitis	Tendinitis
	Tendinitis	Enthesopathy
	Deep tears	Bursitis
	Sever apophysitis (os calcis)	
	Periosteal reaction due to stress fracture	Periostitis at or close to entheses

Adapted from Perry JD: Exercise, injury and chronic inflammatory lesions. Br Med Bull 48:668–682, 1992.

uninjured joint. High mileage (>40 miles per week) may be associated with the development of osteoarthritis in the hip or knee. Long-term prospective studies of high-mileage runners are needed.

REFERENCES

1. Alexander CJ: Osteoarthritis: A review of old myths and current concepts. Skel Radiol 19:327–333, 1990.
2. Allen ME: Arthritis and adaptive walking and running. Rheum Dis Clin North Am 16:887–914, 1990.
3. Altman R, Asch E, Bloch D, et al: Development of criteria for the classification and reporting of osteoarthritis. Arthritis Rheum 29:1039–1049, 1986.
4. Altman RD, Fries JF, Bloch DA, et al: Radiographic assessment of progression in osteoarthritis. Arthritis Rheum 30:1214–1225, 1987.
5. Anderson JJ, Felson DT: Factors associated with osteoarthritis of the knee in the first national Health and Nutrition Examination Survey (Hanes I). Am J Epidemiol 128:179–189, 1988.
6. Baker MD, Swafford D, Paty JG, Jr, et al: Knee effusions in long distance runners. Arthritis Rheum 24:561, 1981.
7. Brandt KD, Fife RS, Braunstein EM, et al: Radiographic grading of the severity of knee osteoarthritis: Relation of the Kellgren and Lawrence grade to a grade based on joint space narrowing, and correlation with arthroscopic evidence of articular cartilage degeneration. Arthritis Rheum 34:1381–1386, 1991.
8. Brandt KD, Slemenda CW: Osteoarthritis; Epidemiology, Pathology, and Pathogenesis. Primer on Rheumatic Diseases, 10th ed. Atlanta, Arthritis Foundation, 1993, pp 184–188.
9. Burke MJ, Fear EC, Wright V: Bone and joint changes in pneumatic drillers. Ann Rheum Dis 36:276–279, 1977.
10. Davis MA, Ettinger WH, Neuhaus JM, et al: The association of knee injury and obesity with unilateral and bilateral osteoarthritis of the knee. Am J Epidemiol 130:278–288, 1989.
11. Devereaux MD, Lachmann SM: Patello-femoral arthralgia in athletes attending a sports injury clinic. Br J Sports Med 18:18–21, 1984.
12. Dickinson JA, Cook SD, Lleinhardt TM: The measurement of shock waves following heel strike while running. J Biomech 18:415–422, 1985.
13. Doherty M, Jones A: Indomethacin hastens large joint OA in humans—how strong is the evidence? J Rheumatol 22:2013–2016, 1995.
14. Dorr LD: Arthritis and athletics. Clin Sports Med 10:343–357, 1991.
15. Ernst E: Jogging—for a healthy heart and worn-out hips? J Intern Med 228:295–297, 1990.
16. Genti G: Occupation and osteoarthritis. Baillieres Clin Rheumatol 3:193–204, 1989.
17. Glyn JH, Sutherland I, Walker GF, et al: Low incidence of osteoarthrosis in hip and knee after anterior poliomyelitis: A late review. Br Med J 2:739–742, 1966.
18. Hadler NM: Industrial rheumatology: Clinical investigations into the influence of the pattern of usage on the pattern of regional musculoskeletal disease. Arthritis Rheum 20:1019–1025, 1977.
19. Hamerman D: The biology of osteoarthritis. New Engl J Med 320:1322–1330, 1989.
20. Hicks JE, Leonard JA, Jr, Nelson VS, et al: Prosthetics, orthotics, and assistive devices. 4. Orthotic management of selected disorders. Arch Phys Med Rehabil 70:S-210–S-217, 1989.
21. Jokl P: Prevention of disuse muscle atrophy in chronic arthritides. Rheum Dis Clin North Am 16:837–844, 1990.
22. Kaiki G, Tsuji H, Yonezawa T, et al: Osteoarthrosis induced by intra-articular hydrogen peroxide injection and running load. J Orthop Res 8:731–740, 1990.
23. Kellgren JH, Lawrence JS: Radiological assessment of osteo-arthrosis. Ann Rheum Dis 16:494–501, 1957.
24. Kohatsu ND, Schurman DJ: Risk factors for the development of osteoarthrosis of the knee. Clin Orthop Rel Res 261:242–246, 1990.
25. Konradsen L, Hansen EM, Sondergaard L: Long distance running and osteoarthrosis. Am J Sports Med 18:379–381, 1990.
26. Korvick DL, Puanowski GJ, Schaeffer DJ: Three-dimensional kinematics of the intact and cranial cruciate ligament-deficient stifle of dogs. J Biomech 27:77–87, 1994.
27. Kujala UM, Kettunen J, Paananen H, et al: Knee osteoarthritis in former runners, soccer players, weight lifters, and shooters. Arthritis Rheum 38:539–546, 1995.
28. Lane NE, Bloch DA, Huberth HB, et al: Running, osteoarthritis and bone density: Initial two year longitudinal study. Am J Med 88:452–459, 1990.
29. Lane NE, Bloch DA, Jones HH, et al: Long-distance running, bone density, and osteoarthritis. JAMA 255:1147–1151, 1986.
30. Lane NE, Bloch DA, Wood PD, et al: Aging, long-distance running, and the development of musculoskeletal disability. Am J Med 82:772–780, 1987.
31. Lane NE, Michel B, Bjorkengren A, et al: The risk of osteoarthritis with running and aging: A 5-year longitudinal study. J Rheumatol 20:461–468, 1993.
32. Leadbetter WB: Cell-matrix response in tendon injury. Clin Sports Med 11:533–578, 1992.
33. Marti B, Knobloch M, Tschopp A, et al: Is excessive running predictive of degenerative hip disease? Controlled study of former elite athletes. Br Med J 299:91–93, 1989.
34. Matheson GO, Macintyre JG, Taunton JE, et al: Musculoskeletal injuries associated with physical activity in older adults. Med Sci Sports Exerc 21:379–385, 1989.
35. McDermott M, Freyne P: Osteoarthrosis in runners with knee pain. Br J Sports Med 17:84–87, 1983.
36. Menard D, Stanish WD: The aging athlete. Am J Sports Med 17:187–196, 1989.
37. Nigg BM, Herzog W, Read LJ: Effect of viscoelastic shoe insoles on vertical impact forces in heel-toe running. Am J Sports Med 16:70–76, 1988.
38. Panush RS: Does exercise cause arthritis? Long-term consequences of exercise on the musculoskeletal system. Rheum Dis Clin North Am 16:827–836, 1990.
39. Panush RS, Lane NE: Exercise and the musculoskeletal system. Baillieres Clin Rheumatol 8:79–103, 1994.
40. Panush RS, Schmidt C, Caldwell JR, et al: Is running associated with degenerative joint disease? JAMA 255:1152–1154, 1986.
41. Paty JG Jr: Diagnosis and treatment of musculoskeletal running injuries. Semin Arthritis Rheum 18:48–60, 1988.
42. Paty JG Jr: Running injuries. Curr Sci 6:203–209, 1994.

43. Perry JD: Exercise, injury and chronic inflammatory lesions. Br Med Bull 48:668–682, 1992.

44. Pretorius DM, Noakes TD, Irving G, et al: Runner's knee: What is it and how effective is conservative management? Physician Sportsmed 14:71–81, 1986.

45. Puranen J, Ala-Ketola L, Peltokallio P, et al: Running and primary osteoarthritis of the hip. Br Med J 1:424–425, 1975.

46. Radin EL, Eyre D, Kelman JL, et al: Effect of prolonged walking on concrete on the joints of sheep. ARA (abstracts), Arthritis Rheum 22:649, 1979.

47. Radin EL, Paul IL, Rose RM: Role of mechanical factors in pathogenesis of primary osteoarthritis. Lancet 1:519–521, 1972.

48. Reimann I: Experimental osteoarthritis of the knee in rabbits induced by alteration of load-bearing. Acta Orthop Scand 44:496–504, 1973.

49. Requa RK, DeAvilla LN, Garrick JG: Injuries in recreational adult fitness activities. Am J Sports Med 21:461–467, 1993.

50. Sohn RS, Micheli LJ: The effect of running on the pathogenesis of osteoarthritis of the hips and knees. Clin Orthop 198:106–109, 1985.

51. Sokoloff L: Natural history of degenerative joint disease in small laboratory animals. Arch Pathol Lab Med 65:118–128, 1956.

52. van Mechelen W, Hlobil H, Kemper H, et al: Prevention of running injuries by warm-up, cool-down, and stretching exercises. Am J Sports Med 21:711–720, 1993.

53. Videman T: The effect of running on the osteoarthritic joint: An experimental matched-pair study with rabbits. Rheumatol Rehabil 21:1–8, 1982.

54. Weiler JM: Medical modifiers of sports injury: The use of nonsteroidal anti-inflammatory drugs (NSAIDs) in sports soft-tissue injury. Clin Sports Med 11:625–643, 1992.

ELLEN J. COLEMAN

CHAPTER FIFTEEN
Nutrition and Running

In addition to heredity, proper nutrition and training are important for running success. Many runners who train hard to excel are defeated by their diets instead of their competitors. Although a balanced diet does not guarantee athletic success, an unbalanced diet can undermine training and competition.

Some runners try any dietary regimen in an effort to improve performance. The desire for the magic bullet may cause them to disregard sound nutrition practices and become victims of nutrition fraud. Unfortunately, nutrition misconceptions may hinder performance and ultimately even endanger health.

Runners can get the most out of their training by following the scientific nutritional practices outlined in this chapter. A brief discussion of fuel use precedes the sections that discuss the nutritional requirements of running. Specific dietary recommendations are provided in these sections to enable runners to perform closer to their potential.

DETERMINANTS OF FUEL USE

Factors that determine fuel use during running include exercise intensity, exercise duration, training status, and dietary composition.[15]

Exercise energetics dictate that carbohydrates are the preferred fuel for high-intensity work. Muscle glycogen supplies nearly all of the energy during a hard workout (>75% $\dot{V}O_2$max). The use of muscle glycogen is most rapid during the early stages of exercise and is exponentially related to exercise intensity.

Fat can be used for fuel up to about only 60% of $\dot{V}O_2$max. Fatty acids from intramuscular triglycerides and adipose supply about half of the energy during exercise of low to moderate intensity (40% to 60% of $\dot{V}O_2$max). Muscle glycogen and blood glucose supply the rest.

Because the oxidation of fat cannot supply energy quickly, muscle glycogen use during intense exercise is an obligatory requirement. The oxidation of carbohydrate also produces more energy per liter of oxygen (5.1 kcal) than does the oxidation of fat (4.62 kcal). This is advantageous during intense exercise, because oxidation of carbohydrate produces lower cardiovascular stress than does oxidation of fat.

As the duration of exercise increases, the intensity must decrease because of the limited supply of stored glycogen. When muscle glycogen stores are low, fat breakdown supplies most of the energy needed for exercise. However, a certain level of carbohydrate breakdown is necessary for fat to be used continuously for energy. To this extent, "fat burns in a carbohydrate flame."

Muscle glycogen is the predominant fuel for running. Most individuals do not run long enough to burn significant amounts of fat as fuel during the exercise itself. Also, many runners train at an exercise intensity of 70% of $\dot{V}O_2$max or above, and thus the use of fat as fuel is limited.

Endurance training increases the $\dot{V}O_2$max and blood lactate threshold, thus allowing runners to perform more aerobically at the same absolute level of exercise. Such training also increases the muscles' capillary density and mitochondrial density, increasing fat oxidation. A higher $\dot{V}O_2$max, blood lactate threshold, and greater fat oxidation enable a runner to use more fat and less glycogen at the same absolute level of exercise.

This glycogen-sparing effect of fat use is advantageous during prolonged exercise because muscle glycogen stores are limited and fat stores are abundant. Endurance training also increases the capacity of the muscles to store glycogen. Untrained individuals have muscle glycogen stores that are approximately 80 to 90 mmol/kg. Trained runners have muscle glycogen stores of 130 to 135 mmol/kg. Endurance training confers a dual performance advantage—the muscle glycogen stores are higher at the onset of exercise and the runner depletes them at a slower rate.

The percentages of carbohydrate and fat in the diet also determine fuel use. A high-carbohydrate diet increases muscle glycogen use. A high-fat diet increases fat use. However, a high-fat diet reduces a runner's ability to sustain high-intensity exercise and decreases endurance owing to low muscle glycogen stores.

RECOMMENDED TRAINING DIET

Building up and maintaining glycogen stores during training requires a carbohydrate-rich diet. Although many runners know the benefits of increasing their muscle glycogen stores before an endurance event, few pay attention to the carbohydrate content of their diet during training. Glycogen depletion can occur over repeated days of heavy training when carbohydrate consumption is inadequate. The feeling of sluggishness associated with muscle glycogen depletion is often referred to as *staleness* and blamed on overtraining.

Glycogen synthesis was evaluated on a 45% carbohydrate diet during three successive days of running 16.1 km at 80% of $\dot{V}o_2max$.[6] Preexercise muscle glycogen levels were approximately 110, 88, and 66 mmol/kg on each of the 3 days. Thus, when adequate carbohydrate is not consumed on a daily basis between training sessions, the preexercise muscle glycogen content gradually declines and training or competitive performance may be impaired.

A diet providing 525 to 648 g of carbohydrate promotes glycogen synthesis of 70 to 80 mmol/kg and provides near maximal repletion of muscle glycogen within 24 hours.[7] This corresponds to a carbohydrate intake of 8 to 10 g/kg daily.

High carbohydrate intake enhances recovery from prolonged exercise. Runners who consumed 8.8 g/kg/day of carbohydrate after a 90-minute run were able to equal their running performance on the next day.[12] The running times of those who consumed only 5.8 g/kg/day of carbohydrate decreased by more than 15 minutes. Runners who train exhaustively on successive days must consume adequate carbohydrate to minimize the threat of chronic fatigue associated with the cumulative depletion of muscle glycogen.

A 1991 review of the literature questions the belief that insufficient dietary carbohydrate during heavy training causes reduced muscle glycogen with subsequent fatigue.[35] However, it is well established that low blood glucose and muscle or liver glycogen concentrations can contribute to fatigue during endurance exercise. Because dietary carbohydrate is necessary for the maintenance of bodily carbohydrate reserves, it makes sense to recommend a high-carbohydrate diet. It is also prudent to watch for signs of staleness and take note of runners whose dietary habits make them more prone to glycogen depletion.

Muscle glycogen stores can be maintained by a carbohydrate-rich diet and periodic rest days to allow for glycogen restoration. Carbohydrate is essential for glycogen synthesis and should provide 6 to 10 g/kg daily (about 60% to 70% of total calories). The typical American diet provides about 4 g/kg (46% of total calories).

A diet containing 8 to 10 g/kg/day of carbohydrate (about 65% to 70% total calories) is recommended for hard workouts (70% of $\dot{V}o_2max$) lasting several hours or more daily. For workouts lasting an hour or less, a diet providing 6 to 7 g/kg/day of carbohydrate (about 60% carbohydrate) is sufficient to replenish muscle glycogen stores.

In addition to providing proper muscle glycogen stores, the diet should help to prevent chronic diseases such as cardiovascular disease and cancer. Both of these objectives can be met by following the 1995 Dietary Guidelines for Americans[37] and the Food Guide Pyramid.[36]

A diet providing 8 to 10 g/kg/day of carbohydrate may require that fat be reduced to 20% to 25% of total calories. A runner's sugar intake may be increased, but at least 50% of the calories should come from complex carbohydrates. Although there appears to be no difference in glycogen storage between complex or simple carbohydrates,[30] complex carbohydrates should be emphasized because they are more nutrient dense. Sugar is nutrient poor, and many sugary baked goods and candies are high in fat as well as sugar.

Some runners train so heavily that they have difficulty eating enough food to obtain the amount of carbohydrate needed for optimum performance. These individuals can use a commercial high-carbohydrate supplement. Such products do not replace regular food but are designed to supply supplemental calories and carbohydrate when needed. High-carbohydrate supplements should be consumed before or after exercise (e.g., with meals or in between meals). Their carbohydrate content (usually 20% to 24%) is too high for use as fluid replacement beverages during exercise.

CARBOHYDRATE LOADING

During endurance events that exceed 90 to 120 minutes (e.g., marathon running), muscle glycogen stores become progressively lower. When they drop to critically low levels (the point of glycogen depletion), high-intensity exercise cannot be maintained. In practical terms, the runner is exhausted and must either stop exercising or drastically reduce pace.

Muscle glycogen depletion is a well-recognized limitation to endurance exercise. Glycogen supercompensation techniques (carbohydrate loading) can nearly double muscle glycogen stores to 200 to 220 mmol/kg. The greater the preexercise glycogen content, the greater the endurance potential.

The classic study on carbohydrate loading compared the exercise time to exhaustion at 75% of $\dot{V}o_2max$ after 3 days of three diets varying in carbohydrate content—a diet with less than 5% carbohydrate, a diet with 50% carbohydrate, and a diet with 82% carbohydrate.[3]

The muscle glycogen stores on the low-carbohydrate diet (38 mmol/kg) sustained only an hour of exercise. The muscle glycogen stores on the mixed diet (106 mmol/kg) sustained 115 minutes of exercise. The muscle glycogen stores on the high-carbohydrate diet (204 mmol/kg) sustained 170 minutes of exercise.

The carbohydrate loading sequence eventually developed into a weeklong sequence. After an exhaustive training session 1 week before competition, the athlete consumed a low-carbohydrate diet for the next 3 days and tapered training. The athlete rested for 3 days before competition and ate a high-carbohydrate diet.

However, 3 days of reduced carbohydrate intake can cause hypoglycemia and ketosis with associated nausea, fatigue, dizziness, and irritability. The dietary manipulations also prove to be too cumbersome for many runners. Furthermore, an exhaustive training session the week before competition increases the risk of injury.

A revised method of carbohydrate loading eliminates many of the problems associated with the classic regimen.[33] Six days before competition, athletes run at 70% to 75% of $\dot{V}o_2max$ for 90 minutes. On that day and the next 2 days, they consume a normal mixed diet (about 4 g/kg of body weight). On the second and third days, training is decreased to 40 minutes at 70% to 75% of $\dot{V}o_2max$.

On days 4 and 5, athletes eat a high-carbohydrate diet (about 10 g/kg of body weight) and reduce training to 20 minutes at 70 to 75 of $\dot{V}o_2max$. On day 6, runners rest but maintain the high-carbohydrate diet. This modified regimen provides muscle glycogen stores equal to those provided by the classic carbohydrate-loading regimen.

Carbohydrate loading enables athletes to maintain high-intensity exercise longer but does not affect pace for the first hour of an event. Runners participated in a 30-k race after eating a normal or high-carbohydrate diet.[20] The high-carbohydrate diet provided muscle glycogen levels of 193 mmol/kg, compared with 94 mmol/kg for the normal diet. All runners covered the 30-k distance faster (by about 8 minutes) when they began the race with high muscle glycogen stores. Carbohydrate loading does not enable runners to start out faster, but they are able to maintain the same pace longer.

PREEXERCISE MEAL

Runners are often advised to eat 2 to 3 hours before exercise to allow adequate time for gastric emptying. Rather than getting up at daybreak to eat, many runners who train or compete in the morning simply forgo food before exercise. This overnight fast lowers liver glycogen stores by about 80% and can impair performance, especially if a person attempts to train or compete in a prolonged endurance event (over an hour) that relies heavily on blood glucose.

Although the preexercise meal does not contribute immediate energy, it can be beneficial when exercise lasts longer than an hour. The carbohydrate in the meal elevates blood glucose to provide energy for the exercising muscles. The meal may also prevent the feeling of hunger, which in itself may impair performance.

Runners are sometimes instructed to avoid high-carbohydrate meals immediately before exercising. The concern is that carbohydrate elevates blood insulin levels at the start of exercise, resulting in subsequent hypoglycemia and fatigue during exercise.[13] Actually, these insulin and glucose responses are transient and probably do not harm performance.[16] A few individuals, however, may be sensitive to lowering of blood glucose. Thus, a runner's response to the preexercise meal should be evaluated during training—not before competition.

Carbohydrate feedings before exercise can help to restore suboptimal liver glycogen stores, thus enhancing performance during prolonged exercise. If muscle glycogen levels are also low, the preexercise meal may increase them as well. If gastric emptying is a concern, liquid meals should be considered.

The pre-event meal should provide 1 to 4 g of carbohydrate per kilogram of body weight and should be consumed 1 to 4 hours before exercise.[32, 34] To avoid potential gastrointestinal distress, the carbohydrate content of the meal should be reduced as the exercise period becomes closer. For example, a carbohydrate feeding of 1 g/kg is appropriate an hour before exercise, whereas 4 g/kg can be safely consumed 4 hours before exercise.

Fat should be limited because it slows food transit time. Carbohydrates provide the quickest and most efficient source of energy and are rapidly digested. Fiber may need to be limited to avoid interrupting exercise for a bathroom stop, which is merely inconvenient during training but can be disastrous during competition. Above all, runners should choose familiar, well-tolerated foods.

Commercially formulated liquid meals satisfy the requirements for preexercise food. They are high in carbohydrate, are palatable, and contribute to both caloric intake and hydration. Liquid meals can be consumed closer to competition than regular meals owing to their shorter gastric emptying time. This may help to avoid precompetition nausea for individuals who are tense and have an associated delay in gastric emptying.

Liquid meals can also provide a convenient alternative to solid meals for athletes competing in ultramarathons and multiple running events. They may also be used for nutritional supplementation during heavy training when caloric requirements are extremely high. Liquid meals supply a significant amount of calories and contribute to satiety.

CARBOHYDRATE INTAKE DURING EXERCISE

Carbohydrate feedings during endurance exercise lasting longer than 60 to 90 minutes may enhance endurance by providing glucose for the muscles to use when their glycogen stores have dropped to low levels. As the muscles run out of glycogen, they take up more blood glucose, placing a drain on the liver glycogen stores.

The longer the exercise session, the greater the use of blood glucose by the muscles for energy. Although a few runners experience central nervous system symptoms typical of hypoglycemia (dizziness, nausea, confusion, and partial blackout), most note local muscle fatigue and have to reduce their exercise intensity.

The improved performance associated with carbohydrate feedings is probably related to the maintenance of blood glucose levels. Dietary carbohydrate supplies glucose for the muscles at a time when their glycogen stores are diminished. Thus, carbohydrate use (and therefore energy production) can continue at a high rate and endurance is enhanced.

The benefits of carbohydrate feedings were first demonstrated during strenuous prolonged bicycling. During the ride without carbohydrate, fatigue occurred after 3 hours and was preceded by a decline in blood glucose.[8] During the ride with carbohydrate feedings, blood glucose levels were maintained and the cyclists were able to ride an additional hour before becoming fatigued. Both groups used muscle glycogen at the same rate, indicating that endurance was improved by maintaining blood glucose levels rather than by glycogen sparing.

Running performances with and without carbohydrate feedings have also been evaluated. During a 40-k run in the heat, a carbohydrate feeding (55 g/hour) increased blood glucose levels and enabled runners to finish the last 5 k significantly faster compared with the run without carbohydrate.[22] In a treadmill run at 80% of $\dot{V}O_2$max, the run with carbohydrate (35 g/hour) was 23 minutes longer (115 minutes) than the run without carbohydrate (92 minutes).[39]

Runners should consume 30 to 60 g of carbohydrate every hour to improve endurance.[9] Liquid carbohydrate feedings encourage the consumption of water needed to maintain hydration during exercise. During exercise, carbohydrate and fluid requirements can be met simultaneously by drinking 600 to 1200 ml/hour of drinks containing 4% to 8% carbohydrate.[1]

The performance benefits of a preexercise carbohydrate feeding appear to be additive to those of consuming carbohydrate during exercise. Cyclists who received carbohydrate both 3 hours before and during exercise were able to exercise longer (289 minutes) than when receiving carbohydrate either before exercise (236 minutes) or during exercise (266 minutes).[41]

It is important to note that the improvement in performance with preexercise carbohydrate feeding is less than when smaller quantities of carbohydrate are consumed during exercise. Therefore, if the goal is to provide a continuous supply of glucose during exercise, runners should consume carbohydrate during exercise.

CARBOHYDRATE FEEDINGS AFTER EXERCISE

An evaluation of glycogen repletion after exercise has demonstrated that the period in which carbohydrate is consumed is also important. Delaying carbohydrate intake for too long after exercise reduces muscle glycogen storage and impairs recovery.

When carbohydrate was consumed immediately after cycling exercise, muscle glycogen synthesis was 15 mmol/kg after 2 hours.[17] When the carbohydrate feeding was delayed for 2 hours, muscle glycogen synthesis fell to 5 mmol/kg. By 4 hours after exercise, total muscle glycogen synthesis for the delayed feeding was still 45% slower than that for the feeding given immediately after exercise.

Runners should consume 1.5 g of carbohydrate per kilogram of body weight within 30 minutes of exercise, followed by additional 1.5 g/kg feedings every 2 hours thereafter.[18] Replenishing muscle glycogen stores after exercise is particularly beneficial for individuals who train hard several times a day. This enables them to get the most out of their second workout.

Runners may have impaired muscle glycogen synthesis after unaccustomed exercise that results in muscle damage and delayed onset of muscle soreness (e.g., downhill running). The muscular responses to such exercise appear to decrease both the rate of muscle glycogen synthesis and the total muscle glycogen content. Although a diet providing 8 to 10 g of carbohydrate per kilogram of body weight usually replaces muscle glycogen stores within 24 hours, the damaging effects of unaccustomed exercise significantly delay muscle glycogen repletion.[31] Furthermore, normalization of muscle glycogen stores does not guarantee normal muscle function after unaccustomed exercise.

HYDRATION BENEFITS AND RECOMMENDATIONS

Consuming cool fluids at regular intervals during exercise is vital for safeguarding health and for optimizing athletic performance. It is well established that during prolonged exercise in the heat, sweat losses constituting as little as 2% of body weight impair athletic performance and temperature regulation.[25] Inadequate fluid intake speeds up dehydration and can ultimately cause a life-threatening heat illness.

At rest, runners need at least 2 liters of fluid daily. Consuming fluids before exercise appears to reduce or delay the detrimental effects of dehydration. The American College of Sports Medicine (ACSM) recommends that individuals prepare for exercise in the heat by drinking 500 ml of fluid 2 hours before exercise.[1] Such hyperhydration helps to lower the body's core temperature and reduce the added stress that heat places on the cardiovascular system.

Drinking during exercise is essential to prevent the detrimental effects of dehydration on body temperature and exercise performance. Runners should drink 150 to 350 ml of cool fluid every 15 to 20 minutes during exercise to replace sweat losses.[1] The actual amount consumed during exercise varies based on the rate of dehydration. The ACSM emphasizes that athletes perform at their best when their fluid intake closely matches their fluid loss from sweating.

There is no safe level of dehydration that can be tolerated before cardiovascular function and temperature regulation are compromised. Fluid replacement was varied to evaluate the effect of different degrees of dehydration on body temperature, heart rate, and stroke volume during 2 hours of cycling in a warm environment.[23] The amount of dehydration that occurred after exercise was the major factor causing elevated body temperature and cardiovascular stress. The loss of every liter of water (about 1.4% of body weight) caused heart rate to be elevated by 8 beats per minute, cardiac output to decline by 1 L/min, and core temperature to increase by 0.3°C.

Inadequate fluid intake is the primary obstacle to fluid replacement. Thirst is not an adequate guide, because runners replace only about 50% of their fluid losses during exercise.[25] Runners can dehydrate by 2% to 6% of their body weight during exercise in the heat despite the availability of fluids.[1] Thus, fluid intake must be regulated by drinking according to a schedule rather than by the perception of thirst.

Runners should weigh before and after exercising (preferably nude) to determine how much fluid they are losing. They should drink 500 ml of fluid for every pound lost.[1] Runners who gradually lose weight during hot weather training may be experiencing chronic dehydration rather than fat loss. Dark-colored urine may also indicate a dehydrated state.

Enhancing the palatability of the fluid replacement beverage is one way to improve the match between fluid intake and sweat losses. In general, fluids that are sweetened, flavored, and cooled to between 15°C and 21°C stimulate fluid intake.[1] Another important consideration is the rate at which the fluid is emptied from the stomach and absorbed from the intestines into the blood. To prevent dehydration, the fluid must be rapidly absorbed.

The gastric emptying rate is influenced by the volume, temperature, and composition of the ingested fluid and by exercise intensity. Of the factors that influence gastric emptying, the glucose concentration and volume of the drink have the greatest impact.[1] The greater the volume of the drink, the greater the gastric emptying rate. However, the rate of gastric emptying is slowed proportionately with increasing glucose concentration above 8%.

Once ingested fluid moves into the intestine, water can be absorbed from the intestine into the blood. The addition of carbohydrate to the beverage enhances intestinal absorption of water. Intestinal absorption of water and 6% and 10% carbohydrate solutions was measured via a multilumen catheter placed in the small intestine during bicycle exercise.[14] The 6% solution was absorbed faster than water, which was absorbed faster than the 10% solution. The 10% solution resulted in fluid secretion into the intestine and gastrointestinal distress.

Carbohydrate's primary role in fluid replacement drinks, however, is to maintain blood glucose concentration and enhance carbohydrate oxidation.[1] Carbohydrate feedings enhance performance during exercise that lasts longer than an hour, especially when muscle glycogen stores are low. Fluid replacement and carbohydrate ingestion independently improve high-intensity exercise lasting an hour, and these beneficial effects are additive.[2] However, water remains an effective and inexpensive fluid replacement beverage for exercise lasting less than an hour.

For optimum absorption and performance, the fluid replacement beverage should contain 4% to 8% carbohydrate in the form of glucose, sucrose, or maltodextrins.[1] Fructose should not be the predominant carbohydrate because it is converted too slowly to glucose to be readily oxidized and thus does not improve performance. Fructose may also cause gastrointestinal distress.

ELECTROLYTES

Sweating results in electrolyte losses (particularly sodium) as well as water losses. However, water losses during sweating are proportionately greater than electrolyte losses, and thus the body's cells actually end up with a greater electrolyte concentration.[26] Also, as runners become acclimated to the heat, the sodium content of sweat decreases.

Runners' electrolyte needs can generally be met by consuming a balanced diet. Although sodium is the major electrolyte lost in sweat, the American diet provides an abundance of salt. The loss of 1 g of sodium, which occurs with a 2-pound sweat loss, can easily be replaced by moderate salting of food. One-half teaspoon of salt supplies 1 g of sodium.

Electrolyte deficits (especially sodium) may occur under several conditions—when acclimating to a hot environment, after repeated workouts in hot weather, and during ultraendurance events such as 50-mile runs.[26]

Consuming only plain water during ultraendurance runs can cause hyponatremia. Sodium losses in sweat during endurance events can be considerable, and consuming only water or low-sodium beverages reduces the amount of sodium left in the blood.[26]

Although heat illnesses are more common, runners should know that hyponatremia may occur during ultraendurance exercise.

Consuming beverages containing sodium during prolonged exercise reduces the risk of hyponatremia. The sodium in such drinks also encourages fluid intake because it makes the drink more palatable. The ACSM recommends that drinks consumed during exercise lasting longer than an hour contain 500 to 700 mg of sodium per liter to enhance palatability and prevent hyponatremia.[1]

PROTEIN

Although carbohydrate and fat provide most of the energy during endurance exercise, protein use may be increased when the body stores of glycogen and glucose are diminished. In this regard, endurance exercise may be comparable to a state of starvation. Protein may contribute as much as 15% of the energy during prolonged exercise.[40]

Leucine, isoleucine, and valine are the primary amino acids oxidized for energy during endurance exercise. These branched-chain amino acids are also important nitrogen sources for alanine, which may be converted to glucose by the liver via the alanine-glucose cycle.

Adequate dietary carbohydrate before and during endurance exercise provides a significant protein-sparing effect by maintaining muscle glycogen levels. When muscle glycogen stores are high, protein use decreases to about 5%.[40] Although protein catabolism may predominate during exercise, protein synthesis is enhanced in the recovery period that follows. Regular training also seems to increase the effectiveness of the protein synthesis that occurs during recovery.

Runners should consume 1.2 g/kg of protein daily and may benefit from as much as 1.4 g/kg during prolonged endurance exercise.[21] Increased protein intake appears to be more important during the early phase of training than later in the training program. Endurance athletes initially need more protein to support increases in myoglobin, aerobic enzymes in the muscle, and red blood cell formation.[40]

Runners can easily meet their protein requirements with diet.[40] The average American consumes about 100 g of protein per day (70% from animal sources, which contain all the essential amino acids), for a total protein intake of about 1.4 g/kg of body weight. A well-balanced vegetarian diet can easily supply enough protein as long as the protein sources are varied and the athlete eats enough calories during the day. Furthermore, runners consume more protein when their caloric intake increases as a result of training.

Runners can obtain 1.2 to 1.4 g/kg of protein with a diet providing 12% to 15% of calories as protein. This amount of protein is consistent with the dietary recommendations for runners—for example, 60% to 70% carbohydrate, 12% to 15% protein, and 20% to 30% fat.

The guidelines for protein assume that a runner is consuming sufficient calories. Protein requirements increase when caloric intake is reduced to maintain a low body weight for performance reasons.[40] When runners fulfill their caloric requirements, they generally take in enough protein.

FAT

Americans typically eat about 37% of their calories as fat—an amount that has been linked to cardiovascular disease, cancer, and obesity. Dietary fat also displaces carbohydrate in the diet and decreases carbohydrate intake. Because muscle glycogen stores cannot be adequately maintained on a low-carbohydrate diet, training and competitive performance may be jeopardized.

Although there is no performance advantage to excess body fat stores or a high-fat diet, there is a performance advantage when fat use is increased through endurance training. The ability to use fat spares muscle glycogen and improves endurance.[15]

Although nutritional strategies to improve endurance usually focus on increasing muscle glycogen stores before exercise, several popularized studies have led some runners to try fat loading in place of carbohydrate loading.

Cyclists were fed a high-fat diet (85% fat) for 4 weeks to evaluate muscle glycogen use and performance.[29] After adaptation to the high-fat diet, muscle glycogen use fell fourfold and glucose use fell threefold on the ride to exhaustion. Fat use rose to make up the difference. However, the exercise time to exhaustion at 63% of $\dot{V}O_2max$ was not significantly different compared with a diet providing 50% carbohydrate. Therefore, adaptation to a high-fat diet did not provide any endurance benefit.

Another study of dietary fat and running performance continues to promote the fallacy that high-fat diets enhance endurance. Running time to exhaustion at 75% to 85% $\dot{V}O_2$max was significantly longer after a high-fat diet (91 minutes), compared with a normal diet (69 minutes) and high-carbohydrate diet (76 minutes).[24] The results of this study were considerably weakened because the order of the diets was not random. Also, the respiratory exchange ratio and blood glycerol response did not support the claim that the high-fat diet produced the improvement in performance.

Ultimately, the potential adverse health effects of a high-fat diet must be considered. Because exercise does not eliminate the health dangers of a high-fat diet, runners should follow current public health recommendations for total fat intake (30% or less of total calories) and saturated fat intake (10% or less of total calories).[37]

VITAMINS AND MINERALS

Many runners take vitamin and mineral supplements to enhance their performance or for nutritional insurance. The principal argument for vitamin supplementation is that exercise increases vitamin requirements. However, the vitamin requirements of runners are not significantly higher than those of sedentary individuals.[38] Also, vitamin supplements at levels exceeding the recommended dietary allowances (RDAs) do not improve the performance of well-nourished runners.[38]

The RDA is the daily amount of a nutrient that is scientifically judged to meet the nutrient needs of practically all healthy people. In general, the nutrient needs for an average person are only about two thirds of the RDA. As long as runners consume at least 67% of the RDA for a given nutrient, they are probably protected from a nutritional deficiency.

Although vitamin deficiencies can impair performance, it is unusual for runners to have such deficiencies. There is a linear relationship between calorie intake and vitamin intake—the more food eaten, the greater the vitamin intake.[38] Runners generally eat more than sedentary people and thus tend to obtain more vitamins in relation to their needs. However, individuals who limit their caloric intake to maintain a low body weight for performance reasons (e.g., female distance runners) can be at nutritional risk.[38] A

vitamin/mineral supplement supplying 100% of the RDA may be appropriate for these individuals.

Antioxidant vitamins (vitamin E, C, and betacarotene) purportedly reduce the amount of muscle damage caused by heavy exercise. Because the available scientific data are limited and equivocal, however, additional research is required before antioxidant supplement recommendations can be established.[19]

The Committee on Diet and Health (Food and Nutrition Board, National Research Council) recommends that people avoid taking vitamin supplements that exceed 100% of the RDA in any 1 day.[5] The toxicity of high doses (five times the RDA) of vitamins A and D is well established. Like fat-soluble vitamins, excess minerals are stored and can gradually build up to toxic levels. Even high doses (10 times the RDA) of water-soluble vitamins are not innocuous. Large doses of vitamin C can cause urinary stone formation and impaired copper absorption, and large doses of vitamin B_6 can cause sensory neuropathy.

Although runners (especially women) may have iron depletion, the incidence of iron deficiency erythropoiesis and iron deficiency anemia is small in the running population.[4] It is well established that iron deficiency anemia compromises endurance performance. However, iron depletion, the early stage of iron deficiency, is not associated with performance decrements.[4]

Women runners are much more likely to suffer from iron deficiency anemia due to menstrual blood losses and inadequate iron intake. However, running may increase iron loss in both genders through foot-strike hemolysis, losses in sweat, and gastrointestinal bleeding.[4] Runners at risk for iron deficiency, particularly menstruating women, should have their iron status checked routinely via measurements of ferritin, serum transferrin, and hemoglobin.

When iron supplements are given to runners with iron deficiency anemia, iron status is improved and so is running performance.[4] Iron supplements, however, do not improve the performance of runners with iron depletion.[4] Furthermore, excessive iron can interfere with the absorption of zinc and can cause iron overload in those individuals (2 to 3 individuals per 1000) who are genetically predisposed to hemochromatosis.

An adequate intake of calcium is an important nutritional strategy in the prevention of osteoporosis, particularly for women. The RDA for calcium for adolescents and young adults up to age 24 years is 1200 mg/day. For adult men and women, the RDA for calcium is 800 mg/day. Half of all adult women consume less than 500 mg of calcium per day.

The National Institutes of Health (NIH) suggests that the calcium needs of adult women are well above the recommended 800-mg level.[28] The NIH recommends that premenopausal adult women and women of any age on estrogen replacement therapy consume 1000 mg/day of calcium. Postmenopausal and amenorrheic women not on estrogen should consume 1500 mg/day.

Because estrogen deficiency is an important risk factor for the development of osteoporosis, amenorrhea may increase a runner's risk of stress fractures and early osteoporosis. Spinal bone density was found to be lower in amenorrheic runners than in eumenorrheic runners.[11] The amenorrheic group's bone density values at a mean age of 24.9 years were equivalent to those of women at a mean age of 51.2 years.

In a follow-up study, spinal bone density increased in the women who were previously amenorrheic but who had resumed menstruation.[10] However, their bone density remained well below the average for their age group, even 4 years after they resumed normal menses. Decreased spinal bone density appears to be more related to disturbances in ovulation than to either amenorrhea or exercise.[27]

Estrogen replacement therapy, weight gain, diet modification, and reduced training may be used to promote the resumption of menstruation. Because the female athlete triad is prevalent in endurance sports, runners who present with amenorrhea should also be evaluated for eating disorders.[27]

REFERENCES

1. American College of Sports Medicine: Position stand: Exercise and fluid replacement. Med Sci Sports Exerc 28:1, 1996.
2. Below PR, Coyle EF: Fluid and carbohydrate ingestion independently improve performance during 1 hr of intense exercise. Med Sci Sports Exerc 27:200, 1995.
3. Bergstrom J, Hermansen L, Hultman E, et al: Diet, muscle glycogen, and physical performance. Acta Physiol Scand 71:140, 1967.
4. Clarkson PW: Minerals: Exercise performance and supplementation in athletes. J Sports Sci 9:91, 1991.
5. Committee on Diet and Health: Diet and Health,
Implications for Reducing Chronic Disease Risk. Washington, DC, National Academy Press, 1989, p 17.
6. Costill DL, Bowers R, Branam G, et al: Muscle glycogen utilization during prolonged exercise on successive days. J Appl Physiol 31:834, 1971.
7. Costill DL, Sherman WM, Fink WJ, et al: The role of dietary carbohydrate in muscle glycogen resynthesis after strenuous training. Am J Clin Nutr 34:1831, 1981.
8. Coyle EF, Coggan AR, Hemmert WK, et al: Muscle glycogen utilization during prolonged strenuous exercise when fed carbohydrate. J Appl Physiol 61:165, 1986.
9. Coyle EF, Montain SJ: Benefits of fluid replacement with carbohydrate during exercise. Med Sci Sports Exerc 24(Suppl):S324, 1992.
10. Drinkwater BL, Bruemner B, Chesnut CH: Menstrual history as a determinant of current bone density in young athletes. JAMA 263:545, 1990.
11. Drinkwater BL, Nilson K, Chesnut CH, et al: Bone mineral content of amenorrheic and eumenorrheic athletes. JAMA 311:277, 1984.
12. Fallowfield JL, Williams C: Carbohydrate intake and recovery from prolonged exercise. Int J Sports Nutr 3:150, 1993.
13. Foster C, Costill DL, Fink WJ, et al: Effects of pre-exercise feedings on endurance performance. Med Sci Sports Exerc 11:1, 1979.
14. Gisolfi CV, Summers RW, Schedl HP, et al: Human intestinal water absorption: Direct vs. indirect measurements. Am J Physiol Gastrointest Liver Physiol 258:G216, 1990.
15. Gollnick PD: Energy metabolism and prolonged exercise. In Lamb DR, Murray R (eds): Perspectives in Exercise Science and Sports Medicine, volume 1. Prolonged Exercise. Indianapolis, Benchmark Press, 1989, p 1.
16. Hargreaves M, Costill DL, Fink WJ, et al: Effects of preexercise carbohydrate feedings on endurance cycling performance. Med Sci Sports Exerc 19:33, 1987.
17. Ivy JL, Katz AL, Cutler CL, et al: Muscle glycogen synthesis after exercise: Effect of time of carbohydrate ingestion. J Appl Physiol 6:1480, 1988.
18. Ivy JL, Lee MC, Broznick JT, et al: Muscle glycogen storage after different amounts of carbohydrate ingestion. J Appl Physiol 65:2018, 1988.
19. Kanter MM: Free-radicals, exercise, and antioxidant supplementation. Int J Sports Nutr 4:205, 1994.
20. Karlsson J, Saltin B: Diet, muscle glycogen, and endurance performance. J Appl Physiol 31:203, 1971.
21. Lemon PRW: Do athletes need more dietary protein and amino acids? Int J Sports Nutr 5(Suppl):S39, 1995.
22. Millard-Stafford ML, Sparling PB, Rosskopf LB, et al: Carbohydrate-electrolyte replacement improves distance running performance in the heat. Med Sci Sports Exerc 24:934, 1992.
23. Montain SJ, Coyle EF: Influence of graded dehydration on hyperthermia and cardiovascular drift during exercise. J Appl Physiol 73:1340, 1992.
24. Munio DM, Leddy JJ, Horvath PJ, et al: Effect of dietary fat on metabolic adjustments to maximal $\dot{V}O_2$ and endurance in runners. Med Sci Sports Exerc 26:81, 1994.
25. Murray R: Fluid needs in hot and cold environments. Int J Sports Nutr 5(Suppl):S62, 1995.
26. Murray R: The effect of consuming carbohydrate-

electrolyte beverages on gastric emptying and fluid absorption during and following exercise. Sports Med 4:322, 1987.

27. Nativ A: The female athlete triad. Clin Sports Med 13:405, 1994.

28. NIH Consensus Development Conference: Optimal Calcium Intake. Bethesda, MD, Office of Medical Application of Research and National Institute of Arthritis and Musculoskeletal and Skin Disease, 1994, pp 19–20.

29. Phinney SD, Bistian BR, Evans WJ, et al: The human metabolic response to chronic ketosis without caloric restriction: Preservation of submaximal exercise capacity with reduced carbohydrate oxidation. Metabolism 32:769, 1983.

30. Roberts KM, Noble EG, Hayden DB, et al: Simple and complex carbohydrate-rich diets and muscle glycogen content of marathon runners. Eur J Appl Physiol 57:70, 1988.

31. Sherman WM: Recovery from endurance exercise. Med Sci Sports Exerc 24(Suppl):S336, 1992.

32. Sherman WM, Brodowicz DA, Wright WK, et al: Effects of 4 hr preexercise carbohydrate feedings on cycling performance. Med Sci Sports Exerc 12:598, 1989.

33. Sherman WM, Costill DL, Fink WJ, et al: The effect of exercise and diet manipulation on muscle glycogen and its subsequent use during performance. Int J Sports Med 2:114, 1981.

34. Sherman WM, Peden MC, Wright DA: Carbohydrate feedings 1 hr before exercise improves cycling performance. Am J Clin Nutr 54:866, 1991.

35. Sherman WM, Wimer GS: Insufficient dietary carbohydrate during training: Does it impair athletic performance? Int J Sports Nutr 1:28, 1991.

36. US Department of Agriculture and US Department of Health and Human Services: Food Guide Pyramid: A guide to daily food choices, Washington, DC, US Government Printing Office, 1992.

37. US Department of Agriculture and Department of Health and Human Services: Nutrition and Your Health: Dietary Guidelines for Americans, 4th ed. Washington, DC, US Government Printing Office, 1995.

38. Van Der Beek EJ: Vitamin supplementation and physical exercise performance. J Sports Sci 9:77, 1991.

39. Wilber RL, Moffatt, RJ: Influence of carbohydrate ingestion on blood glucose and performance in runners. Int J Sports Nutr 2:317, 1993.

40. Williams MH: The role of protein in physical activity. In Nutrition for Fitness and Sport, 4th ed. Dubuque, William C Brown Communications, 1995, p 158.

41. Wright DA, Sherman WM, Dernbach AR: Carbohydrate feedings before, during, or in combination improves cycling performance. J Appl Physiol 71:1082, 1991.

PAUL J. KIELL

━━━ **CHAPTER SIXTEEN**

Running and Mood Disorders

That running (or its equivalent) helps make for both a healthy body and soul is a truism known to poets and philosophers through the ages. About 2500 years ago, Plato, writing in *The Republic,* decried the remedies of his day: "Our present system of medicine," he contended, "may be said to educate diseases." The solution, he opined, would lie in educating the youth. He advocated that for the first 10 years, education should be predominantly physical and that every school should have a gymnasium and a playground where play and sport would be the entire curriculum. In so doing, enough health would then be generated and stored to make all medicine unnecessary.

Extending this philosophy to late first century, we have satirist Juvenal's prayer for a sane mind and healthy body ("mens sana in corpore sano").

Jumping to the seventeenth century, poet John Dryden ("To My Honor'd Kinsman, John Driden") penned:

By chase our long-liv'd fathers earn'd
  their food,
Toil strung the nerves and purified the
  blood:
But we, their sons, a pamper'd race of
  men,
Are dwindled down to three score years
  and ten.
Better to hunt in fields for health
  unbought
Than fee the doctor for a nauseous
  draught.
The wise for cure on exercise depend;
God never made his work for man to
  mend.

The intuitive prescient thoughts of philosophers and poets have been vindicated through the epidemiologic studies of Paffenbarger and associates, whose contributions have been legion, the most recent attesting to the value of vigorous exercise in terms of both quality of life and life span.[29, 44, 46]

A century ago, the poet/philosopher Thoreau, who is our case study here, had a few things to say about exercise not only for the body but also for the soul and mind, proclaiming the unity of body, mind, and soul:

I never feel that I am inspired unless my body is also. They are fatally mistaken who think while they strive with their minds that they may suffer their bodies to stagnate in luxury and sloth. The body is the first proselyte the soul makes. The whole duty of man may be expressed in one line . . . make to yourself a healthy body.

(Thoreau: From his *Journal,* June 21, 1840)

Reviewing medical literature through the early 1990s, Anthony[2] documented the salutary effect of exercise on psychologic states such as anxiety, depression, and coronary-prone behavior, which have indeed been helped by regular aerobic exercise. Exercise, according to his medical literature review, seems to elevate mood and increase intellectual function, including self-concept.[2]

Physicians can more effectively motivate patients by following certain psychologic principles to obtain compliance and adherence. Physicians should also be role models. An exercise program should be individualized, convenient, and fun. Excessive exercise, however, can lead to states of stress (e.g., exercise addiction and burnout).[2]

First, then, does exercise truly help, and what psychologic benefits can be earned? If exercise does work, what is the physiologic rationale supporting the exercise prescription? What is the right dose? What are the possible side effects of overdose? Finally, what are those psychologic principles underlying a physician's prescription that can lead to a unifying theory of why running benefits the soul?

BENEFITS OF EXERCISE

Greist and colleagues were among the first to hint at the restorative effect of running for those with mild to moderate mood depressions.[22, 23] They randomly assigned 18 depressed people to a running group or to a group that used two kinds of time-limited conventional forms of psychotherapy. The running group exercised for 12 weeks; another group underwent traditional forms of psychotherapy. After the 12 weeks, those in the running group and those in the psychotherapy group were significantly improved, and the improvement in the running group was superior to one of the traditional psychotherapies and equal to the other.[22, 23]

More importantly, only one person from the running group returned for treatment a year later, compared with half the psychotherapy subjects.[22, 23] Furthermore, in the general population, this form of treatment is most effective for those with mild to moderate depressions. In that general subgroup, the antidepressant drugs usually have less effect than they do with those with more severe depressions, so the economics are obvious. (It is emphasized later that most of the studies of depression are confined to the mildly to moderately depressed population.)

As for the economics, even earlier, deVries demonstrated that exercise was comparable to meprobamate, a muscle relaxer, in reducing muscle tension, as measured by electromyographic testing.[16] The rationale is that the best way to relax muscles is to exhaust them through exercise.

Around the same time as Greist, Brown and his group showed that the more vigorous activities from running at one extreme to softball at the other extreme produced the best results in depression.[8] Their study included 167 subjects, high-school and university students. Six did not exercise and were the controls. Activities were softball, wrestling, jogging, and tennis, with at least 30 minutes of activity three times a week. On entering the study, all were given the Jung Depressive Inventory, the Eysenck Personality Inventory, and Human Figure Drawings.[8]

Significant reductions in depression were noted for those who jogged, played tennis, or wrestled but not for softball players or nonexercisers.[8]

In the second phase of the study, 561 university students made choices to jog three or five times a week or not to exercise at all. Testing was more comprehensive. Of 561 subjects, 101 were clinically depressed based on these pretests. Ten weeks later, a significant reduction in depression scores was noted for both depressed and normal subjects who exercised but not for depressed and normal subjects who did not exercise. Those who jogged the most had the greatest reduction in depression. The only fault with the study was that the subjects were not randomly assigned; rather, the most depressed chose the most vigorous exercise.[8]

About 5 years later, in a well-controlled study, 43 depressed women were randomly assigned to aerobic exercise or to a placebo group where relaxation exercise was practiced and to a no-treatment group as controls. After 10 weeks, those in the aerobic group showed greater improvement in aerobic capacity than those in the other two groups, and those in the aerobic exercise group had reliably lower depression scores than those in the other two groups. The effective treatment was achieved within the first 5 weeks. The second 5 weeks did not add substantially to the effect.[35]

Published about a year later was a study of inpatients with Diagnostic and Statistical Manual criteria for major depression, controlled for medication and psychotherapy, with patients randomly assigned to exercise or nonexercise groups. Mean reductions in Beck Inventory and comprehensive psychopathologic rating scale scores were greater in those who trained. In this study, compared with other studies, a one-to-one correlation between increase in $\dot{V}o_2$max and degree of improvement was observed. Furthermore, with the patients meeting the criteria for a major depression, this may be one of the few studies correlating vigorous exercise with improvement in a more severe type of depression.[34]

Critically reviewing the subsequent literature of 1985 to 1990, LaFontaine and coworkers point out that the studies differ widely on variables, such as the type of mood, the methods of comparisons, and the criteria.[28] Nevertheless, the great majority of the researchers of aerobic exercise and mood unanimously conclude that aerobic exercise vis-à-vis depression and anxiety are related in an inverse and consistent manner. Most researchers also consistently report that aerobic exercise affects the treatment of mild to moderate forms of depression and anxiety. In fact, several researchers thought that aerobic exercise was as effective as more traditional methods, and it was consistently reported that the increased benefits were greater in those who were more depressed and more anxious.

To be more specific, in anxiety states, Casper's review of the literature[11] on anxiety (an uneasy apprehension over impending or unknown ill or danger, more common in women) shows that in normal populations, exercise has been shown to have the most benefit on transitory or "state" anxiety (a subjective sense of apprehension associated with autonomic nervous system activation) as compared with much lesser relief of "trait" anxiety (a more stable and permanent disposition to experience anxiety).

Another consistent conclusion was that an increase in cardiovascular fitness was not necessary for mood enhancement,[28] even though some studies found a one-to-one relationship.[33]

Aerobic exercise is better than no treatment but not significantly different from other forms of therapy, including psychotherapy, in treatment of mood disorders.[9] Byrne and Byrne also conclude from their review that aerobic and anaerobic forms are equally effective. The results are restricted to patients with mild to moderate forms of unipolar depression. They found two studies showing that exercise does have a preventive effect on depression. In comparing exercise with medication, one study demonstrated that exercise and medication were no better than exercise alone. The second study showed that combined exercise and medication were superior to exercise alone, and although exercise does have an effect on unipolar depression, its value may be limited and may be more of a supplement.[9]

Others, too, have reviewed articles, summarizing the studies of depressed patients and physical activity.[33] Aerobic exercise, they conclude, is more effective than no treatment but not significantly different from other forms of psychotherapy. Aerobic and anaerobic forms are equally effective. Again, aerobic fitness is not necessary for improvement in mood, although some studies do indicate that aerobic exercise gives even better results than an-

aerobic.[33] For example, Martinsen and colleagues conducted their own study and found a one-to-one correlation between increase in $\dot{V}o_2$max and degree of improvement.[33]

Both aerobic and anaerobic exercise help lower scores on the Beck Depression Inventory. Martinsen and associates find in their review that most investigations are restricted to patients with moderate to mild forms of unipolar depression. Whether in outpatients or inpatients, males or females, or with ages ranging from 17 to 60 years, the trend is the same, showing the beneficial antidepressant effect associated with exercise in general.[34] Few well-conducted studies, however, show intervention in psychotic depression or melancholia.[33]

Experiments have addressed another aerobic sport, swimming. Berger and Owen studied 100 Brooklyn College students between the ages of 17 and 50 years who were novice and intermediate swimmers. The primary focus was on the short-term influence of swimming on the participants' mood. The swimmers swam twice a week for 40-minute sessions during a 14-week span. Swimmers felt better before and after the study than did controls in terms of depression, anger, vigor, confusion, and tension, but not fatigue. The Profile of Mood States (POMS) scale was used. Women had less tension, anxiety, depression, anger, and confusion to begin with. There were no gender differences in improvements.[6]

In another investigation, the mood-enhancing effects of swimming were compared with those of hatha yoga.[7] Eighty-seven college students formed two swimming classes; also included were yoga classes and a lecture control class. Each person completed mood and personality inventories before and after class on three occasions. Graded decreases in scores on anger, confusion, tension, and depression were found among the first two groups compared with the controls. In men, the immediate decreases in tension, fatigue, and anger after yoga were significantly greater than those with swimming. Women reported similar mood benefits after swimming and yoga.[7]

The researchers also reviewed articles showing that swimmers swimming either on uncomfortably warm days or in warm pools felt that extreme heat detracted from the mood benefits of swimming. They have concluded that, in general, the exercise must be of low intensity to obtain psychologic benefits. Hatha yoga involves a gentle form of stretching, balancing, and breathing routines. Both hatha yoga and swimming facilitate abdominal breathing, which in turn is included in many stress reduction techniques.[7]

At the risk of belaboring the point that aerobic fitness is not a sine qua non for mood enhancement, Doyne and group studied 40 women who were clinically depressed.[17] They were randomly assigned to 8 weeks of running (aerobic), weightlifting, or a wait-list control. Depression was monitored by the Beck Depression Inventory, Lubin's Depression Adjective Check List, and the Hamilton Scale for Depression. Both exercise modalities significantly reduced depression as compared with the controls, and the findings were that both types of exercise significantly reduced depression, with the results not dependent on achieving an aerobic effect.[17]

EXERCISE IN PREVENTION OF DEPRESSION

If exercise is good for someone whose emotional state—mood, if you will—is impaired, does it also have the property of preventing the malady? Camacho and associates[10] monitored 8023 nonhospitalized adults older than age 20 years, beginning in 1965, with data analyzed again in 1974 and again in 1983. They found that those who reported a low activity level at the onset were at a greater risk for depression in the first follow-up, compared with those who reported high levels of activity at baseline. This held after factoring in of possible confounding variables. Furthermore, the risk of depression at these three junctures can be altered by changes in exercise habits, but the associations, after adjustment for confounding variables, were not statistically significant. In fact, it seemed that of those who were chronically inactive and probably more at risk for depression, their inactivity was related more to their basic state of physical health.[10]

A question again is whether the benefits of physical activity hold also for more severe forms of depressive disorder. The beneficial association of physical activity seems again to apply only for the milder forms.[10]

In another study from their ongoing observation of Harvard Alumni ages 35 to 74 years, in a 23- to 27-year follow-up, Paffenbarger and colleagues found 387 first attacks of depression among 10,201 alumni and 129 suicides among 21,569 alumni surviving through 1988. Depression rates were lower among those physically active. Suicide, however, was unrelated to antecedent physical activity but was substantially higher among men reporting personality traits that predicted increased rates of depression.[45]

After the probable suicide of Meriwether Lewis (of Lewis and Clark), Thomas Jefferson wrote the following:

> Governor Lewis had, from early life, been subject to hypochondriac affections. It was a constitutional disposition in all the nearer branches of the family of his name, and was more immediately inherited by him from his father. They had not, however, been so strong as to give uneasiness to his family. While he lived with me in Washington I observed at times sensible depressions of mind; but knowing their constitutional source, I estimated their course by what I had seen in the family. During his Western Expedition, the constant exertion which that required of all the faculties of body and mind, suspended these distressing affections; but after his establishment at St. Louis in sedentary occupations, they returned upon him with redoubled vigour, and began seriously to alarm his friends.[7a]

Running may possibly have a role in the prevention of cancers as a byproduct of its beneficial effect on mood disorders. Shephard reviewed literature and found that occupational surveys and studies of recreational activity show an association between sedentary living and risk of colon cancer.[53] A more limited study suggests that a history of active leisure correlates with a reduced risk of all-cause cancer and, in women, of breast and reproductive system cancers. It does, however, portend an apparent increase in the risk of prostate cancer in active men.[53]

A study of five bereaved and severely depressed cancer patients with initial progression-free disease found that they had a tendency toward early onset of decreased natural killer cell activity and reduced binding affinity of β-endorphin to peripheral blood lymphocytes.[58] In another study of cancer patients, plasma levels of β-endorphin and mood depression were inversely correlated in cancer patients faring well clinically. Physical activities may counteract possible day-to-day depressive disorders, leading to speculation that for a definable subgroup of cancer patients, physical activities raise endorphin levels and psychologic well-being, both of which might modulate the activity of the immune-competent cells, leading to an extended period of progression-free disease.[58]

From all of the foregoing studies, it should be obvious that running (generic) helps certain types of mood disorders and tends to help prevent them. The recent mention here of β-endorphin[58] prompts the question of what are the physiologic underpinnings to this benefit? The reasons, however interesting, fascinating, or intriguing, perhaps are not yet as clear-cut as we would like them to be, but you be the judge.

PHYSIOLOGIC RATIONALE

As will be seen, surveys and experiments focus on exercise and the concomitant response of two classes of chemicals that exist in the brain and the rest of the body—endogenous opiates and the brain monoamines. Some brief background is necessary.

It has long been known that natural receptor sites for morphine existed in the neurons of the brain.[14] Scientists inferred from this that natural morphine-like chemicals existed within the central nervous system (CNS). They were first detected, inadvertently, when researchers were using a new technique to cut up animal pituitary glands to extract adrenocorticotropic hormone (ACTH). From this, new proteins other than ACTH were found. Later work isolated these substances, and depending on their peptide configuration, they were classified into one of three groups: the endorphins, the enkephalins, or the dynorphins.[14]

They fulfilled the definition of an opiate by their ability to inhibit stimulation of the vas deferens or myenteric plexus in guinea pigs. Also, the effect of endorphins on pain can be nullified by the opioid antagonist naloxone.[15]

The important substances to study are the endorphins and met-enkephalin, because both of their concentrations in plasma increase with exercise. (Enkephalin comes from *en-*, "in," and *cephalo-*, "head.")

β-endorphin is always coreleased with ACTH from the anterior pituitary in both rats and humans, and thus any stimulus that modulates the release of circulating ACTH similarly alters plasma β-endorphin. Both β-endorphin and ACTH are derived from a common molecule. β-endorphin is present in the cerebrospinal fluid (CSF) in higher concentrations than in the plasma. It poorly penetrates the blood-brain barrier. Endorphinergic neurons are found within the arcuate nucleus of the hypothalamus. Opiate receptors are found in the limbic system, the area thought to be the center of emotion, as well as the hippocampus, amygdala, cerebellum, medulla, and other parts of the brainstem.[24]

The endogenous opiates act as messengers within the CNS and as hormones in the peripheral circulation. The belief is that most circulating met-enkephalin originates in the sympathetic nervous system. Whether this is mediated through the endorphins is conjectural; some studies show that it is, and some that it is not. Opioid receptors are also located in the brainstem and carotid body, and these receptors have an inhibitory role in respiration at high-intensity exercise.[24]

Plasma and tissue levels of the endorphins are measured by radioimmunoassay. The important hormonal actions that have been identified are that they probably lead to elevations in circulating prolactin and growth hormones and may slightly stimulate the release of thyroid-stimulating hormone. Growth hormone and prolactin secretion is also stimulated by physical exercise. High concentrations of enkephalins are coreleased with catecholamines in the adrenal medulla.

One very important consideration vis-à-vis the body's own opiate system is that the neurotransmission function is largely inhibitory (e.g., inhibition of pain impulses). They have, however, an indirect stimulatory function on the pyramidal cells of the hippocampus, where they inhibit the inhibitory transmitters, thus producing a double-negative type of effect, resulting in stimulation.

Given this brief introduction to the body's intrinsic opiate system, what then is its response to running/aerobic exercise and what effect does that response, in turn, have on running and on the mood?

ENDORPHINERGIC RESPONSE TO RUNNING

LITERATURE REVIEW

The CNS studies of exercising rats consistently demonstrate an increase in enkaphalin in brain homogenates.[1] Obviously, there can be few if any such studies of humans. All of such studies of humans have been of peripheral venous blood samples in exercising subjects. For example, studies do show elevated levels of endorphins in venous blood samples from exercising subjects, particularly those in long, strenuous events such a marathons,[3] with largest elevations at descents in high mountain runs, where it was speculated that the heat loads encountered at drops in elevation in turn cause a change in permeability of the blood-brain barrier. A possible relationship between plasma and CSF is thus postulated.[3]

Other research shows similar blood plasma results.[25, 27] Some studies also show a decrease in resting plasma endorphin levels with training[3] and failure to increase—in fact a decrease—with resistance training.[36, 47] A positive correlation was found in another study, although the amount of exercise involved a maximum effort.[26]

The best indication of CNS stimulation of endorphins with exercise is probably derived from indirect circumstantial evidence. These studies involve the subjective responses, along with objective test responses, of exercisers given agents that block opiate receptors before, during, and after exercise. The responses are then compared with the responses of exercisers being given a placebo.

For example, in a double-blind crossover study of 12 recreational male runners, mood changes were tested before, during, and after treatment.[1] The subjects exercised 45 minutes once a week for 4 weeks. Intravenous naloxone was given before, during, and after, versus placebo. Dosage was important, and the researchers cite references of studies that failed to show a positive effect, presumably because lower doses of naloxone were administered.[1] Significant trends toward calmness were noted on the POMS scale and the Visual Analogue Scale in those administered placebo versus naloxone.[1]

The calmness was blocked by preloading with 5 mg of naloxone beforehand, then an intravenous drip of an additional 5 mg during the exercise. No changes were noted in anger scale score, possibly because it was at low range to begin with. The biggest change was in fatigue in the placebo group, with fatigue diminishing after 45 minutes of running on a treadmill.[1]

In another study of 13 women and 6 men, aerobic class participants ages 20 to 46 years were given naltrexone (another opiate receptor blocker) and placebo in randomized double-blind crossover on two separate occasions and in the same 75-minute high-intensity aerobics class. POMS was used along with a mood adjective checklist and a visual analog scale measuring mood in relation to several emotional changes. Using the placebo, mood states became calmer, more relaxed and pleasant, tending away from depression, anger, and confusion. Positive mood shifts did not occur when subjects were preloaded with naltrexone. This result again suggests that activity-generated mood changes are mediated—at least in part—through endorphinergic mechanisms.[15]

STIMULATION AND LOCUS OF ENDORPHINERGIC SYSTEM

Thoren's group, in reviewing the literature, proposes that prolonged rhythmic exercise can activate central opioid systems by triggering discharge from mechanosensitive afferent nerve fibers that are contracting in the skeletal muscles, particularly stimulation for 30-minute intervals of rats' sciatic nerves, activating these somatic afferents and in turn stimulating central mechanisms for activation of the opioid system. An increased pain threshold persisted long after the 30 minutes, and this increase in pain threshold could be blocked by naloxone, thus again offering circumstantial evidence for involvement of a central opioid system activated by stimulating the leg muscles.[56]

The β-endorphin system is involved with pain perception and the control of body temperature. Those particular fibers are found in the hypothalamic area, midbrain, and back of the medulla, the cell bodies of these fibers also being involved in the autonomic outflow.[56]

In the anterior pituitary, β-endorphin and ACTH are synthesized from a common precursor molecule. Both β-endorphin and ACTH are secreted in equivalent amounts from the anterior pituitary in response to exercise and other stressful stimuli. The researchers emphasize that the peripheral concentration of β-endorphin would not be expected to modify the central activity because of the poor penetration of the blood-brain barrier. Their hypothesis is that CNS opioids are activated by prolonged exercise. In animals in which the central effects could be studied, prolonged submaximal exercise—as contrasted to brief strenuous exercise—increased the brain β-endorphin content and increased the pain threshold.[56]

Further review of articles finds that rats trained to run spontaneously show an increase in β-endorphin concentration in their CSF.[1, 12]

As for endorphin blood concentration peripherally, review articles show an increase in peripheral blood endorphin concentration after exercise, but most of the plasma endorphin reflects pituitary corelease with ACTH in response to stressful stimuli rather than activation of a specific CNS β-endorphin pathway.[56]

ENDORPHINS: POSSIBLE LINK TO HEART DISEASE

The role of endorphins and the implications that regular exercise has a role in decreasing pain sensitivity prompt now a brief side discussion of symptomatic angina and silent ischemia. In a review of the literature, Droste found that patients with symptomatic and asymptomatic myocardial ischemia have significantly different plasma β-endorphin levels at rest and during physical exercise.[18, 19]

Elucidating further, Droste[18] notes from the literature that reduced sensitivity to pain is demonstrable after long-distance running, such as a marathon, and after intensive physical exercise on a laboratory ergometer. Elevation of the pain threshold is most pronounced during maximal exertion, and the hypoalgesia remains present after exercise is stopped, with the preexercise pain threshold returning about 1 hour after the exercise.[18, 19]

Droste believes that the plasma β-endorphin is not directly involved in the exercise-induced hypalgesia but is rather a marker for the activating of central analgesic mechanisms. The same stress-induced hypalgesia may also have a role in coronary heart disease, when the myocardial ischemia is silent, and patients with complete asymptomatic myocardial ischemia show a generalized hypalgesia demonstrable independent of exercise stimulus, indicating a central set-point change in the antinociceptive system.[18, 19, 30]

In one particular study of 45 patients with a history of coronary heart disease and documented myocardial ischemia during exercise testing, the investigators looked for the possible relationship between psychologic factors, such as depression and type A behavior, plasma and β-endorphin response, and pain during maximal exercise-induced ischemia.[29] The Minnesota Multiphasic Personality Inventory subscale was used to assess depressions. Type A behavior was evaluated in a structured interview. Ischemia was defined by the ST segment depression. Eighteen reported anginal pain. Those with high depression scores showed lesser increases in plasma and β-endorphin levels, tended to report more anginal pain, and rated pain more severe during exercise than those with the low depression scores.[29]

The hemodynamic response in severity of ischemia did not differ between depression groups, and depression was significantly associated with a lesser β-endorphin response among those who reported angina.[29] They also had earlier pain onset and greater pain duration and severity. Type A compared with type B groups showed no differences in pain, β-endorphin response, or measures of ischemia. The experimenters concluded that the depressed patients may have a blunted or absent β-endorphin response accounting for their anginal pain, given the preexisting ischemic heart disease.[29]

Elsewhere, the symptomatic, hemodynamic, and opioid responses of cardiac patients to exercise testing and a public speaking task were determined at rest and after stress. Nineteen of 50 had angina during exercise. Thirty-one of 50 had asymptomatic ischemia. None had angina during the speech; two had electrocardiographic changes, and 39% had radionuclide changes of ischemia. Patients with asymptomatic ischemia on exercise had a significantly greater β-endorphin response than those with angina. Public speaking actually evoked a larger β-endorphin increase "relative to change in double product" (an index of stress) than did exercise. Therefore, patients with silent ischemia seem to have a greater outpouring of β-endorphin relative to exercise than those with painful ischemia related to exercise. β-endorphin response to the stressor of speechmaking is greater than that to exercise (when controlled for an index in stress), and the increased β-endorphin response to a speech stressor may partially explain the silent ischemia during psychologic stress such as making a speech.[41]

As always, other researchers do not agree. In another study, endorphin plasma levels were similar in patients with both painful and silent ischemia. Naloxone infusion had no effect on anginal symptoms. It was suggested that endogenous opiates do not have an important role in modulating symptoms of myocardial ischemia and that the increase in β-endorphin is just part of the physiologic stress response coinciding with increase in plasma cortisol from the anterior pituitary's outpouring of ACTH.[32]

Nevertheless, pro or con, whatever the underlying physiology, depression is reasonable to anticipate in patients with myocardial infarction. The drugs that are commonly used in treating mood depressions react with the brain monoamines, another system involved not only in mood disorder but in an aerobic exercise such as running.

MONOAMINES

For a brief review, the brain monoamines are involved in neurotransmission (impulse from one neuron to another) and have been implicated in the pathogenesis and in the treatment of depression.

Chaouloff[12] cites studies having to do with brains of exercising rats, eschewing at the same time other studies involved with urinary metabolites of noradrenaline, dopamine, and serotonin because there is no evidence that urinary monoamine metabolite levels closely reflect central monoaminergic activity.[12]

Marked increases in CSF levels of homovanillic acid (HVA) were found in running rats. HVA is the metabolite of serotonin. The metabolism of dopamine, another neurotransmitter, is accelerated in running mice as compared with sedentary in terms of stress (e.g., acute treadmill exercise and exposure to cold). The areas where it is accelerated are the midbrain and to a lesser extent the frontal cortex and striatum. Also found has been an increase in the metabolite of dopamine in the hypothalamus of exercising rats.[12]

A preponderance of experimental investigations shows evidence that physical exercise affects the central dopaminergic systems with increased synthesis and metabolism. Dopamine is converted to noradrenaline (NA) by the enzyme dopamine β-hydroxylase. NA, in turn, is metabolized by various enzymes, among them a monoamine oxidase. Exercise tends to increase central NA synthesis and metabolism.[12]

All of the monoamines are broken down by monoamine oxidase, and the action of antidepressant drugs is either to inhibit the action of monoamine oxidase or to prevent resorption of the monoamine into the cell so that it remains at the synapse, where it facilitates transmission. (The neurotransmitters, in effect, "grease" the transmission of impulses.) Thus anything that increases the levels of the monoamines at the synapses (drugs, exercise) theoretically affects mood.

Another monoamine, serotonin, is the neurotransmitter regulated by a new family of drugs, (selective serotonin uptake inhibitors.) The breakdown metabolite of serotonin is 5-hydroxyindoleacetic acid (5-HIAA). Here too monoamine oxidase is involved. Exercise also accelerates this system in animals.[12]

Of note is the work of Post and colleagues in 1973, showing increases in lumbar CSF of 5-HIAA and HVA in depressed patients asked to participate in moderate exercise.[49] Patients were evaluated for depression and mania. Baseline lumbar punctures were performed, and 5-HIAA was measured before and after simulation of mania in the patients who were moderately depressed. They were asked to be hyperactive and hyperverbal; to run up and down corridors; to play Ping-Pong, tennis, and pool; to dance, sing, and tell jokes; and to do light calisthenics. Two other patients were asked only to be physically hyperactive and to make no attempt to imitate mania or manic mood. As a result, most of the patients experienced some mood elevation and regarded the experience as positive. Of those who simulated mania, the levels of CSF amine metabolites were higher than at bed rest, and the ones who were physically hyperactive also had elevated levels in the same order of magnitude as the patients who simulated mania. 5-HIAA and HVA were significantly elevated in the CSF. MHPG (the main metabolite of noradrenaline, 3-methoxy-4-hydroxyphenylethyglycol) levels increased, approaching but not reaching statistical significance because in one patient the results were the opposite.[49]

The depressed patients in this study had low levels of psychomotor activity and the lowest CSF amine metabolite levels. Hypermanic and manic patients had intermediate levels. The patients who simulated mania and who were most intensely active for a brief period had the highest levels of CSF amine metabolites. Among the total group of depressed patients, the agitated ones did not have significantly higher levels of amine metabolites than did the predominantly retarded patients, and no significant relationship was found between CSF amine metabolite levels and the severity of the depression.[49]

Another researcher summarized the literature, finding a preponderance of studies showing that vigorous exercise has beneficial effects on depression,[50] and cited other studies of depressed patients demonstrating increased postexercise urinary excretion of the metabolites of NA, serotonin, and dopamine in the urine[20] and CSF.[49]

If, based on careful controlled studies, we are now convinced of the usefulness of exercise on mood disorders, then how much exercise is good? What is the optimal dosage, and what are the side effects?

DOSAGE AND SIDE EFFECTS

I think that I cannot preserve my health and spirits, unless I spend four hours a day at least—and it is commonly more than that—sauntering through the woods and over the hills and fields, absolutely free from all worldly engagements.

(Thoreau: From his *Journal,* April 26, 1841)

Was it his endorphins or his brain monoamines or both or neither? It seems that not much impetus is needed to activate the brain monoamines, as shown in the experiment in which just a little exercise and simulation of manic activity brought about an elevation of mood with a concomitant increase in the CSF metabolites of the monoamines.[50] Results of other reviews of works on CSF monoamines that have to do with exercising rats[12, 50] are hard to extrapolate to humans.

For our case study, as best as can be determined, the Bard of Walden would daily walk a half mile from his cabin to the road, then another mile into Concord Village, making a round trip of 3 miles. Most afternoons he'd walk, pen and notebook in hand, from 2:30 to 5:30 p.m. "to see what I've caught in my traps which I set for facts." Assuming this regimen for 6 days a week, the poet-philosopher would earn 36 aerobic points a week, 6 above what Dr. Kenneth Cooper considered necessary for fitness.

Thoreau jotted down his observations of the countryside, and here we may have the first description of the "runner's high." Thoreau wrote,

The fashions of the wood are more fluctuating than those of Paris. Snow, rime, ice, green and dry leaves incessantly make new patterns. There are all shapes and hues of

the kaleidoscope. . . . Every time I see a nodding pine top, it seems as if a new fashion of wearing plumes has come into vogue.

Compare this with a description of the runner's high, a "euphoric sensation experienced during running, usually unexpected, in which the runner feels a heightened sense of well-being, enhanced appreciation of nature, and transcendence of barriers of time and place."[51]

What, again, is the dosage? It is best studied in terms of duration of effort rather than in distance. In his book *The Joy of Running,*[25a] psychiatrist Thaddeus Kostrubala observed that when one runs for about 30 minutes, "the senses seem to increase in alertness." He emphasized that "the first one was visual." Was that what Thoreau was describing or what the poet Charles McSorley described in "The Song of the Ungirt Runners," whose last two lines read

And we run because we like it
Through the broad bright land.

Does the land look bright because of the run? Such a perception is probably quite subjective and the province of the very sensitive. For most of us, the feeling is calmness, a sense of freedom, relaxation, and perhaps mild euphoria—but again, for how long?

In a double-blind crossover study of 12 recreational male runners, 45 minutes of running brought about a significant state of calm, and at the same time, fatigue diminished.[1] Naloxone inhibited these positive effects, implicating the endorphinergic system.[1] Swimmers who swam twice a week for 40-minute sessions over 14 weeks, compared with controls, improved on all scales except fatigue.[6]

Positive mood changes may not necessarily even require exercise, and by further inference, neither may the endorphin response. For example, students using hatha yoga enjoyed equivalent benefits in mood as those who swam for 45 minutes.[7]

Remember too Thoreau's "sauntering . . . absolutely free from all wordly engagements." Although the poet was aerobically fit, he emphasized a kind of peaceful isolation from all mundane considerations, reminiscent of a study in which benefits comparable to those earned by a similar group with exercise were obtained without exercise. Seventy-five men and women were randomly assigned to exercise, meditation, or what was considered the placebo, consisting of isolation in a quiet, sound-filtered room. The exercisers walked on a motor-driven treadmill for 20 minutes at 70% $\dot{V}o_2$max. The meditators practiced 20 minutes of Benson's Relaxation Response in the same sound-filtered room. Positive benefits were found in all three groups.[4]

It might be said that Thoreau availed himself of at least two (exercising and isolation) and perhaps even the third modality (meditation) if his sauntering was rhythmic.

Where exercise itself was the key ingredient in mood improvement, most studies show that when benefit occurs, it is equal among men and women. Aerobic exercise for 20 to 60 minutes at least three times a week reduced anxiety levels for 30 minutes to 2 hours even in the elderly, and, by and large, cardiovascular fitness has been found to be associated with an even greater sense of well-being and reduced anxiety.[11]

Casper cited one study showing that those who experienced the cognitive concomitants of anxiety (e.g., worry and lack of concentration) sought out vigorous exercise, whereas those who experienced the more physiologic signs (e.g., palpitations and sweating) sought out relaxation programs. As for depression, most studies showed 1 hour of postexercise alleviation of *temporary* depressive symptoms.[11]

MARATHONS AND RESISTANCE TRAINING

Some other studies have investigated duration of activity and benefits and their biochemical correlations. Appenzeller and his group conducted a longitudinal study of runners repeatedly completing high-altitude marathon runs in consecutive years from 1979 to 1982. The most significant increases in β-endorphins were at the finish line. Through the years, however, the resting levels of their and other subjects' plasma levels of β-endorphins actually decreased.[3, 31]

Heitkamp studied 16 healthy athletes, endurance runners who volunteered for exhausting incremental graded treadmill exercise and a marathon run. Various blood samples were taken at 30, 60, and 120 minutes during the recovery phase. In the marathon race, venous blood was collected before, after 1 and 2 hours of running, and at the very end, then at $\frac{1}{2}$, 1, 2, and 24 hours during the recovery phase. Both the incremental graded treadmill exercise and the marathon run led to significant increases in levels of β-endorphin and ACTH (similarly raised), and the β-endorphin level tended to be higher after the marathon run. The decrease of both of these was slower during the recovery from the marathon than from the incremental test; concentrations of β-endorphins and ACTH increased exponentially during the marathon run.[25]

What really seems to activate the endorphinergic systems is intense and long exercise leading to anaerobic metabolites (i.e., lactic acid). Kraemer and associates studied plasma β-endorphin concentrations as challenged by varying heavy-resistance exercise protocols.[26] They found that by lightening the weights but increasing the number of repetitions and decreasing the rest period, the patterns of response of plasma β-endorphin and serum cortisol were similar to that during heavy exercise.[26] That is, with heavy-resistance exercise, the force needed was 10 repetitions maximum with 1 minute of rest. The greater total workload produced a greater increase in β-endorphin than did the fewer repetitions and longer rest period protocols.[26] Lactate concentrations were correlated with plasma β-endorphin concentration. They concluded that the duration of force production and the length of rest periods between sets are key exercise variables influencing increases in plasma β-endorphin and serum cortisol and that significant challenges to the acid-base balance of the blood, in turn due to marked increases in whole blood lactate, may correlate with mechanisms modulating peripheral blood concentrations of β-endorphin and cortisol.[26]

In another study, researchers compared plasma levels of β-endorphin, ACTH, and cortisol in three different training programs: sprint intervals, endurance runs, or a combination of the two. The study spanned a 10-week period, and blood samples were taken before the training, after 10 weeks, and before, immediately after, and at 5 and 15 minutes after maximum exercise testing. The sprint interval group showed significant post-training increases and 5-minute postexercise blood lactate concentration increases in response to maximal exercise, but no training-induced hormonal changes were observed for the endurance group. The researchers believe that aerobic exercise that includes a substantial anaerobic component, which in turn raises the blood lactate levels, is the single important factor in influencing endorphin, ACTH, and cortisol release.[27]

Is activation of the endorphinergic system necessary for mood enhancement? McGowan's group found that resistance exercise actually brings about a decrease in β-endorphins, possibly because of the intermittent nature of the exercise.[36] This observation was consistent with other research showing no significant changes in β-endorphin immunoreactivity after resistance exercise.[47] They also found no relationship between β-endorphin levels and total mood disturbance or Profile of Mood States subscores.[37] We have already mentioned that resistance exercise can contribute to mood enhancement,[17] despite the findings that resistance exercise can actually bring about a decrease in β-endorphins[36, 47] whereas maximal resistance training seems to elevate levels of endorphins.[26]

In another work, McGowan's group also studied mood alterations with a single bout of physical activity.[37] Seventy-two college age students participated in one of three 75-minute activity classes (running, karate, weightlifting), and the lecture class was the control. The running class was required to run a minimum of 2 miles and to walk for the remainder of the 75 minutes. The karate class participants showed no significant difference between preexercise and postexercise scores. The POMS indicated that a single bout of exercise (75 minutes) significantly reduced total mood disturbance, tension, depression, anger, and confusion.[37]

To increase plasma levels of β-endorphins, very strenuous activity is apparently necessary. For example, in one study, 10 men and 10 women exercised on a bicycle ergometer with varying degrees of intensity.[38] The duration of exercising on the bicycle ergometer was 20 minutes. The intensity was to 40%, 60%, and 80% maximal oxygen uptake to determine the relationship between plasma β-endorphin, catecholamines, and exercise intensity. Plasma β-endorphin level was not significantly elevated during the 40% and 60% workloads, but 80% of the maximal oxygen uptake significantly elevated levels of endorphins. Plasma NA levels correlated significantly with endorphins, but not with epinephrine. Anaerobic activity produced the most significant endorphin response. The researchers believed that the increase in lactate at the 80% level may have been the stimulus for the β-endorphin elevation.[37]

Schwarz's group also produced data indicating that strenuous anaerobic effort is needed to cause an increase in lactate concentration and that β-endorphin levels increase when the anaerobic threshold is exceeded or at a point where a disproportionate increase in lactate occurs. Blood β-endorphin levels do not increase until exercise duration exceeds approximately 1 hour.[52]

Taylor and associates described the role of acidosis, showing a correlation between acidosis, in turn associated with high-intensity exercise, as a primary stimulus for β-endorphin release. Buffering of the blood attenuated the rate of β-endorphin release.[54]

Another rationale for the role of endorphins in exercise and general stress is that β-endorphin inhibits respiration during exercise. β-endorphin values peak during the 10-minute recovery period, paralleling the appearance of lactic acidosis. Acidosis does stimulate respiration, acting on chemosensitive neurons in the medullary respiratory control center. The role of β-endorphin may be to prevent hyperventilation during respiratory challenge; thus, acidosis would be an ideal stimulus. Acidosis would stimulate respiration and concurrently stimulate β-endorphin as a feedback inhibitor.[54]

The relationship between acidosis and high-intensity exercise is in the realm of excess of, even addiction to, running.

ADDICTION, DEPENDENCE

One can obviously overdo a good thing. Morgan first called attention to the negative effects.[42] He cited cases of runners who fulfilled criteria for addiction (requiring daily and increasing doses of running, experiencing withdrawal symptoms if deprived of the exercise, and running when otherwise contraindicated, e.g., when injured). Those overdoing it experienced symptoms of depression (e.g., insomnia, anorexia, restlessness, anhedonia[42]), symptoms also noted in his study of swimmers when their daily regimen was doubled from 4000 to 9000 meters per day at 94% of $\dot{V}o_2$max.[43]

The question of addiction, when it exists, may in turn relate to the endorphins. Already mentioned was the decrease in resting levels of β-endorphin–β-lipotropin in highly trained athletes and the 14 runners who ran this marathon for 3 years in a row, showing significant reductions in the run-induced elevation of β-endorphins.[3] It is speculated that adaptive mechanisms account for this.[3]

This adaptive mechanism may be analogous to what is postulated in heroin addicts, who may suffer a reduction in absolute number of opiate receptors.[21] Perhaps some athletes may suffer the same because of repeated surges of endogenous opiates, leading to desensitivity of the receptor sites, so that greater endorphin levels are needed to reach prior levels of opiate receptor activity.[3]

To determine whether the β-endorphin response to endurance exercise has any relationship to exercise dependence, eight women first completed a written test on exercise-dependence assessment. Plasma β-endorphin level was measured before their 45 minutes of continuous aerobic dance and after the routine. Although the β-endorphin levels were significantly higher after the aerobics routine, the percent changes were not significantly correlated with scores on the exercise-dependence survey, indicating that at least the scores on exercise dependence are not related to changes in plasma β-endorphin levels after exercise.[48]

That dependence is not correlated with increases in the plasma endorphins may confirm the hypothesis that those addicted do not have a desensitivity of the receptor sites.[3]

Running addiction (a drive or push) *was* found to be associated with frequent runs, which in turn did not contribute to mood enhancement, whereas mood enhancement was positively correlated with fewer but longer runs.[13] Positive addiction scores and high run frequencies were associated with low interpersonal sensitivity, low phobic anxiety, and low psychoticism. Run duration was negatively associated with interpersonal insecurity, depression, anxiety, hostility, paranoid ideation, and obsessive-compulsive tendencies. Therefore, in this study, the prescription would be for few but long runs to improve mood but to avoid addiction.[13]

UNIFYING THEORY AND IMPLICATIONS FOR TREATMENT

Know then thyself, presume not God to scan
The proper study of mankind is man

(Alexander Pope, *An Essay on Man,* 11.i.)

Before treating, a physician should know the patient and diagnose the illness. What then is human nature? Without implying any dichotomy, what is the physiologic and psychic makeup of humans? The best approach to these questions follows the teleologic—at least that is how the poets saw it. In Dryden's first line, "By chase our long-liv'd fathers earn'd their food," he was no doubt alluding to humans of the hunter-gatherer stage, whose heritage was embodied in the hominid *Australopithecus africanus,* found in Tanzania's Olduval Gorge. The hominid's ancestors, in turn, had survived the terrible droughts and swirling dust storms of the Pliocene for millions of years. Our hominid, whom the Leakeys studied, was determined to have weighed between 80 and 100 pounds, was both carnivorous and herbivorous, and was highly predatory, even against his own species. *A. africanus* was a hardy runner who outwitted and outfought fierce predators in packs and ran down and slaughtered for food the lesser creatures that roamed the plains.

Such was the body that evolved over millions and millions of years. It was and is a body suited for running long distances and for surviving nature's capricious cataclysms. In only the past 15,000 years have agricultural humans begun to replace the hunter-gatherers, and in only the past 50 years have we particularly partaken of the benefits, along with the ills, of technology. But we have not had the time to evolve and adapt to the comfortable life. Rather, our bodies still crave the long run, the chase, the challenge.

To meet any challenge, physical or psychic, we have evolved physiologic and psychic mechanisms to combat stress. Physiologically, the body responds by overreacting (e.g., the buildup of muscle in response to demand). At the same time, homeostatic mechanisms restore the organism to its regular state (e.g., the pituitary/adrenocortical axis to conserve sodium and glucose and to quell the excesses of the inflammatory reaction, among many other functions). The psyche has analogous mechanisms to maintain the status quo, the status quo here being the function of mental mechanisms (e.g., repression, rationalization, sublimation, reaction formation) to preserve the self-esteem.

The psyche has a type of immunologic homeostasis akin to the body's formation of antibodies to foreign protein (e.g., bacteria). That which is foreign to one's self-conception, self-esteem, or integrity, if you will, is fought with internal mental forces—the mental mechanisms—that defend the ego. Overwhelm these mental mechanisms and a mixture of insecurity, fear, and depression ensues. Specifically, with loss of self-esteem, depression fills the vacuum. All of these—fear, anxiety, tension, depression—are types of mood disorders.

Important to any therapy of mood disorder is to provide a sense of control, of mastery. Mastery is another theory of why exercise helps, depression then being a loss of control.[39] Accordingly, Greist and colleagues recommended that each run be so gentle and comfortable that patients look forward to the next run, that runners finish with more energy than they had at the beginning, and that concerns with pace and competition with others be minimized.[22]

Thoreau, our case study, thoroughly advocated the aerobic way of life ("Of all ebriosity," he wrote in *Walden,* "who does not prefer to be intoxicated by the air he breathes."), as did Dryden ("Toil strung the nerves and *purified the blood.*"). The poet also cautioned about pace ("If a man does not keep pace with his companions, perhaps it is because he hears a different drummer. Let him step to the music he hears, however measured or far away."). Remember that patients tend to pick their own form of exercise, depending, in the case of anxiety, on whether the symptoms are cognitive or physiologic. Those who need to run longer distances and stimulate the endorphins will naturally do so.[11]

Thoreau also warned about overdoing it in *Walden*: "If the condition of things which we were made for is not yet, what were any reality which we can substitute. We shall not be shipwrecked on a vain reality." He was presaging sports medicine literature, which concludes that the adverse effects of staleness, compulsivity, or the "athlete's neurosis" occur because self-esteem is based on physical prowess, therefore making participants vulnerable to injury and loss of the overvalued aspect of the self.[11]

Thoreau was therefore cautioning against the possibility of addiction or injury in some. Exercise regimens that are rigid and inflexible breed boredom and dropout. Thoreau's close friend and colleague, Emerson, cautioned against those compulsive regimens that did not contain a good degree of fun and variety when he wrote that "a foolish consistency is the hobgoblin of little minds."

The feeling of control and mastery is im-portant enough that a scale with a name showing a positive correlation with exercise adherence has been devised, called the *locus of control.*[57] Its premise is that individuals who view themselves as having more control over their destiny are more likely to have an optimistic attitude about the benefits of exercise.[55] Greist's prescription clearly fulfills this test.[22]

Emotional benefits, earned from the pain and lactate acidosis of very long-distance running and of maximal-repetition resistance exercise, stimulating endorphinergic response, can also be obtained from meditation and quiet rest. Their benefits were shown to have a physiologic basis by reducing plasma levels of epinephrine, NA, and lactate.[40]

The endorphinergic response and the monoamine response are part of evolutionary adaptive and homeostatic mechanisms that empower our bodies to be effective hunter-gatherers. Facilitation of the levels of monoamines that may, in turn, allow us to feel relatively happy when we are in pain and of the endorphinergic neurotransmitter response that, along with ACTH, calms the pain and other distress of the challenge all are part of adaptation. In fact, one of the roles of the endogenous opiates, incidentally stimulated by acidosis, is actually to inhibit the compensatory hyperventilation of acidosis, allowing for more efficient respiration and prevention of overcompensation to alkalosis. These responses all are part of the efficient system of checks and balances that make up homeostasis and response to stress, that marvelous inherent system that exercise such as running can awaken.

A prominent neurologist (who, by the way, was the first to break the 4-minute mile barrier) years ago offered poetic thoughts and words that through the years have gained scientific validity:

I have always been reluctant to dragoon people into boring fitness routines. I have wanted them to choose activities they find exciting. . . . Even at noncompetitive levels, running, or jogging, has swept America, becoming the only healthful addiction I know. . . . Stemming at first from fear of coronary heart disease, it is now mainly sustained—and this is the important fact—because it is enjoyable for its own sake.[5]

He hinted too at a runner's high and the importance of distraction. He writes how each season, because of the publicity attached to his appearances, "I almost hated athletics . . . it left me no freedom to run as I pleased. So in August of 1951, I lost myself in Scotland for two weeks, walking and climbing and sleeping in the open." He describes running across a moor when it began to rain, giving him the "feeling that I was cradled in the rainbow arc as I ran. I felt I was running back to the primitive joy that my season had destroyed."[5]

He reminded all of us how we are the beneficiaries of bodies that have evolved through millenia with enough strength and resilience to confront major physical and mental struggles. In our modern electronic age, we are robbed of many of the demands our parents and grandparents had to face. Given the bodies that crave challenge, we re-create them in the guise of sport or play, and in so confronting the challenge, we feel good about ourselves. Bannister says,

> We run not because we think it is doing us good, but because we enjoy it and cannot help ourselves.
>
> It also does us good because it helps us do other things better. It gives a man or woman the chance to bring out the power that might otherwise remain locked inside. The urge to struggle lies latent in everyone. The more restricted our society and work become, the more necessary it will be to find some outlet for this craving for freedom. No one can say, 'You must not run faster than this, or jump higher than that.' The human spirit is indomitable.[5]

Substitute endorphins, monoamines, adaptation, and homeostasis for spirit, and then we can truly believe that the human spirit *is* indomitable. It just needs a stimulus such as running to spark it to life and remind us of the words of a poet who told us that "God never made his work for man to mend."

CONCLUSION

It should be a certainty that running (or its equivalent) has a salubrious effect on mood disorders. The biochemical concomitant of this effect is partly related to stimulation of the brain's neurotransmitters. Its psychic concomitant involves the ability of running to restore self-esteem. The dosage of exercise is quite variable, from 20 minutes three times a week to 100 miles per week, and should be monitored, flexible, playful, fun, and individually tailored. The rationale of this benefit is best understood as a thrust to use our bodies as they were meant to be—that is, to be hunter-gatherers. Running, in effect, is a bodily expression of that stage and evokes all the adaptive mechanisms to bring this about. These mechanisms have to do with homeostasis and allow us to perform near-herculean tasks while mobilizing our physiologic and mental resources. These in turn modulate and neutralize distress of body and mind, making us feel good at times when reason would dictate that we should feel bad.

REFERENCES

1. Allen ME, Coen D: Naloxone blocking of running-induced mood changes. Ann Sports Med 3:190–195, 1987.
2. Anthony J: Psychologic aspects of exercise. Clin Sports Med 10:171–180, 1991.
3. Appenzeller O, Appenzeller J, Standefer J, et al: Opioids and endurance training; longitudinal study. Ann Sports Med 2:22–25, 1984.
4. Bahrke MS, Morgan WP: Anxiety reduction following exercise and meditation. Cognit Ther Res 2:323–334, 1978.
5. Bannister R: The Four-Minute Mile. New York, Lyons and Burford, 1994.
6. Berger BG, Owen DR: Mood alteration with swimming—Swimmers really do "feel better." Psychosom Med 45:425–432, 1983.
7. Berger BG, Owen DR: Mood alteration with yoga and swimming: Aerobic exercise may not be necessary. Percept Mot Skills 75:1331–1343, 1992.
7a. Biddle N, Allen P: History of the Expedition Under the Command of Captains Lewis and Clark. Philadelphia, Bradford and Inskeep, 1814.
8. Brown RS, Ramirez DE, Taub JM: The prescription of exercise for depression. Physician Sportsmed 6:34–45, 1978.
9. Byrne A, Byrne DG: The effect of exercise on depression, anxiety and other mood states: A review. J Psychosom Res 37:565–574, 1993.
10. Camacho TC, Roberts RE, Lazarus NB, et al: Physical activity and depression: Evidence from the Alameda County Study. Am J Epidemiol 134:220–231, 1991.
11. Casper RC: Exercise and mood. World Rev Nutr Diet 71:115–143, 1993.
12. Chaouloff F: Physical exercise and brain monoamines: A review. Acta Physiol Scand 137:1–13, 1989.
13. Chapman CL, DeCastro JM: Running addiction: Measurement and associated psychological characteristics. J Sports Med Phys Fitness 30:283–290, 1990.
14. Chung S-H, Dickenson A: Pain, enkephalin and acupuncture. Nature 283:243–244, 1980.
15. Daniel M, Martin AD, Carter J: Opiate receptor blockade by naltrexone and mood state after acute physical activity. Br J Sports Med 26:111–115, 1992.
16. deVries HA, Adams GM: Electromyographic compari-

son of single doses of exercise and meprobamate as to effects on muscular relaxation. Am J Phys Med 51:130–141, 1972.

17. Doyne EJ, Ossip-Klein DJ, Bowman ED, et al: Running versus weight lifting in the treatment of depression. J Consult Clin Psychol 55:748–754, 1987.

18. Droste C: Influence of opiate system in pain transmission during angina pectoris. Z Kardiol (Germany) 79(Suppl):31–43, 1990.

19. Droste C: Transient hypoalgesia under physical exercise—relation to silent ischaemia and implication for cardiac rehabilitation. Ann Acad Med Singapore 21:23–33, 1992.

20. Ebert MH, Post RM, Goodwin FK: Effect of physical activity on urinary MHPG excretion in depressed patients. Lancet 2:766, 1971.

21. Gold MS, Pottash ALC, Extein I, et al: Evidence for an endorphin dysfunction in methadone addicts; lack of ACTH response to naloxone. Drug Alcohol Depend 8:257–262, 1981.

22. Greist JH, Eischens RR, Klein MH, et al: Antidepressant running. Psychiatr Ann 9:23–33, 1979.

23. Greist JH, Klein MH, Eischens RR, et al: Running as treatment for depression. Compr Psychiatry 20:41–53, 1979.

24. Grossman A, Sutton JR: Endorphins: What are they? How are they measured? What is their role in exercise? Med Sci Sports Exerc 17:74–81, 1985.

25. Heitkamp H-CH, Schmid K, Scheib K: β-endorphin and adrenocorticotropic hormone production during marathon and incremental exercise. Eur J Appl Physiol 66:269–274, 1993.

25a. Kostrubala T: The Joy of Running. New York, JB Lippincott, 1976.

26. Kraemer WJ, Dziados JE, Marchitelli LJ, et al: Effects of different heavy-resistance exercise protocols on plasma β-endorphin concentrations. J Appl Physiol 74:450–459, 1993.

27. Kraemer WJ, Fleck SJ, Callister R, et al: Training responses of plasma beta-endorphin, adrenocorticotropin, and cortisol. Med Sci Sports Exerc 21:146–153, 1989.

28. LaFontaine TP, DiLorenzo TM, Frensch PA, et al: Aerobic exercise and mood—a brief review, 1985–1990. Sports Med 13:160–170, 1992.

29. Lee I-M, Hsieh C-C, Paffenbarger RS Jr: Exercise intensity and longevity in men: The Harvard Alumni Health Study. JAMA 273:1179–1184, 1995.

30. Light KC, Herbst MC, Bragdon E, et al: Depression and type A behavior pattern in patients with coronary artery disease: Relationships to painful versus silent myocardial ischemia and beta-endorphin responses during exercise. Psychosom Med 6:669–683, 1944.

31. Lobstein DD, Rasmussen CL: Decreases in resting plasma beta-endorphin and depression scores after endurance training. J Sports Med Phys Fitness 31:543–551, 1991.

32. Marchant B, Umachandran V, Wilkinson P, et al: Reexamination of the role of endogenous opiates in silent myocardial ischemia. J Am Coll Cardiol 23:645–651, 1994.

33. Martinsen EW: Physical activity and depression: Clinical experience. Acta Psychiatr Scand 377 (Suppl):23–27, 1994.

34. Martinsen EW, Medhus A, Sandvik L: Effects of aerobic exercise on depression: A controlled study. Br Med J 291:109, 1985.

35. McCann L, Holmes D: Influence of aerobic exercise on depression. J Pers Soc Psychol 46:1142–1147, 1984.

36. McGowan W, Pierce EF, Eastman N: Beta-endorphins and mood states during resistance exercise. Percept Mot Skills 76:376–378, 1993.

37. McGowan RW, Pierce EF, Jordan D: Mood alterations with a single bout of physical activity. Percept Mot Skills 72:1203–1209, 1991.

38. McMurray RG, Forsythe WA, Mar MH, Hardy CJ: Exercise intensity-related responses of β-endorphin and catecholamines. Med Sci Sports Exerc 19:570–574, 1987.

39. Mellion MB: Exercise therapy for anxiety and depression: Does the evidence justify its recommendation? Postgrad Med 77:59–62, 1985.

40. Michaels RR, Huber MJ, McCann DS: Evaluation of transcendental meditation as a method of reducing stress. Science 192:1242–1244, 1976.

41. Miller PF, Light KC, Bragdon EE, et al: Beta-endorphin response to exercise and mental stress in patients with ischemic heart disease. J Psychosom Res 37:455–465, 1993.

42. Morgan WP: Negative addiction in runners. Physician Sportsmed 7:57–70, 1979.

43. Morgan WP, Costill DL, Flynn MG, et al: Mood disturbance following increased training in swimmers. Med Sci Sports 20:408–414, 1988.

44. Paffenbarger RS Jr: 40 Years of Progress: Physical Activity, Health and Fitness. American College of Sports Medicine—40th Anniversary Lectures. Indianapolis, IN, American College of Sports Medicine, 1994.

45. Paffenbarger RS Jr, Lee I-M, Leung R: Physical activity and personal characteristics associated with depression and suicide in American college men. Acta Psychiatr Scand 377(Suppl):16–22, 1994.

46. Paffenbarger RS Jr, Kampert JB, Lee I-M, et al: Changes in physical activity and other lifeway patterns influencing longevity. Med Sci Sports Exerc 26:857–865, 1994.

47. Pierce EF, et al: Resistance exercise decreases β-endorphin immunoreactivity. Br J Sports Med 28:164–166, 1994.

48. Pierce EF, Eastman NW, Tripathi HL, et al: Beta-endorphin response to endurance exercise: Relationship to exercise dependence. Percept Mot Skills 77:767–770, 1993.

49. Post RM, Kotin J, Goodwin FK, Gordon EK: Psychomotor activity and cerebropinal fluid amine metabolism in affective illness. Am J Psychiatry 130:67–72, 1973.

50. Ransford CP: A role for amines in the antidepressant effect of exercise: A review. Med Sci Sports Exerc 14:1–10, 1982.

51. Sachs ML: The runner's high. In Sachs ML, Buffone GW (eds): Running as Therapy: An Integrated Approach. Lincoln, NE, University of Nebraska Press, 1984.

52. Schwarz L, Kindermann W: Changes in β-endorphin levels in response to aerobic and anaerobic exercise. Sports Med 13:25–36, 1992.

53. Shephard RJ: Exercise in the prevention and treatment of cancer. An update. Sports Med 15:258–280, 1993.

54. Taylor DV, Boyajían JG, James N, et al: Acidosis stimulates β-endorphin release during exercise. Am Physiol Soc 77:1913–1918, 1994.

55. Thompson CE, Wankel LM: The effects of perceived activity choice upon frequency of exercise behavior. J Appl Soc Psychol 10:436–444, 1980.

56. Thoren P, Floras JS, Hoffmann P, Seals DR: Endorphins and exercise: Physiological mechanisms and clinical implications. Med Sci Sports Exerc 22:417–428, 1990.

57. Wallston BS, Wallston KA, Kaplan GD, Maides SA: Development and validation of the health locus of control scale. J Consult Clin Psychol 44:580, 1976.

58. Zanker KS, Kroczek R: Looking along the track of the psychoneuroimmunologic axis for missing links in cancer progression. Int J Sports Med 12:58–62, 1991.

ANNETTE M. ZAHAROFF

CHAPTER SEVENTEEN

The Female Athlete Triad in Runners

In the past 25 years, the participation of women in athletics and running has made dramatic advancements historically as well as medically. It was in 1967 that Kathrine Switzer (the future winner of the 1974 New York City marathon) entered the Boston marathon as K. Switzer. Women were not allowed to compete in the event at that time, and when officials learned K. was a woman, physical attempts were made to remove her from the course (Fig. 17–1). She eventually completed the marathon in 4 hours and 20 minutes. In 1995, 9106 women officially entered the New York City marathon and 6470 completed it. Tegla Loroupe, the first black woman to win a major marathon, won the 1995 New York City marathon for the second year in a row, with a time of 2 hours and 28:06 minutes.

Because women's participation in running has increased, more information on female runners has emerged. Data on the physiologic, medical, and psychologic implications of physical activity and female athletes are now being examined. Although running has been found to have many health benefits for women, when taken to the extreme, it may place female athletes at risk for developing significant health-related problems. One such health issue recognized is a potentially fatal triad of medical disorders described in the literature as the female athlete triad. Al-

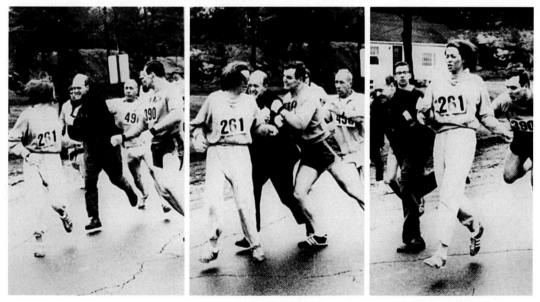

Figure 17–1

Hopkinton, Mass., April 19, 1967. Who says chivalry is dead? A woman listed only as "K. Switzer of Syracuse" found herself about to be thrown out of the normally all-male Boston marathon today when a husky companion, Thomas Miller, of Syracuse, threw a block that tossed a race official out of the running instead. The photos show Jock Semple, official, moving in to intercept Switzer, then being bounced himself by Miller. (Photos by Harry Trask of Boston Traveler.)

though the disorder is not unique to female runners, the characteristics of endurance athletes, such as long-distance runners, place women at risk for the development of the female athlete triad. Consequences of the triad may lead to psychologic, medical, and orthopedic problems; therefore, recognition of the triad becomes essential to anyone working with the female running population.

This chapter reviews the prevalence, risk profile, and components of the triad as they relate to running, and it includes information on its evaluation, treatment, and prevention.

GENERAL CONSIDERATIONS

The female athlete triad comprises three distinct yet interrelated disorders that often affect active women and girls: disordered eating, amenorrhea, and osteoporosis (Fig. 17–2).[63]

Disordered eating refers to a spectrum of abnormal patterns of eating. Anorexia nervosa and bulimia are at the extreme end, with other, less severe abnormal eating behaviors at the other end. In athletes, any degree of disordered eating poses a risk of progressing in severity along the spectrum. Disordered eating of any degree can lead to adverse effects on health, with morbidity and the risks of mortality increasing as the severity of the disorder increases. The mortality rate in treated anorectic women (nonathletes) is 10% to 18%.[40]

Amenorrhea (secondary) has been defined as the absence of 3 to 12 consecutive menstrual periods in women who have already begun menstruating. In female athletes who begin training before puberty, delayed menarche, defined as not having menstrual periods by 16 years of age, may occur. The menstrual irregularities encountered in athletes range along a spectrum from the extreme of hypoestrogenic amenorrhea to periods of oligomenorrhea (menstrual cycles greater than 36 days). One medical concern arising from the presence of amenorrhea and hypoestrogenism in athletes is the development of osteoporosis and premature bone loss.

Osteoporosis in premenopausal athletes refers to premature bone loss or inadequate bone formation. In young athletes, approximately 60% of final bone mass is accumulated during the pubertal growth spurt, making an adolescent's bony structure particularly vulnerable to any disorder affecting bone formation. If an athlete has a reduced capability to fully develop skeletal mass, attain peak bone mass, and maintain bone mass, she may be at increased risk of stress fractures and premature osteoporotic fractures.[48]

The etiology of the female athlete triad is believed to be multifaceted. Young female athletes who are driven in their sport may attempt to fit a specific athletic body image in order to reach performance goals. They may develop patterns of disordered eating in order to control their weight.[60] The disordered eating may lead to menstrual dysfunction,[39, 50, 56] which in turn leads to premature osteoporosis (Fig. 17–3).[1, 27, 30, 33] Each disorder of the triad may occur alone and represents a significant medical concern. In combination, however, the triad of disorders may lead to significant morbidity and even a high rate of mortality,[40, 63] and patients may incur lifelong psychologic, medical, and physical consequences.

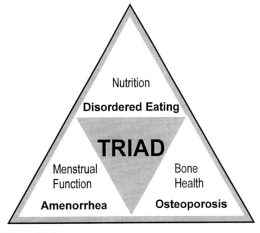

Figure 17–2

Relation among disordered eating, amenorrhea, and osteoporosis.

RISK PROFILE

Long-distance runners share many common features with the risk profile identified for the development of the female athlete triad. Any factor that serves to increase the risk of abnormal eating behaviors may serve as an impetus to disordered eating and the development of the triad (Fig. 17–4). It is believed that individual sports (e.g., gymnastics, figure skating, distance running, and other sports that focus on low body fat and

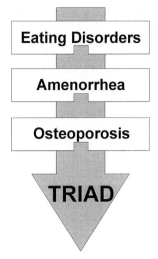

Figure 17–3

Development of the female athlete triad.

weight) pose a higher risk for the development of the triad.[7, 63] Much of today's popular running literature encourages good runners to try to achieve 12% to 18% body fat, with less than 10% being ideal. Although this information is unfounded, female runners may strive to attain such standards through abnormal eating behaviors in order to lose body weight and fat. The drive and intensity of elite marathon runners and the desire to fit the lean, thin profile emphasized in marathon running are risk factors for the development of the triad. Adolescent and young adult runners are also at greater risk, because this age group has been found to be highly susceptible to abnormal eating patterns and to be very sensitive to body image.[35, 37]

Other factors also predispose athletes to the development of the triad. The pressure to excel and to win at all costs may have a significant psychologic impact on athletes and may further emphasize body image and weight.[37, 60] Coaching techniques with negative reinforcement for weight gain or poor performance may also be a factor predisposing to disordered eating patterns. Athletes with overcontrolling coaches or parents may use their food intake as a means of compensation to gain control over their structured lives. Athletes socially isolated from their peers and having narrow goals and life interests, focused only on their sport and winning, may incorporate severely regimented diets into their lives. Athletes with a family history of disordered eating are also found to develop abnormal eating behaviors more commonly, predisposing them to the subsequent triad of disorders.[24]

PREVALENCE

At present, the prevalence of the female athlete triad is unknown. Because of the secretive nature of disordered eating, accurate data become difficult to obtain. Much of the information currently available is collected through self-report questionnaires. The female athlete triad may develop in nonathletes, but certain athletic populations demonstrate higher rates of prevalence.[44, 45, 54, 59, 63] Females are at higher risk of developing disordered eating patterns than are males (10:1 female-to-male ratio), and a focus on thinness and body weight often serves as the initial impetus. In the athletic population, studies have reported disordered eating patterns in young female athletes at rates of 15% to 62%.[44, 45]

The prevalence of amenorrhea is also higher in athletes than in the general population. Amenorrhea occurs at rates of 10% to 20% in runners, compared with 5% in the general population and as high as 50% in elite female runners.[50, 55, 56] Certain sports such as running appear to be associated with consistently higher rates of amenorrhea (Fig. 17–5). The incidence of eating disorders has

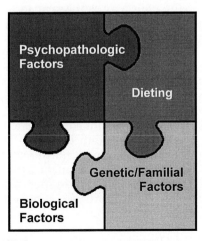

Figure 17–4

Risk factors for eating disorders. (Adapted from Wilson GT, Eldredge K: Pathology and development of eating disorders: Implications for athletes. In Brownell KD, Rodin J, Wilmore JH [eds]: Eating, Body Weight, and Performance in Athletes. Philadelphia, Lea & Febiger, 1992, p 115.)

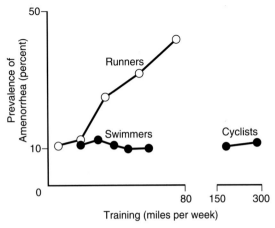

Figure 17–5

The prevalence of amenorrhea in runners, swimmers, and cyclists, relative to training mileage. (From Sanborn CF, Martin BJ, Wagner WW: Is athletic amenorrhea specific to runners? Am J Obstet Gynecol 143:860, 1982.)

also been shown to be higher in amenorrheic runners.[4, 20, 30] Gadpaille and colleagues identified diagnosable eating disorders in 62% of the amenorrheic population in their study.[20]

The prevalence of premature osteoporosis in young female athletes is not known. Assessing bone health in active women has demonstrated the positive effects that weight-bearing exercise may have on increasing bone mass.[5, 52] The potentially negative effects of exercise and menstrual dysfunction on bone health are now being brought to light. Clear evidence in the past 20 years has demonstrated the presence of premature osteoporosis and decreased bone mineral density (BMD) in 100% of amenorrheic runners compared with their eumenorrheic counter-

parts.[13, 30, 32, 34, 45] This alarming revelation has spurred more research in this area, which should provide a better understanding of the prevalence of premature osteoporosis in female athletes in the future. An increased incidence of musculoskeletal injuries and stress fractures, which may be a result of premature osteoporosis, has been identified in runners with menstrual dysfunctions.[4, 15, 27, 30, 33, 43] Lloyd and colleagues reported four times as many stress fractures in amenorrheic versus eumenorrheic runners.[27] An alarmingly high prevalence of eating disorders has also been noted in amenorrheic groups of runners with stress fractures.[4, 20]

COMPONENTS OF THE FEMALE ATHLETE TRIAD

DISORDERED EATING

Types of Disorders

The most severe forms of disordered eating behavior are the recognized clinical diagnoses of anorexia nervosa and bulimia nervosa.[2] The new concept of disordered eating emphasizes a spectrum of abnormal eating patterns with poor nutritional habits at one end and anorexia and bulimia at the other. Various abnormal eating behaviors and thought patterns related to eating have been identified (Table 17–1).

Although a number of different patterns of disordered eating may be present in and related to the female athlete triad, female runners may demonstrate some specific tendencies.[6, 54, 59] Emphasis on low body fat and weight in running may provoke female runners to begin various abnormal eating behaviors and weight control measures as described. Low body weight may also be caused by insufficient caloric intake combined with the high energy expenditure of long-distance running.[3, 20, 29, 30] Other poor nutritional habits such as insufficient calcium intake are known to be characteristic of young runners and may have a role in the disturbance of bone health in young athletes.[3, 13, 30, 33]

Effects of Disordered Eating

These poor nutritional patterns may have negative effects not only on athletic performance but on the athletes' health as well. Undereating and weight loss can contribute to

TABLE 17–1   Spectrum of Disordered Eating

Behaviors	Thought Patterns
Binging with / without purging	Preoccupation with food
Food restriction	Dissatisfaction with one's body
Prolonged fasting	Fear of becoming fat
Loss of control over eating	Distorted body image
Purging by use of diet, pills, laxatives, diuretics, self-induced vomiting, and/or excessive exercise	Overconcern with body weight and fat

Adapted from Nattiv A, Yeager K, Drinkwater B, et al: The female athlete triad. In Agostini R (ed): Medical and Orthopedic Issues of Active and Athletic Women. Philadelphia, Hanley & Belfus, 1994, p 169.

chronic fatigue, which can result in decreased endurance, strength, reaction time, speed, and ability to concentrate.[16, 29] Medical consequences may be far reaching and may affect numerous physiologic functions. One of the concerns specific to the female athlete triad is the effect of disordered eating on menstrual function. Almost 100% of the women who meet criteria for anorexia nervosa experience loss of menses or do not achieve menarche if the disorder begins prepubertally and remains untreated.[24] Caloric deprivation has been proposed to have a significant role in the development of amenorrhea in female athletes.[20, 23, 38, 56] Amenorrheic runners have been found to demonstrate lower caloric intake than their eumenorrheic counterparts, as well as other nutritional differences.[13, 33, 38] It is proposed that the low energy intake leads to an energy drain resulting in disturbances to hypothalamic function and subsequent amenorrhea.[48, 50] How these disturbances contribute to the development of amenorrhea is discussed in the next section.

Evaluation and Treatment

Although information on screening for the female athlete triad is presented in a following section, some basic information about the evaluation and treatment of eating disorders is provided here. Once an athlete is suspected of having an eating disorder, she should be approached gently and not accused of wrongdoing. Concerns about her health and well-being should be addressed. A team approach, including a nutritionist and a psychologist or psychiatrist, may work most effectively.

A physician may monitor the athlete's medical status and athletic participation and may also coordinate her care. Follow-up should include a thorough diagnostic evaluation along with a detailed history and physical examination. The physical examination should include an evaluation for signs of starvation such as bradycardia, fat and muscle loss, dry hair and skin, cold and discolored hands and feet, and lanugo (baby-fine hair over the body). Signs of purging include parotid gland enlargement, so-called chipmunk cheeks, face and extremity edema, and tooth enamel erosion from self-induced vomiting. Dehydration may also cause orthostatic blood pressure changes.

Laboratory evaluation should include a urinalysis, complete blood count, and sedimentation rate to screen for infection, malignancy, inflammatory processes, and anemia. If the athlete's pulse is less than 50, she may have an electrolyte abnormality or frequent purging behavior. An electrocardiogram (ECG) should be performed to assess for bradycardia, low voltage, low or inverted T waves, and possibly prolonged QT intervals.

The athlete's participation in exercise should be determined by a physician. Factors to take into consideration may include appropriate weight gain if the athlete is losing weight and correction of abnormal laboratory and ECG findings.

The nutritional and psychologic evaluation and treatment are beyond the scope of this chapter, but excellent information on nutrition is provided in Chapter 15 of this book, and several other references are recommended for more information.[7, 22, 24] Each health care team member should have experience in managing eating disorders as well as an understanding of sports participation to provide the most benefit to female athletes. Although treatment is directed toward outpatient care, if an athlete's condition is severe enough, hospitalization may be indicated. Criteria for hospitalization include weight loss of 30% or more of normal body weight, cardiac compromise, hypotension, dehydration, electrolyte abnormalities, failure to improve, or worsening of symptoms after 3 months of outpatient treatment.

Prognosis

The long-term prognosis for athletes with disordered eating behaviors is unknown at this time. Information about nonathletes estimates that 40% of treated patients with disordered eating recover; approximately 30% show some improvement but struggle with weight, body image, and relapses; and 30% suffer a chronic debilitating course that includes a 10% to 18% mortality rate in treated anorectic, nonathletic women.[22, 24, 53]

AMENORRHEA

Definitions

A spectrum of menstrual dysfunctions is known to occur in female athletes. The three principal types observed with endurance runners are delayed menarche or primary amenorrhea, secondary amenorrhea, and more subtle cycle phase abnormalities such as prolonged follicular and shortened luteal phases.[55] For the purpose of this chapter, the focus is on amenorrhea because it is the menstrual dysfunction included in the female athlete triad. Amenorrhea has been defined as the absence of 3 to 12 consecutive menstrual periods.[16] Other definitions are given in the literature, however, and in an effort to standardize future studies, the International Olympic Committee has agreed on one period or less per year as the definition.[31] Primary amenorrhea is an absence of menstrual bleeding by age 16 years, and secondary amenorrhea is defined as at least one episode of menstrual bleeding before amenorrhea occurs.

Etiology of Amenorrhea

Many factors are believed to contribute to the development of amenorrhea in athletes. With respect to the female athlete triad, diet and nutritional statuses have been shown to influence the reproductive system. Female athletes with disordered eating patterns that result in diets low in calories, fat, and protein, as well as vegetarian diets, have been associated with a higher rate of amenorrhea.[50] Changes in weight and body composition, as well as physical and emotional stress, may also promote the development of amenorrhea.[48, 50]

Hypothalamic amenorrhea is the most common cause of secondary amenorrhea in athletes and can also be a cause of primary amenorrhea or delayed menarche.[26, 39] The effects of disordered eating patterns and the other factors mentioned are proposed to provide negative feedback to the hypothalamic-pituitary-gonadal axis, impairing gonadotropin-releasing hormone secretion, thereby resulting in decreased pulsatile luteinizing hormone and follicular-stimulating hormone and deficient production of estrogen by the ovaries.[28, 31] Women who participate in endurance sports such as running and who have menstrual bleeding less frequently than every 4 months or are totally amenorrheic are probably hypoestrogenic.[50]

Effects of Amenorrhea

Amenorrhea in athletes was originally thought to be simply reversible when training was reduced or discontinued, with no short-term or long-term health risks. It is now believed that hypoestrogenic amenorrhea may have a major impact on the health of female athletes. One of the most significant consequences of hypoestrogenic amenorrhea is disruption of normal calcium metabolism and uncoupling of bone formation and bone resorption. This disruption leads to decreased bone mineral content and premature osteoporosis in premenopausal women. In young runners, menarche may be delayed, leading to a prolonged hypoestrogenic state. This may contribute to bone loss and osteopenia at an age when bone density should ideally be increasing.[3, 50] A lower peak bone mass may result, thus facilitating earlier osteoporosis in subsequent years. The clinical effects of this premature osteoporosis are discussed shortly.

The effects of amenorrhea on performance, measured by metabolic parameters, have not been as well studied. One such study did measure oxygen uptake, minute ventilation, heart rate, respiratory exchange ratio, rating of perceived exertion, and time to fatigue, comparing amenorrheic and eumenorrheic runners. Results were identical for the two groups.[9]

Evaluation and Treatment

A screening evaluation of female athletes may reveal amenorrhea. Athletes with amenorrhea should be more thoroughly evaluated to assess factors relating to exercise and to rule out other pathologic conditions. A thorough history, a physical examination, including a pelvic examination, and blood tests should be performed to screen for more serious conditions (Table 17–2). Based on the findings of these tests and the serum estradiol levels detected, a specific treatment plan can be formulated. Therapy for hypoestrogenic amenorrheic women, excluding other serious pathology, includes hormonal replacement primarily for skeletal protection. The treatment protocols may vary depending on

TABLE 17–2   Diagnostic Evaluation of Amenorrhea

History, including dietary intake
Physical examination, including pelvic examination
Prolactin, free thyroxine, thyroid-stimulating hormone, follicle-stimulating hormone, luteinizing hormone, dehydroepiandrosterone sulfate, testosterone, β-human chorionic gonadotropin estradiol
Progestin challenge test

From Shangold MM: Menstruation and menstrual disorders. In Shangold MM, Mirkin G (eds): Women and Exercise, 2nd ed. Philadelphia, FA Davis, 1994, p 299.

TABLE 17–3 Treatment of Hypoestrogenic Amenorrhea

If fertility desired: clomiphene citrate
If contraception needed or preferred: oral contraceptives
If contraception and fertility not of concern: cyclic
  estrogen and progestin therapy
If diet inadequate: correct deficiencies
If very thin: weight gain?
If exercising very heavily: less exercise?

From Shangold MM: Menstruation and menstrual disorders. In Shangold MM, Mirkin G (eds): Women and Exercise, 2nd ed. Philadelphia, FA Davis, 1994, p 300.

whether or not the athlete wishes to become pregnant (Table 17–3).

Evaluation of young athletes with delayed menarche should include a similar assessment (Table 17–4). Therapy depends on the cause of the problem. Readers are referred to several excellent references for further information on evaluation and treatment of amenorrhea, as well as the advantages and disadvantages of hormonal replacement therapy for athletes.[31, 49, 50]

Prognosis

There is no evidence that all cases of secondary amenorrhea or primary amenorrhea related to the female athlete triad are reversible. Therefore, regular follow-up to monitor the effects of treatment to restore normal menstruation and prevent more serious resultant pathology is essential to promote a more successful outcome.

OSTEOPOROSIS

Effects of Estrogen and Calcium

Osteoporosis in the female athlete triad is related to premature bone loss and inade-

TABLE 17–4 Diagnostic Evaluation of Primary Amenorrhea

History, including dietary intake
Physical examination, including pelvic examination
Prolactin, free thyroxine, thyroid-stimulating hormone,
  follicle-stimulating hormone, luteinizing hormone,
  testosterone, estradiol, dehydroepiandrosterone
  sulfate, β-human chorionic gonadotropin
Progestin challenge test
If uterus not palpable on pelvic examination: sonogram
If uterus absent: testosterone, karyotype
If follicle-stimulating hormone high: karyotype

From Shangold MM: Menstruation and menstrual disorders. In Shangold MM, Mirkin G (eds): Women and Exercise, 2nd ed. Philadelphia, FA Davis, 1994, p 301.

quate bone formation. Numerous studies have established the correlation between the presence of hypoestrogenic amenorrhea and the development of premature osteoporosis in female athletes.[8, 10, 12, 13, 15, 30, 44, 46] Lower bone mineral densities and reduced levels of estradiol have been measured in amenorrheic runners compared with their eumenorrheic counterparts.[13, 30, 31, 39, 55] The loss of estrogen is thought to reduce bone mass in two ways. First, renal and intestinal calcium homeostasis is disrupted, and increased amounts of calcium are thus needed to maintain calcium balance. Second, evidence suggests that estrogen has a direct effect on bone cell function, and a deficiency in estrogen allows osteoclasts to reabsorb bone with greater efficiency. The end result is a loss in bone mass.[18]

The role of nutrition and calcium should also be emphasized with regard to bone health. Disordered eating patterns may lead to inadequate intake of dietary or supplemental calcium, which has an important role in the development of peak bone mass. Because the 2 to 3 years of pubertal growth spurt are associated with deposition of 60% of final bone mass, a dietary insufficiency of calcium may have a severe effect on bone formation during this time.[51] Calcium undernutrition can have a significant role in reducing a young female athlete's ability to reach her potential peak bone mass. In the third through fifth decades of life, the effect of calcium deficiency and age-related bone loss is less clear-cut; more research in this population is needed.

Although total body BMD has been shown to be lower in amenorrheic runners, a preferential loss of bone appears to occur in skeletal areas with a high proportion of trabecular bone.[30, 34] Bone loss in the spine, particularly in the lumbar vertebrae,[13, 15, 30, 41, 46] has been reported. Others have found peripheral sites such as the femoral neck to be involved (Fig. 17–6).[10, 32]

Rate of Bone Loss

The extent of bone loss may be rapid and severe in amenorrheic runners. Spinal bone density has been reported to decrease from 1% to 3% per year,[19, 42] with the most significant loss occurring in the first 3 to 4 years of amenorrhea.[8] The spinal bone density of amenorrheic athletes has been found to be around 10% to 20% below the levels expected according to age.[62] Drinkwater re-

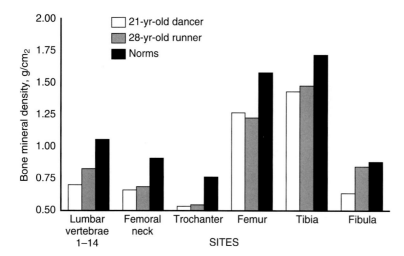

Figure 17–6

Bone mineral density of an amenorrheic 21-year-old dancer and a 28-year-old runner compared with mean values at six sites for eumenorrheic athletes, mean age 26 years. (From Drinkwater BL: Amenorrhea, body weight, and osteoporosis. In Brownell KD, Rodin J, Wilmore JH [eds]: Eating, Body Weight, and Performance in Athletes. Philadelphia, Lea & Febiger, 1992, p 240.)

ported that 20-year-old amenorrheic athletes have BMDs equivalent to that of 60-year-olds.[12, 13, 15]

Clinical Effects of Osteoporosis

The potential consequences of lower BMD are an increased risk of musculoskeletal injuries and stress fractures. Stress fractures have been found to occur more commonly in amenorrheic runners than in their eumenorrheic counterparts.[4, 27, 30, 33, 43] A rate of stress fractures as high as 54% in athletes with amenorrhea compared with 17% in athletes without amenorrhea has been reported.[57] The most commonly reported sites include the metatarsals and tibia,[4, 30] with less frequent reports of femoral stress fractures.[4, 15, 33] Because these skeletal sites are less frequently reported to demonstrate lower BMD in amenorrheic athletes, other variables such as nutrition may need to be combined to fully understand the etiology of the stress fractures noted in this population. For interested readers, an excellent review of the evaluation and treatment of stress fractures is provided in Chapter 4.

In both adolescent and adult runners, lower BMD may lead to an increased risk of osteoporotic fractures noted when bone mineral decreases to below a certain level referred to as the fracture threshold. The age at which this fracture threshold occurs is directly correlated with age-related bone loss and peak bone mass. The latter is most likely to be influenced in amenorrheic runners. In adolescents, a prolonged hypoestrogenic state reduces the peak bone mass, leading to lower

bone density at the time of menopause and an increased risk of fracture in subsequent years. Reports also describe premenopausal amenorrheic runners with bone density levels below the fracture threshold,[13, 61] which may increase their risk of vertebral compression fractures.

Evaluation and Treatment

Further evaluation of bone density measurements in female athletes suspected of having osteoporosis depends on the clinician's findings on history taking and physical examination. No published reports offer specific guidelines about when to obtain bone measurement assessments of young athletes with amenorrhea. A baseline measurement may be helpful for women who have been amenorrheic for longer than 6 to 12 months in order to determine current bone status and to help make informed decisions about treatment. One of the more accurate and precise techniques for measuring bone density is dual-energy x-ray absorptiometry (DEXA). The use of DEXA allows assessment of trabecular and cortical bone as well as whole-body and regional areas.

Treatment to reverse bone loss is directed toward increasing circulating reproductive hormones either naturally through resumption of menses or by hormonal replacement therapy.[51] Because decreased BMD appears to have many causes, treatment is directed at several areas. A reduction in training intensity accompanied by increased body weight has been observed to reestablish normal menstrual cycles in amenorrheic runners, with a resultant increased BMD.[10, 14, 25] If menses does not resume or the athlete refuses to alter her training schedule or dietary patterns, estrogen replacement therapy is recommended.[49, 50] At present, it is assumed that doses prescribed to postmenopausal women would be adequate to reduce bone loss in amenorrheic athletes, although precise information about young female athletes is not available. Increasing calcium intake to 1500 mg daily is suggested if the athlete is amenorrheic, although data about the effect of increasing dietary calcium on vertebral BMD are conflicting. Several studies investigated increased calcium intake (1500 mg daily) among amenorrheic athletes and reported no change in BMD at the proximal femur or lumbar spine after 12 and 24 months of intervention.[12, 58] Other studies have reported an increase in cortical BMD in the high-calcium-intake amenorrheic group, perhaps indicating a site-specific response to an area of greatest mechanical stress rather than a systemic response.[12, 17] It appears as though calcium by itself is not effective enough to override the detrimental effects of low estrogen.

Prognosis

How much bone mass can be regained is still in question. Evidence suggests that at least some bone can be regained if an athlete resumes normal menses. An average increase of 6% in vertebral BMD was reported over a 14-month period in female athletes who resumed menses.[10, 12, 25] The amount of bone mass that can be restored may be limited, however. Follow-up investigation of these athletes revealed that increases in BMD slowed to 3% the following year and ceased during the next 2 years.[10, 11, 14] Even with treatment and normal menses, the previously amenorrheic athletes continued to demonstrate lower BMDs than their eumenorrheic counterparts.

SCREENING FOR THE FEMALE ATHLETE TRIAD

A high index of suspicion, along with increased awareness of the existence of the problem, is required by an athlete's health care team in order to diagnose one or all of the components of the female athlete triad. Physicians who treat female runners should be aware of the presenting signs and symptoms of the components of the triad. A female runner may present to the treatment team in any number of ways, ranging from complaints of fatigue related to inadequate caloric intake and poor nutrition to a stress fracture.[43] Clinicians need to be aware that the presenting symptoms may be a result of factors (disordered eating, amenorrhea, and osteoporosis) that produce the triad. Evaluation of female runners should be expanded to include a screening for components of the female athlete triad along with the appropriate evaluation of the presenting problem.

A *nutritional screening* is important to detect the presence of disordered eating in female athletes. Because disordered eating patterns are often kept secret, clinicians should establish good rapport with athletes and should ask very specific questions about dietary and body weight patterns, diet pills and laxative use, and binging and purging behaviors. An athlete's nutritional intake should be documented in a diet and training log for at least 1 week. Body fat may be assessed with skinfold calipers, and although low body fat has not been identified as the single factor causing amenorrhea, it may reflect poor nutritional status.[46] If an athlete is identified to be at risk for an eating disorder, further follow-up should be arranged with a nutritionist as well as a psychologist or psychiatrist.

An *exercise history* should be taken to determine if exercise is excessive, with a comparison between the athlete's caloric intake and estimated energy expenditure.

A *menstrual history* should be taken, including questions about the onset of menarche and menstrual patterns. Irregular or absent periods require further investigation, as previously outlined in the section discussing amenorrhea.

Other screening information should include a history of musculoskeletal injuries to determine the frequency of overuse and stress fracture problems, a family history to determine any familial tendencies toward disordered eating behaviors, and a social history to outline an athlete's stress level and stress relievers.

TREATMENT AND PREVENTION

On completion of the evaluation, an appropriate treatment plan can be outlined to address the specific problems identified in the female athlete. Basic information, along with references, has been discussed for each of the components of the triad. The best treatment for the female athlete triad, however, is prevention and early detection.

Preparticipation examinations may offer an ideal opportunity for screening female athletes and identifying disordered eating patterns, amenorrhea or menstrual irregularities, and a history of stress fractures or other pathologic fractures.[21, 39, 63] Education and awareness about the disorders are also important for prevention, using widespread efforts to reach athletes, parents, coaches, training staff, and physicians. An action plan for future prevention and treatment of the female athlete triad was developed by the American College of Sports Medicine Ad Hoc Task Force on Women's Issues in Sports Medicine.[1, 35, 37, 63] Information about the effects of disordered eating, appropriate nutrition and weight control methods, and increased medical awareness of the interrelatedness of the triad of disorders all are part of the prevention program.

No long-term studies have investigated the morbidity and mortality of the female athlete triad. The short-term and long-term effects may involve psychologic, medical, and orthopedic consequences and at the extreme may lead to premature death. It is believed, however, that the earlier intervention starts, the better the chance for recovery and reduced morbidity.[36]

CONCLUSION

The information provided in this chapter is not meant to imply that every long-distance runner is at high risk for developing the female athlete triad. Running and exercise provide many health benefits for women. At some point, however, the risks outweigh the benefits of running. Those involved with the care of female runners should be aware of their potential risk of developing the triad, because long-distance runners share many features of its risk profile. The goal for a female runner and her medical team should be for her to participate and succeed in her sport safely and in the most healthy manner possible.

REFERENCES

1. American College of Sports Medicine: The female athlete triad: Disordered eating, amenorrhea, osteoporosis: Call to action. Sports Med Bull 27:4, 1992.
2. American Psychiatric Association: Diagnostic and Statistical Manual of Mental Disorders, 4th ed. Washington, DC, American Psychiatric Association, 1994.
3. Baer J, Taper JL: Amenorrheic and eumenorrheic adolescent runners: Dietary intake and exercise training status. J Am Diet Assoc 92:89, 1992.
4. Barrow GW, Subrata S: Menstrual irregularity and stress fractures in collegiate female distance runners. Am J Sports Med 6:209, 1988.
5. Brewer V, Meyer BM, Kiele MS, et al: Role of exercise in prevention of involutional bone loss. Med Sci Sports Exerc 15:445, 1983.
6. Brownell KD, Rodin J: Prevalence of eating disorders. In Brownell KD, Rodin J, Wilmore JH (eds): Eating, Body Weight, and Performance in Athletes. Philadelphia, Lea & Febiger, 1992, p 128.
7. Brownell KD, Rodin J, Wilmore JH (eds): Eating, Body Weight and Performance in Athletes. Philadelphia, Lea & Febiger, 1992.
8. Cann LE, Martin MC, Genant HK, et al: Decreased spinal mineral content in amenorrheic women. JAMA 51:626, 1984.
9. DeSouza MJ, Maguire MS, Rubin KR, et al: Effects of menstrual phase and amenorrhea on exercise performance in runners. Med Sci Sports Exerc 22:575, 1990.
10. Drinkwater BL, Bruemmer B, Chestnut CH III: Menstrual history as determinant of current bone density in young athletes. JAMA 263:545, 1990.
11. Drinkwater BL: Amenorrhea, body weight and osteoporosis. In Brownell KD, Rodin J, Wilmore JH (eds): Eating, Body Weight, and Performance in Athletes. Philadelphia, Lea & Febiger, 1992, p 235.
12. Drinkwater BL, Chestnut CH III: Site specific skeletal response to increased calcium in amenorrheic athletes. Med Sci Sports Exerc 24:545, 1992.
13. Drinkwater BL, Nilson K, Chestnut CH III, et al: Bone mineral content of amenorrheic and eumenorrheic athletes. N Engl J Med 311:277, 1984.
14. Drinkwater BL, Nilson K, Ott S, Chestnut CH III: Bone mineral density after resumption of menses in amenorrheic athletes. JAMA 256:380, 1986.
15. Dugowson CE, Drinkwater BL, Clark JM: Nontraumatic femur fracture in an oligomenorrheic athlete. Med Sci Sports Exerc 23:1323, 1991.
16. Eichner ER: General health issues of low body weight and undereating in athletes. In Brownell KD, Rodin J, Wilmore JH (eds): Eating, Body Weight, and Performance in Athletes. Philadelphia, Lea & Febiger, 1992, p 191.
17. Elders PJ, Lips P, Netelenbos JL, et al: Calcium reduces lumbar bone loss in pre- and perimenopausal women, but not in early postmenopausal women. Bone Miner 17:73, 1992.
18. Eriksen EF, Colvard DS, Berg NJ, et al: Evidence of estrogen receptors in normal human osteoblasts. Science 241:84, 1988.
19. Firooznia H, Golimbu C, Rafii M, Schwartz MS: Rate of spinal trabecular bone loss in normal perimenopausal women: CT measurement. Radiology 161:735, 1986.
20. Gadpaille WJ, Sanborn CF, Wagner WW: Athletic amenorrhea, major affective disorders and eating disorders. Am J Psychiatry 144:939, 1987.
21. Johnson MD: Tailoring the preparticipation examination to female athletes. Physician Sportsmed 20:61, 1992.
22. Johnson MD: Disordered eating in active and athletic women. Clin Sports Med 13:355, 1994.

23. Kaiserauer S, Snyder AC, Sleeper M, et al: Nutritional, physiological, and menstrual status of distance runners. Med Sci Sports Exerc 21:120, 1989.

24. Katz J: Eating disorders. In Shangold MM, Mirkin G (eds): Women and Exercise, 2nd ed. Philadelphia, FA Davis, 1994, p 292.

25. Lindberg JS, Powell MR, Hunt MM, et al: Increased vertebral bone mineral in response to reduced exercise in amenorrheic runners. West J Med 146:39, 1987.

26. Liu JH: Hypothalamic amenorrhea: Clinical perspectives, pathophysiology, and management. Am J Obstet Gynecol 163:1732, 1990.

27. Lloyd T, Triantafyllou SJ, Baker ER, et al: Women athletes with menstrual irregularity have increased musculoskeletal injuries. Med Sci Sports Exerc 18:374, 1986.

28. Loucks AB, Mortola JF, Gerton L, et al: Alterations in hypothalamic-pituitary-ovarian and hypothalamic-pituitary-adrenal axes in athletic women. J Clin Endocrinol Metab 68:402, 1989.

29. Lutter JM: Health concerns in women runners. Clin Sports Med 4:671, 1985.

30. Marcus R, Cann C, Madvig P, et al: Menstrual function and bone mass in elite women distance runners. Ann Intern Med 102:158, 1985.

31. Marshall LA: Clinical evaluation of amenorrhea in active and athletic women. Clin Sports Med 13:371, 1994.

32. Myburgh KH, Bachrach LK, Lewis B, et al: Low bone mineral density at axial and appendicular sites in amenorrheic athletes. Med Sci Sports Exerc 25:1197, 1993.

33. Myburgh KK, Hutchins J, Fataar AB: Low bone density is an etiologic factor for stress fractures in athletes. Ann Intern Med 113:754, 1990.

34. Myerson M, Gutin B, Warren MP, et al: Total body bone mineral density in amenorrheic runners. Obstet Gynecol 79:973, 1992.

35. Nattiv A, Agostini R, Drinkwater B, et al: The female athlete triad: The interrelatedness of disordered eating, amenorrhea, and osteoporosis. Clin Sports Med 13:405, 1994.

36. Nattiv A, Lynch L: The female athlete triad—managing acute risk to long term health. Physician Sportsmed 22:60, 1994.

37. Nattiv A, Yeager K, Drinkwater B, et al: The female athlete triad. In Agostini R (ed): Medical and Orthopedic Issues of Active and Athletic Women, Philadelphia, Hanley & Belfus, 1994, p 169.

38. Nelson ME, Fisher EC, Catsos PD, et al: Diet and bone status in amenorrheic runners. Am J Clin Nutr 43:910, 1986.

39. Otis CL: Exercise-associated amenorrhea. Clin Sports Med 11:351, 1992.

40. Palla B, Litt IF: Medical complications of eating disorders in adolescents. Pediatrics 81:613, 1988.

41. Prior TC, Vigna YM, Schechter MT, et al: Spinal bone loss and ovulatory disturbances. N Engl J Med 323:1221, 1990.

42. Riggs BL, Wahner HW, Melton LJ III, et al: Rates of bone loss in appendicular and axial skeletons of women: Evidence of substantial vertebral bone loss before menopause. J Clin Invest 77:1487, 1986.

43. Roberts WO: Primary amenorrhea and persistent stress fractures. Physician Sportsmed 23:33, 1995.

44. Rosen LW, Hough DO: Pathogenic weight-control behavior of female college gymnasts. Physician Sportsmed 16:141, 1988.

45. Rosen LW, McKeag DB, Hough DO, et al: Pathogenic weight-control behavior in female athletes. Physician Sportsmed 14:79, 1986.

46. Sanborn CF, Albrecht BH, Wagner WW: Athletic amenorrhea: Lack of association with body fat. Med Sci Sports Exerc 19:207, 1987.

47. Sanborn CF, Martin BJ, Wagner WW: Is athletic amenorrhea specific to runners? Am J Obstet Gynecol 143:859, 1982.

48. Schwartz B, Cumming DC, Riordan E, et al: Exercise-associated amenorrhea: A distinct entity? Am J Obstet Gynecol 141:662, 1981.

49. Shangold MM: Menstruation and menstrual disorders. In Shangold MM, Mirkin G (eds): Women and Exercise, 2nd ed. Philadelphia, FA Davis, 1994, p 152.

50. Shangold MM, Rebar RW, Wentz AC, et al: Evaluation and management of menstrual dysfunction in athletes. JAMA 263:1665, 1990.

51. Snow-Harter CM: Bone health and prevention of osteoporosis in active and athletic women. Clin Sports Med 13:389, 1994.

52. Snow-Harter CM, Bouxsein ML, Lewis BT, et al: Effects of resistance and endurance exercise on bone mineral status of young women: A randomized exercise intervention trial. J Bone Miner Res 7:761, 1992.

53. Steinhauser H, Rauss-Mason C, Seidel R: Follow-up studies of anorexia nervosa: A review of four decades of outcome research. Psychol Med 21:447, 1991.

54. Sundgot-Borgen J: Risk and trigger factors for development of eating disorders in elite female athletes. Med Sci Sports Exerc 26:414, 1994.

55. Warren MP: Amenorrhea in endurance runners. J Clin Endocrinol Metab 75:1393, 1992.

56. Warren MP: Eating, body weight, and menstrual function. In Brownell KD, Rodin J, Wilmore JH (eds): Eating, Body Weight, and Performance in Athletes. Philadelphia, Lea & Febiger, 1992, p 222.

57. Warren MP, Brooks-Gunn J, Hamilton LH: Scoliosis and fractures in young ballet dancers: Relation to delayed menarche and secondary amenorrhea. N Engl J Med 314:1348, 1986.

58. Weltman A, Snead DB, Weltman JY, et al: Effects of calcium supplementation on bone mineral density (BMD) in premenopausal women. Med Sci Sports Exerc 24:S12, 1992.

59. Wilmore JH: Eating and weight disorders in female athletes. Int J Sport Nutr 1:104, 1991.

60. Wilson GT, Eldredge K: Pathology and development of eating disorders: Implications for athletes. In Brownell KD, Rodin J, Wilmore JH (eds): Eating, Body Weight, and Performance in Athletes. Philadelphia, Lea & Febiger, 1992, p 115.

61. Wolman RL, Clark P, McNally E, et al: Dietary calcium as a statistical determinant of spinal trabecular bone of the appendicular and axial skeleton with aging: Relationship to spinal osteoporosis. J Clin Invest 67:328, 1981.

62. Wolman RL, Reeve J: Exercise and the skeleton. In Harris W, Williams C, Stanish WD, Micheli LJ (eds): Oxford Textbook of Sports Medicine, New York, Oxford University Press, 1994, p 267.

63. Yeager KK, Agostini R, Nattiv A, et al: The female athlete triad: Disordered eating, amenorrhea, osteoporosis (commentary). Med Sci Sports Exerc 25:775, 1993.

GUY G. SIMONEAU ▪ KEVIN E. WILK ▪ WILLIAM G. CLANCY, JR.

CHAPTER EIGHTEEN

Strengthening and Flexibility Concepts for Runners

Running athletes, competitive or recreational, can fall victim to numerous injuries. The majority of these injuries involve the lower extremities and lower back as a result of the repetitive weight-bearing forces applied to these parts of the body during training or racing. Most running injuries are a result of repetitive microtraumas and can be classified as overuse injuries resulting in nagging, persistent, painful conditions that restrict the runner's performance. Among the most commonly recognized factors contributing to these injuries are muscle weakness, poor flexibility, training errors, poor/abnormal lower extremity biomechanics, and poor running shoes. Injuries that have been specifically linked to inadequate muscle flexibility or strength include Achilles tendinitis, iliotibial band syndrome, patellar tendinitis, posterior tibial tendinitis, and plantar fasciitis.[19] The highly repetitive nature of the sport and the magnitude of the forces applied to the lower extremities at each step of a run mean that over time, even relatively small deficits in flexibility or strength can cause microtraumas, culminating in an injury that excludes a runner from participation.

The average running athlete places tremendous stresses on the lower extremities during a 1-mile run. Mann[24] has calculated that an average 150-pound man with a step length of 3.5 feet would take 1175 steps in a 1-mile run. At initial ground contact, the impact force between the foot and the ground is approximately 2.5 times the runner's body weight. Thus, a total of 440,625 pounds is imparted to the lower extremities during a 1-mile run (110 tons for each lower extremity). For runners who run at least 1 mile at least three times per week, the stresses applied to the muscular and bony structures of the

lower extremities are indeed significant. Therefore, the muscles of the lower extremities must be strong enough and flexible enough to absorb and control these repetitive stresses in order to prevent the numerous types of microtrauma injuries recognized to afflict recreational and competitive runners.

The most common site of injury to a runner is the knee.[19, 22] Posterior tibial tendinitis and Achilles tendinitis are also extremely common.[22] Tendinitis most often develops with a gradually worsening course, and the runner continues to run despite the increasingly significant discomfort. Medical attention is often sought only after the tendinitis is well established and after running has become extremely difficult and often impossible because of pain. Welsh and Clodman[33] surveyed 50 track and field athletes diagnosed with Achilles tendinitis. The researchers reported that 54% of the athletes could continue to compete but with considerable duress and a reduced level of performance; 16% were forced to abandon sports participation permanently. As with many sports injuries, prevention and early intervention through an adequate flexibility and strengthening program may be the best treatment approach.

Tendinitis is one of the most common injuries encountered by running athletes. Clancy[3] has reported that the term *tendinitis* is confusing and perplexing. He has suggested a classification of tendon injury that includes tenosynovitis, tendinitis (acute and chronic), and tendonosis. The treatment of each type of tendon injury is based on the duration of symptoms and the location and classification of the injury. The treatment most commonly consists of a nonoperative approach based on a series of specific stretching and strengthening rehabilitation exercises. Ice, heat, ultrasound, and corticosteroids all can be used as possible adjuncts to this rehabilitation program. Only when the conservative approach has been exhausted should surgical interventions be considered.

The purpose of this chapter is to review and discuss rehabilitative exercises for running athletes. The initial section of this chapter specifically discusses general flexibility and strengthening principles. The second section of this chapter focuses on descriptions of specific strengthening and stretching exercises for the lower extremities and lumbar spine. These exercises can be implemented as an injury-preventing strategy or included as part of a rehabilitation program. Although some aspects of the biomechanics of running are mentioned, readers are referred to other chapters of this book for a comprehensive discussion of the topic. Similarly, detailed information about the evaluation and treatment of selected specific injuries related to running is provided in other chapters of this book.

PRINCIPLES OF STRETCHING

Adequate and necessary joint range of motion to perform athletic activities, without undue stress, requires proper muscle flexibility. Two types of flexibility have been described by deVries,[10] static and dynamic. Static flexibility is a measure of the range of motion available at a joint or over a series of joints. Dynamic flexibility relates to the resistance to active motion at the joint. Both aspects of flexibility have an important role in minimizing the occurrence of injuries during participation in leisure activities and sports, including running.[6, 37] Although a few people are inherently very flexible, most individuals must participate in a regular stretching program in order to acquire and maintain the flexibility necessary for injury-free sports participation. For runners, the flexibility program should focus on the muscles of the lower extremities, particularly the ankle plantar flexors (posterior calf muscles), the hamstrings, the iliotibial band, the quadriceps, and the hip flexors.

An effective stretching technique must take into account muscle morphology as well as muscle function. Morphologically, muscles are composed of contractile and noncontractile fibers. The contractile component of the muscle consists of the muscle fibers themselves, which are made up of myosin and actin filaments that interact to shorten the muscle actively. When elongated, these muscle fibers can provide passive resistance to stretching. Just as important, they can also provide active resistance to stretching through a voluntary muscle contraction or involuntary reflex action. The noncontractile component of the muscle consists of collagen fibers (endomysium, perimysium, and epimysium), which surround the muscle fibers and provide them with a support matrix. The noncontractile muscle component, typically accountable for determining muscle flexibility, also provides passive resistance to stretching. Therefore, an effective stretching technique must meet two requirements. First, it must elongate the muscle without triggering a voluntary or involuntary muscle response of the contractile fibers. Second, based on the viscoelastic properties of biologic tissues, it must maintain a tension of appropriate intensity and duration to promote plastic deformation (without causing damage through tearing) of the noncontractile fibers.[23, 30]

BENEFITS OF STRETCHING

Many clinicians and researchers have suggested that increased flexibility may decrease the incidence of sports (including running) injuries,[4, 11–13, 16, 19, 21, 28, 36, 37] minimize postexercise muscle soreness,[7, 9] and possibly (the literature is inconclusive in this regard) enhance athletic performance.[9, 15, 17, 18, 35] The following discussion focuses on the benefits of stretching in reducing the incidence of injuries.

Stretching is believed to reduce the incidence of muscle strains during sports participation because increased extensibility allows the muscle to stretch to a greater length before tearing.[27] Therefore, preparticipation stretches, although not necessarily aimed at achieving permanent lengthening of the muscle, are intended to elongate the muscle temporarily to decrease its resistance to elongation. This allows a runner to run with less effort, better muscular dynamic flexibility, and better biomechanics. In addition, the increased range of motion provides the flexibility necessary to avoid muscle strains that often occur as a result of unexpected or excessive motion of the joint, such as when a long-distance runner slips on an icy surface or when a sprinter overstrides. This aspect of injury prevention is relatively well known in the athletic community.

Perhaps not as well recognized by the athletic community is the fact that inadequate flexibility often induces abnormal body mechanics, which can lead to injuries as a result of excessive and abnormal repetitive microstresses applied on muscular as well as nonmuscular structures. This particular aspect of injury mechanism is especially relevant for long-distance runners, who need optimal lower extremity biomechanics to avoid injuries such as Achilles tendinitis, plantar fasciitis, iliotibial band syndrome, chondromalacia patellae, and posterior tibialis tendinitis, which are usually a result of repetitive microtraumas. Davis[6] reported that 92% of the runners seen in the physical therapy clinic exhibited tightness of one or more lower extremity muscles (specifically, the hamstring and gastrocnemius muscle groups). In the majority of cases, lack of muscle flexibility was found to be a factor contributing to the running-related injuries. A stretching program addressing specific muscles known to lack flexibility may help in preventing repetitive motion injuries such as those listed earlier.

The gait and running literature specifically points to lack of flexibility of the Achilles tendon as a factor contributing to several common running injuries of the lower extremities.[19] Achilles tendon tightness may lead to, among other gait deviations, excessive foot pronation, which results in abnormal stresses placed across the foot and knee region. These abnormal stresses can lead to ailments such as Achilles tendinitis, plantar fasciitis, posterior tibialis tendinitis, and chondromalacia patellae. Other muscle groups whose lack of flexibility may participate in the etiology of running-related injuries include the hip flexors, the hamstrings, and the iliotibial band.[19] The increased lumbar lordosis resulting from a lack of flexibility of the hip flexors may lead to lower back pain as a result of the excessive stresses applied on the lumbar spine when running. Similarly, a direct relationship is believed to exist between hamstring inflexibility and anterior knee pain and between iliotibial band tightness and lateral knee pain. In cases in which tightness causes abnormal lower limb mechanics during running, it is important for athletes not only to precede running with a session of stretching but also to participate in a regular stretching program with the ultimate goal of permanently lengthening the tight muscle.

The work by Wallin and colleagues[32] suggests that it is necessary to engage in a stretching program three to five times per week to increase flexibility. Once flexibility is gained, as little as one session per week of stretching is needed to maintain the gains achieved. Note, however, that interruption of the stretching program results, over several weeks, in a progressive loss of the gains made.[40]

A specific and controlled flexibility program is often implemented as part of the rehabilitation program for various running injuries. This flexibility program, which must be tailored to the particular injury and the runner, aims to optimize the likelihood of recovery and minimize the chances of reinjury. Zachazewski[39] gives a detailed account of the soft tissue healing process and the role of stretching in this process.

PREPARATION FOR STRETCHING

A preliminary warm-up routine to increase intramuscular temperature should be an integral part of a stretching program because increased tissue temperature results in increased elasticity and decreased stiffness of the connective tissue, making it more extensible.[27] It is suggested that this increase in temperature is best achieved with 10 to 15 minutes of light general exercise, such as cycling, fast walking, or stair climbing, to bring the muscle's tissue temperature to approximately 39°C.[23] Clinically, using stretching exercises soon after sports participation has also been found to be beneficial in increasing flexibility because the muscle is maximally warmed up. In addition, postexercise stretches can be useful in preventing the muscle soreness (delayed-onset muscle soreness) sometimes related to excessive physical activity.

METHODS OF STRETCHING

The three most common methods of stretching described in the literature are static stretching, ballistic stretching, and stretching using proprioceptive neuromuscular facilitation (PNF) concepts. All three techniques increase the flexibility of the muscle-tendon unit. The literature identifying the most effective technique remains inconclusive because of the general lack of control of stretching time and stretching force among the three methods.[23]

Static Stretching. Static stretching involves maintaining a constant amount of tension on a muscle for a given period of time in order to create a progressive deformation of the tissues and increase their length. The passive force can be provided by an external force such as another individual or a weight. Through static stretching, stimulation of the Golgi tendon organs, located in the myotendinous junction, is achieved, resulting in decreased muscle tone.[28] Additionally, a slowly applied stretch helps reduce muscle tone by reducing the degree of myotatic reflex contraction.[2, 28, 32] Both neurophysiologic responses participate in the effectiveness of this technique to elongate a muscle through both elastic and plastic deformation of its noncontractile components.

The effectiveness of this type of stretching in increasing flexibility is determined by the duration as well as the intensity (load) of the stretch. Basic and clinical research appears to support the use of low-load, prolonged-duration stretches as being most efficacious.[1] The results from the work by Bandy and Irion[1] on hamstring flexibility suggest that the optimum duration of time to stretch a muscle for each repetition is approximately 30 seconds, with no advantage to holding the stretch for a longer time. Although the optimal number of repetitions is not agreed on, most clinicians believe that three to five stretches per muscle or muscle group are appropriate before participation in physical activity. In addition, Taylor and colleagues[31] suggest that long-lasting increase in flexibility can be achieved with three to five stretches, with minimal additional gain achieved with a greater number of stretches.

Static stretching is often favored over other types of stretching techniques for the following reasons: It is simple, it is nontraumatic, it requires minimal energy, it does not result in muscle soreness, and the force application is well controlled, minimizing the danger of exceeding the extensibility limits of the tissues being stretched. This stretching technique is based on the viscoelastic properties of collagen tissues, which elongate through plastic deformation when a prolonged mild stretch is applied. Although this method is effective at increasing flexibility, Zachazewski[38] suggests that the passive nature of static stretching does little to train the muscles to respond actively when a stretch beyond safe limits is applied. This lack of active response may possibly contribute to traumatic muscle strains.

In summary, to be effective, a static stretching program should be performed at least three to five times per week and should consist of three to five low-load stretches of 30 seconds for each muscle or muscle group to be stretched. Stretching should not traumatize the muscle tissue. Although low load is difficult to define, stretching should be perceived as a low to mild stretch. The "no pain, no gain" mentality does not apply to the practice of stretching for sports participation.

Ballistic Stretching. With this technique, quick, repetitive stretches (bouncing) are applied to the muscle to be stretched.[26, 32] Essentially, the runner "bounces" at end of range, against the resistance to the stretch. This method of stretching, once popular among the general population, is typically discouraged by the sports medicine and health care communities.[2] Ballistic stretching may be less effective than other forms of stretching in increasing muscle flexibility.[32] Additionally, ballistic stretching places a runner at a greater risk of exceeding the extensibility of the tissues being stretched and is more likely to cause muscle soreness.

Neurophysiologically, ballistic movements are less than optimal for stretching because the abrupt stretch of the muscle stimulates the intrafusal muscle spindles, in turn causing a reflex muscle contraction that shortens the muscle—a response contrary to the desired elongation effect.[2, 32] Although ballistic stretching is not recommended as a means to increase flexibility, Malone and associates[23] point to the considerable resemblance between the movement of ballistic stretching and the intermittent stretches that occur during the course of athletic activities. These investigators suggest that training with this type of stretching, only after appropriate warm-up and static stretching has been performed, may carry over to protect against injury by improving the protective muscle response to excessive stretches. Zachazewski[38] emphasizes that the use of ballistic stretches should be limited to athletes who perform ballistic-type movement as part of their sports, for example, karate.

Proprioceptive Neuromuscular Facilitation Stretching. Two types of stretching are typically performed when using PNF principles. These two techniques aim to facilitate the action of the Golgi tendon organs in inhibiting the muscle being stretched. They also use the concept of reciprocal inhibition, in which the muscle being stretched is inhibited by the active action of its antagonists. The hold-relax technique involves a three-step process. First, the muscle is stretched to the limit of motion. Then, the individual performs a 7- to 8-second isometric muscle contraction of the muscle being stretched against an unyielding object or resistance. Finally, the individual relaxes and a further stretch is applied for 7 to 8 seconds.[32] The contract-relax with agonist contraction method can also be used.[14] With this technique, the muscle is first stretched to a comfortable position. Then, the individual isometrically contracts the muscle being stretched for a 6-second period. This is followed by contraction of the antagonist muscles for 3 seconds. As the muscle contracts, inhibition of the muscle being stretched occurs, allowing better elongation. PNF techniques are very effective methods of stretching. However, because of the time and expertise required to use these techniques, they are most likely to be impractical for recreational runners.

STRETCHING PROGRAM FOR RUNNERS

Targeted muscles of the lower extremity for stretching in runners are the hip flexors, quadriceps, hamstrings, iliotibial band, and ankle plantar flexors (Achilles tendon). All of these muscles, when lacking adequate flexibility, have been identified as participating in the etiology of some of the most common running injuries. Specific stretching techniques addressing each of these muscles are provided later in this chapter.

Although the generic principles of stretching presented earlier apply to any individual wanting to increase his or her flexibility, individualized stretching programs can be developed only after a runner's flexibility and biomechanics have been assessed thoroughly. Some muscle groups are typically recognized as needing increased flexibility, but each individual has particular needs based on his or her body type, occupation, and leisure activities. Stretching of joints that already have excessive flexibility may lead to joint instability and injuries.

To summarize, three to five repetitions of a mild static stretch lasting approximately 30 seconds performed three to five times a week are necessary to increase muscle flexibility. Once achieved, a certain level of muscle flexibility can be maintained with as little as one stretching session per week. Stretching should be performed before sports participation but after a 10- to 15-minute general light warm-up program.

PRINCIPLES OF STRENGTHENING

The muscles of the lower extremities and trunk need to be not only flexible but also strong. Adequate muscle strength is required to assist in dissipating the large magnitude of ground reaction forces during running. This section briefly discusses various aspects of muscle strength and its application to a strengthening program. This chapter focuses on exercise principles used in rehabilitation of injuries. Because implementation of a safe and effective strengthening program can be rather complex (and is beyond the scope of this chapter), readers are referred to other sources for detailed information.[34]

MUSCLE STRENGTH AND ENDURANCE

Muscle strength can be defined as the maximum force or tension generated by a muscle or group of muscles.[25] Enhancing muscle strength is often a primary goal of rehabilitation programs. Six interdependent factors influence the strength in normal muscle tissue:

- The cross-sectional area of the muscle
- The length-tension relationship
- The motor unit recruitment pattern
- The type of muscle contraction (concentric, eccentric, isometric)
- The speed of muscle contraction
- Motivational factors

The two most cited changes in the muscular system leading to strength gains are muscle hypertrophy and motor unit recruitment. Hypertrophy is a complex physiologic phenomenon resulting in an increase in myofibril (actin and myosin fibers) size. Because the strength-generating capacity of muscle tissue is directly related to its cross-sectional area, hypertrophy leads to muscle strength gains. Strength gains can also be achieved by recruiting a greater number of motor units simultaneously, thus increasing the force-generating capacity of the muscle. Hypertrophy results from high-intensity, low-repetition muscular exercise.[20]

Adequate muscle endurance, in order to sustain repeated loading of the lower extremities, is also vital to running athletes. Endurance is typically defined as the ability to perform a given workload for an extended time. Therefore, muscle endurance is the ability of a muscle or muscle group to perform an action repeatedly against a given load or to sustain a given tension for a period of time. Improved muscle endurance is a result of increased mitochondria density and number, faster redistribution of blood flow, and increased oxidative enzyme content of the muscle. In addition, increased muscle endurance results from angiogenesis (increased number of blood vessels), which decreases oxygen diffusion distance and capillary diffusion time, increasing the speed of oxygen delivery and waste removal. Muscle endurance is improved through the use of low-intensity, high-repetition muscle exercise.[20]

STRENGTHENING EXERCISES

There are several forms of resistive exercise, including isotonic concentric, isotonic eccentric, isometric, isokinetic, and plyometric. Although all can be used in a rehabilitation program for runners, this discussion is limited to isometric and isotonic exercises.

Isotonic exercises are a dynamic form of exercise carried out against a fixed resistance as a muscle lengthens or shortens through the available range of motion. Examples of isotonic exercises are listed later. During isotonic resistance, the resistance is fixed and the speed of muscle contraction is variable. The term *isotonic* literally denotes the same or constant tension. In fact, when a muscle contracts dynamically against a fixed load (resistance), the tension produced in the muscle varies as it shortens and lengthens through the available range of motion, and maximum muscle tension develops at only one point in the range of motion.

Isotonic exercises can be divided into two phases: concentric and eccentric muscle loading. Concentric muscle loading involves a shortening muscle contraction in which the muscle origin and insertion approximate. Conversely, eccentric muscle loading involves a lengthening muscle contraction in which the muscle origin and insertion separate. More force can be generated during an eccentric muscle action than during a concentric muscle action. Some researchers have advocated the use of eccentric muscle training for the treatment of tendinitis.[5] Isotonic strengthening is the most commonly used form of resistance exercise for muscle training and is most often performed through resistance machines, free weights, or body weight exercises.

Isometric resistance exercise is a static form of exercise occurring when a muscle contracts without appreciable change in length of the muscle or without visible joint motion. Although no physical work is done, a great amount of tension and force output is produced by the muscle. Because no joint movement occurs, isometrics are often implemented early in the rehabilitative process after an injury or during the subacute inflammation phase. Advantages of isometrics include safety, ease of application, prevention of muscle atrophy, and lack of need for equipment. In contrast, a major disadvantage of isometrics is that strength gains are fairly specific to the joint angles at which the exercise was performed, with physiologic carryover of only 20 degrees. Additionally, isometric exercise is often boring, and compliance with this type of exercise thus may be poor.

The type of resistance exercise program developed for a specific muscle or muscle group is often dictated by an athlete's pain and the available equipment; ultimately, however, the muscle should be trained in the way in which it functions. For example, during running, the knee flexion angle is approximately 25 to 40 degrees at ground contact. In this degree of knee flexion, the quadriceps and hamstrings contract to stabilize the joint. Therefore, isometric exercises can be specifically used to enhance dynamic joint stability through co-contraction of the musculature surrounding the joint.

Other muscles or muscle groups active during running include the gluteus maximus, hip adductors, hip abductors, and posterior calf muscles. The gluteus maximus is active during the first 40% of the stance phase during running and assists in controlling hip extension. The hip adductors function during the terminal swing phase and throughout the first 50% of the stance phase of running. The hip abductors function to stabilize the stance leg side of the pelvis during ground contact and thus maintain a level pelvis. The posterior calf muscles are active at the end of the swing phase and undergo a rapid eccentric contraction at the time of initial ground contact. The posterior calf muscles continue to be active for about 60% of the stance phase. In the latter part of the stance phase, the posterior calf muscles provide some degree of propulsion, but the exact amount is yet undetermined.

Of these muscles, the hip abductors have a key role in providing stability to the lower leg during stance. Clinically, the hip abductors are often found to be functionally weak, resulting in poor control of the hip and knee in the frontal plane. This poor control leads to excessive hip adduction and internal rotation shortly after foot contact, which leads to increased valgus at the knee and an increased Q angle, which has been linked to an increased incidence of chondromalacia patellae.[19]

STRENGTHENING PROGRAM FOR RUNNERS

Targeted muscles of the lower extremity for strengthening in runners include the hip extensors, quadriceps, hamstrings, hip abductors, ankle dorsiflexors, and ankle plantar flexors. Specific exercises addressing each of these muscles are described later. As with any strengthening program, strength gains are better achieved by using high loads and keeping the number of repetitions low. On the other hand, endurance gains are better achieved by lifting lighter loads through a high number of repetitions. Most programs aimed at increasing muscle strength should be performed three times a week.[34]

A strengthening exercise program targeting the muscles listed earlier is likely to be useful in increasing overall lower extremity strength. As with muscle flexibility, specific deficits in strength of the lower extremity musculature vary from one individual to another based on body type, occupation, and leisure activities. It is not uncommon to find a weak muscle to be opposed by a muscle lacking flexibility—for example, runners with tight hamstrings may be found also to have weak quadriceps. To establish an individualized strengthening program, a thorough evaluation of strength and running biomechanics is required.

Strengthening exercises are often used in a rehabilitation program for running-related injuries. Low-intensity isometric exercises are useful in the early stages of rehabilitation in order to maintain or increase strength while minimizing irritation of the injured structures. Isotonic exercises are useful in addressing specific muscle deficits. Clinical emphasis has been progressively shifting toward the use of functional exercises that resemble or mimic the activity the athlete will return to.

SPECIFIC CONSIDERATIONS FOR THE LUMBAR SPINE

Although the lower extremities receive most of the focus in terms of mechanics, the lower back also sustains significant stresses during running. In the age group of 30 to 50 years, the degree of repetitive motion in the lumbar spine during distance running is unparalleled in other sports.[29] Most of the lumbar spine pain and radicular symptoms are attributed to the hyperextension repetitive motion. As the foot strikes, the lumbar spine moves from the flat-backed position to an extended lordotic position as the trailing leg leaves the ground. As the back leg trails, in running, hyperextension of the lumbar spine occurs.

To meet the demands of the repetitive hyperextension motion of the lumbar spine and the increased load on the intervertebral discs, it is important to strengthen the transverse spinal system of the lumbar spine, the abdominal musculature, and the erector spinae. The transverse spinal system (multifidus, interspinales, and intertransversarii) is the tonic stabilizer of the spine, working in coordination with the rectus abdominus, external obliques, internal obliques, and erector spinae. The muscles of the hips and pelvis are also important in maintaining a healthy back and preventing the dysfunctions associated with running.

SPECIFIC STRETCHING EXERCISES FOR RUNNERS

As mentioned earlier, specific muscles that generally need stretching in runners include the hip flexors, quadriceps, hamstrings, iliotibial band, and ankle plantar flexors. Stretching exercises for these muscles as well as other commonly useful muscle stretches are included in the exercise program described next.

1. *Trunk flexion (double knees to chest):* Lie on your back with your knees bent and your feet flat on the floor. Contract your lower abdominals and press your lower back against the floor. Then bring one knee at a time to your chest and gently pull your knees toward your chest for 5 to 10 seconds. This exercise provides a gentle stretch of the lumbar musculature.

2. *Trunk rotation:* Sit in a chair with your arms crossed in front of you. Turn your shoulders to one side and hold for 5 seconds. Then return to the starting position before turning to the other side. This exercise provides a gentle stretch to the lumbar spine in rotation.

3. *Hip flexor stretch:* Assume a lunge position with the leg to be stretched extended behind you. Shift your hips forward to stretch the hip flexors. Be sure to keep the trunk erect and to use the abdominal musculature to prevent excessive arching of the back. Hold for 30 seconds (Fig. 18–1).

4. *Hip adductor stretch:* This stretch is performed standing with the legs relatively wide apart. In this position, shift your pelvis in the opposite direction to the leg being stretched.

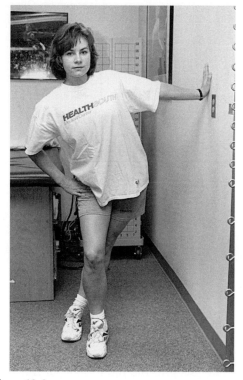

Figure 18–2

Iliotibial band stretch.

Keep your toes facing straight ahead. Hold for 30 seconds.

5. *Iliotibial band stretch:* Cross the foot of the leg to be stretched behind the other foot. Then lean your hips toward the side being stretched while leaning your shoulder in the opposite direction. Hold for 30 seconds (Fig. 18–2).

6. *Hamstring stretch:* Lie on your back with your legs straight. Bring one knee up toward your chest and grab the leg behind the thigh with both hands just above the knee. While maintaining the thigh so that it points straight up toward the ceiling, extend the knee until you feel a stretch behind your thigh. Hold this position for 30 seconds (Fig. 18–3).

7. *Quadriceps stretch:* While standing, bend your knee and grab your ankle behind you with the hand on the same side. The quadriceps is stretched by bringing the heel as close as possible to your buttocks while keeping the hip extended back. This exercise can also be done while lying on your stomach. Hold this position for 30 seconds.

8. *Gastrocnemius stretch:* Stand with both feet shoulder width apart. Step back with the leg to be stretched. Bend the opposite leg

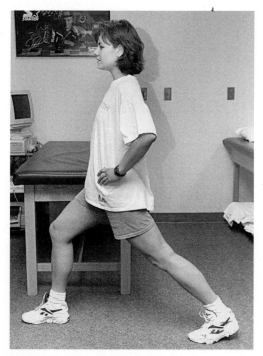

Figure 18–1

Hip flexor stretch.

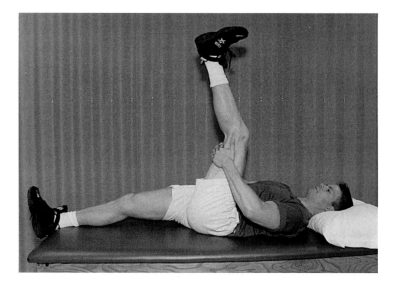

Figure 18–3

Hamstring stretch.

down; keep the trunk erect, the knee of the leg being stretched fully extended and the heel on the floor. Hold this stretch for 30 seconds. With this stretch, special attention must be given to the orientation of the back foot in order to get an effective stretch that is not causing undue stresses across the plantar aspect of the foot. It is important to keep the foot pointing straight ahead and to avoid flattening the arch of the foot. You must posi-

tion the foot so that your leg will be lined up just over the second toe, and make sure the weight under the foot is distributed mostly on the lateral aspect of the foot. A common error with this stretch is to have the lower leg and foot turned out, resulting in flattening and stretching of the arch of the foot instead of stretching of the gastrocnemius (Fig. 18–4).

9. *Soleus stretch:* The gastrocnemius stretch can also be performed for the soleus. In this

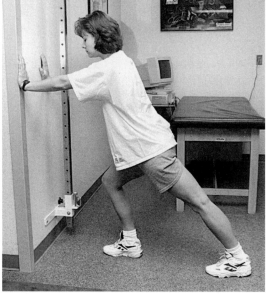

Figure 18–4

Gastrocnemius stretch.

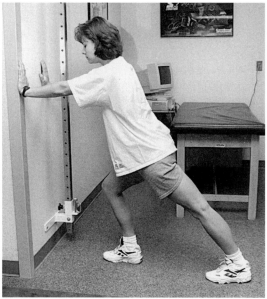

Figure 18–5

Soleus stretch.

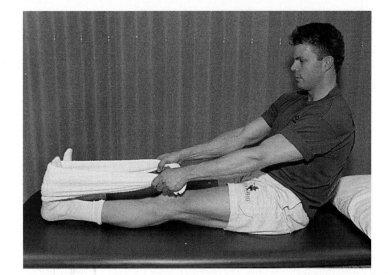

Figure 18–6

Towel stretches.

case, because the soleus inserts below the knee, the knee is bent to alleviate the stretch on the gastrocnemius and to focus on the soleus. Again, a static stretch of 30 seconds is recommended. As for the gastrocnemius stretch, proper foot position is important (Fig. 18–5).

10. *Towel stretches:* The ankle plantar flexors can be stretched using a towel. Sit with your knee extended in front of you. Place a towel under the ball of your foot. Holding both ends of the towel in your hands, pull the towel toward you to stretch the posterior calf musculature. Hold the stretch for 30 seconds. This stretch can be done with the ankle in a neutral position and with the ankle in a slight amount of inversion or eversion to stretch

all sections of the posterior calf musculature (Fig. 18–6).

11. *Plantar fascia stretch:* Sit with your knees bent. With your ankle dorsiflexed, passively pull your toes back toward your ankle with your hand. Hold for 30 seconds (Fig. 18–7). Mild stretching of this structure before running may help prevent injuries by increasing the ability of the plantar fascia to sustain the stresses associated with running. Stretching of the plantar fascia may not be a good practice for all runners. For those with "flat feet" or excessive foot pronation during running, stretching the plantar fascia could actually be contraindicated because the structure is already overstretched. In this case, runners should focus on strengthening the foot intrin-

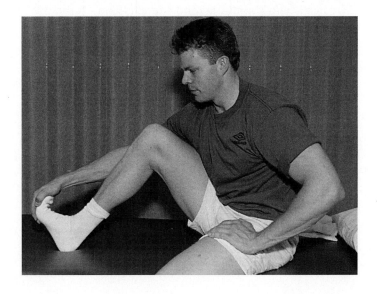

Figure 18–7

Plantar fascia stretch.

sic musculature and on stretching related structures such as the ankle plantar flexors.

SPECIFIC STRENGTHENING EXERCISES FOR RUNNERS

Muscle groups commonly found to be weak in runners include the ankle dorsiflexors, the hip abductors, and the quadriceps. The following exercises address these specific muscles. In addition, other exercises often used in the rehabilitation of running injuries are also presented.

1. *Pelvic tilt:* Lie on your back with your knees bent and your feet flat on the floor. Relax your arms at your sides. Contract your lower abdominals and press your lower back against the floor. Hold this position for 5 to 10 seconds and then relax. This exercise is beneficial in providing a gentle stretch of the lumbar musculature and strengthening the abdominals.

2. *Abdominal crunches:* Lie on your back with your knees bent. Place your hands behind your head with elbows in a wide position and focus on the ceiling. Pull in your abdominals and tilt your pelvis, flattening your lower back against the floor. Lift your head, neck, and shoulders off the floor. Do not curl your neck by bringing your chin to your chest. Your hands are supporting—not pulling—your head/neck forward. Hold this position for 5 seconds and slowly return to the starting position. This exercise helps strengthen the abdominals.

3. *Oblique crunches:* Lie on your back with your knees bent and place your hands behind your head with thumbs behind the ears and elbows wide, looking toward the ceiling. Pull in your abdominals and tilt your pelvis, flattening your lower back against the floor. Lift your shoulder blades up off the floor and rotate your torso to bring the right shoulder toward the left knee. Keep focused up at the ceiling and do not use your hands to bring your head forward and the chin to the chest. Hold this position for 5 seconds and slowly return to the starting position. Repeat, bringing the left shoulder toward the right knee. This exercise helps strengthen the abdominals.

4. *Shoulder blade squeezes:* In a sitting position, squeeze your shoulder blades together, hold for a few seconds and relax. Keep your chin slightly tucked and do not push your head forward as you squeeze the shoulder blades together. This exercise helps strengthen the posterior upper back musculature.

5. *Quadriceps sets:* Sit on a flat surface with your legs straight in front of you. Tighten the muscle on the front of your thigh as you push the back of your knee into the table or floor. Hold for 5 seconds. This isometric exercise can be performed at various angles and is an easy exercise for athletes to perform in the early stages of rehabilitation after an injury.

6. *Straight-leg raise:* Perform a quadriceps set as described above, then raise the entire leg from the table or floor approximately 6 inches, while keeping the knee straight. Hold for 5 seconds, then lower to the starting position. The straight-leg raise combines an isometric quadriceps contraction with an isotonic hip flexor contraction. This exercise is also beneficial in the early stages of rehabilitation. Added resistance may be obtained with the use of ankle weights.

7. *Hip abduction:* Lie on the uninvolved side. Raise the injured leg until it is slightly higher than the level of your hip, keeping the knee straight. Hold for 5 seconds, then lower to the starting position. This exercise helps strengthen the hip abductors without requiring the use of exercise equipment. Added resistance may be obtained with the use of ankle weights (Fig. 18–8).

8. *Hip adduction:* Lie on the injured side. Place the uninvolved leg in a chair or bend the uninvolved knee and cross the leg over so the foot rests in front of the involved leg. Raise the injured leg approximately 5 inches and hold for 5 seconds. Return to the starting position. This exercise isolates the hip adductors. Added resistance may be obtained with the use of ankle weights (Fig. 18–9).

9. *Hip flexion:* In a standing position, raise the knee of the injured leg toward your chest, keeping the upper body upright. Hold for 5 seconds, then lower to the starting position. This exercise strengthens the hip flexors and simulates the function of those muscles during the swing phase of running. Added resistance may be obtained with the use of ankle weights.

10. *Hip extension:* In a standing position, bring the injured leg back, keeping the knee straight and lifting the entire leg toward the ceiling. Lift only as high as your trunk can be maintained upright. Hold for 5 seconds, then lower to the starting position. This exercise strengthens the gluteus maximus. Added resistance may be obtained with the use of ankle weights.

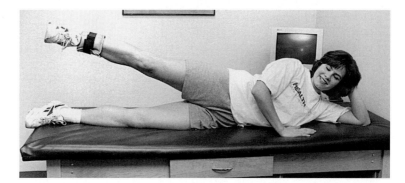

Figure 18–8

Hip abduction strengthening.

11. *Knee extension:* Sitting on the edge of a chair or on a knee extension machine, bring the foot of the injured leg up as far as is comfortable. Slowly lower to the starting position. The quadriceps muscle is isotonically strengthened during this exercise. Added resistance may be obtained with the use of ankle weights.

12. *Hamstring curl:* Lie on your stomach or on a hamstring curl machine. Lift the heel of the injured leg toward your buttocks, then slowly lower to the starting position. This exercise may also be performed in a standing position. The hamstring curl strengthens the hamstring muscles to help in deceleration of the lower leg at terminal swing. Added resistance may be obtained with the use of ankle weights.

13. *Squats:* Start in a standing position, with your feet shoulder width apart and your knees directed over your toes. Slowly lower into a squatting position but do not allow your knees to move ahead of your toes. Hold for 5 seconds, then return to the starting position. Squats are important in strengthening the gluteus maximus, quadriceps, and hamstrings in a functional weight-bearing position. Make sure that as you bend your knees,

each knee remains above its corresponding foot.

14. *Lunges:* Start in a standing position with your feet shoulder width apart. Take one step forward with the injured leg, then slowly lower your body down, allowing the back leg to bend. Keep the knee of the front leg over the ankle and do not allow it to bend more than 90 degrees. Slowly rise and return to the starting position. This exercise may also be performed by moving forward onto the lead leg as you rise up and then alternating lead legs. The musculature of the hip and thigh is strengthened during a lunge (Fig. 18–10).

15. *Side lunges:* Take one step sideways with the injured leg, then return to the starting position. Performing a lunge in this manner emphasizes strengthening of the hip abductors and adductors.

16. *Step-ups:* Stand sideways on a 2- to 8-inch step with the uninvolved leg hanging off the edge of the step. Slowly lower the body until the heel of the uninvolved leg touches the floor, allowing the knee of the injured leg to bend and keeping the upper body upright. Return to the starting position. Although this exercise is useful in strengthening the musculature of the hip and thigh, it is particularly

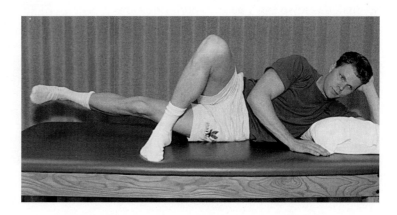

Figure 18–9

Hip adduction strengthening.

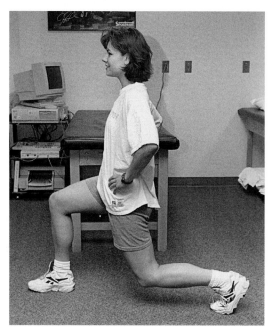

Figure 18–10

Lunges.

useful in strengthening the hip abductors to control the pelvis as in the stance phase of running (Fig. 18–11).

17. *Wall squats:* Lean against a wall and then step both legs out approximately one step length, keeping the upper body against the wall. Slowly slide down into a squat position but do not allow the knees to go past the toes. Hold for 20 to 60 seconds, then return to the starting position. This exercise helps build endurance in the quadriceps muscle.

18. *Leg press:* Lie on the leg press so that the knees are bent to about 90 degrees. Push until the knees are almost fully straightened but not locked out. Slowly lower to the starting position. This exercise may be performed so that the lowering phase is performed on the injured leg only. The leg press can be used to strengthen the quadriceps, hamstrings, and gluteus maximus in the early stages of rehabilitation when weight-bearing exercise is indicated but squat and lunge exercises cannot be tolerated.

19. *Pool running:* During injury rehabilitation, you may be able to run in a swimming pool. Running can be performed in shallow water (4 feet) or in the deep water area (7 feet) with a wet vest. Pool running may diminish contact stresses on your legs and back, and you may be able to train without pain

and exacerbation of your symptoms while maintaining cardiovascular fitness.

20. *Ankle plantar flexors (with towels):* Similar to the exercise for stretching, a towel placed around the ball of the foot can be used to strengthen the posterior calf musculature. In this instance, use the towel to provide resistance with your arms as you point your foot and toes down. The exercise must be done through the full range of motion (Fig. 18–12).

21. *Heel raises:* Stand with the balls of both feet on the edge of a step or curb. Lower your body slowly to stretch the ankles in dorsiflexion. Then raise your body up through full range of motion at the ankle. Be careful to avoid placing excessive stresses on the plantar aspect of the foot by excessively flattening the arch of the foot when lowering your body.

22. *Toe (towel) curls:* Do this exercise with bare feet. Place a towel on a smooth floor. Place your foot on the towel with your heel closest to the edge. Bunch the towel under your foot by using your toes. The exercise can be made more challenging by placing a weight at the end of the towel. This exercise

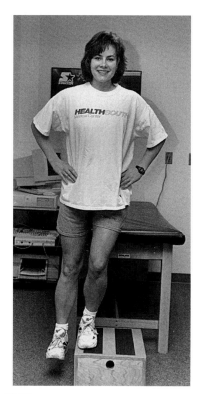

Figure 18–11

Step-ups.

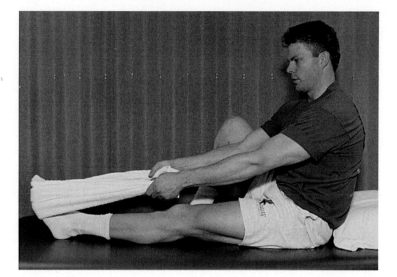

Figure 18–12

Ankle plantar flexors strengthening.

helps strengthen the intrinsic musculature of the foot and may help in controlling excessive pronation (Fig. 18–13).

23. *Picking up marbles:* Do this exercise with bare feet. Small objects, including marbles, are placed on the floor. The goal is to pick up these objects with your toes. Again, this exercise helps strengthen the foot intrinsic musculature.

24. *Ankle dorsiflexors:* This particular exercise requires the use of a Theraband. Sit on the floor with the Theraband circling the dorsal aspect of your foot. The other end of the Theraband must be attached to a heavy object

(the leg of a dresser, for example). Slide away from the heavy object to stretch the Theraband. Then bring your foot up against the resistance of the Theraband (Fig. 18–14).

CONCLUSION

The flexibility and strengthening concepts discussed in this chapter apply to runners as well as to any individuals involved in sports. However, only a thorough, personalized evaluation of flexibility, strength, and running biomechanics can provide the necessary information to design an individualized program of flexibility and strengthening for each athlete. This evaluation must be performed by a person who is knowledgeable about running biomechanics, injuries, and treatment concepts. A proper balance of flexibility, strength, and endurance of the muscle groups of the lower extremities must be achieved for proper injury prevention.

Although this chapter focuses on flexibility and strengthening, it is important to point out that a large percentage of running-related injuries can be attributed to other factors such as training intensity (distance, speed, terrain), training errors (rapid changes in training regimen), and improper footwear. Therefore, adequate flexibility and strength are only two of many interactive factors that must be taken into consideration for successful prevention and rehabilitation of running-related injuries.

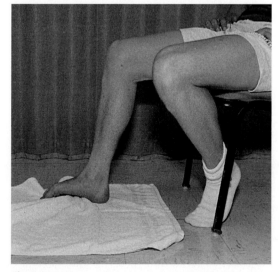

Figure 18–13

Toe (towel) curls.

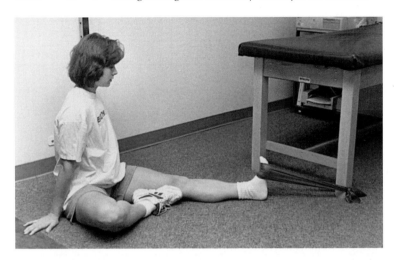

Figure 18–14

Ankle dorsiflexors strengthening.

REFERENCES

1. Bandy WD, Irion JM: The effect of time on static stretch on the flexibility of the hamstring muscles. Phys Ther 74:845–850, 1994.
2. Beaulieu J: Developing a stretching program. Physician Sportsmed 10:137–140, 1981.
3. Clancy WG: Tendinitis and plantar fasciitis in runners. In D'Ambrosia RD, Drez D (eds): Prevention and Treatment of Running Injuries, 2nd ed. Thorofare, NJ, Slack, 1989, pp 121–132.
4. Corbin CB, Noble L: Flexibility: A major component of physical fitness. J Phys Educ 51:23–60, 1980.
5. Curwin S, Stanish WD: Tendinitis: Its Etiology and Treatment. Lexington, MA, DC Heath & Co, 1984.
6. Davis VB: Flexibility conditioning for running. In D'Ambrosia RD, Drez D (eds): Prevention and Treatment of Running Injuries, 2nd ed. Thorofare, NJ, Slack, 1989, pp 221–231.
7. deVries HA: Electromyographic observation of the effects of static stretching on muscular distress. Res Q Exerc Sport 32:468–479, 1961.
8. deVries HA: Prevention of muscular distress after exercise. Res Q Exerc Sport 32:177–185, 1961.
9. deVries HA: The "looseness" factor in speed and oxygen consumption of an anaerobic 100 yard dash. Res Q Exerc Sport 34:305–313, 1963.
10. deVries HA: Flexibility. In deVries HA (ed): Physiology of Exercise for Physical Education and Athletics, 3rd ed. Dubuque, IA, Wm C Brown, 1980, pp 462–472.
11. Ekstrand J, Gillquist J: The frequency of muscle tightness and injury in soccer players. Am J Sports Med 10:75–78, 1982.
12. Ekstrand J, Gillquist J, Lilzedahl S: Prevention of soccer injuries: Supervision by doctor and physiotherapist. Am J Sports Med 11:116–120, 1983.
13. Ekstrand J, Gillquist J: The avoidability of soccer injuries. Int J Sports Med 4:1124–1128, 1983.
14. Etnyre BR, Abraham LD: Antagonist muscle activity during stretching: A paradox reassessed. Med Sci Sports Exerc 20:285–289, 1988.
15. Gleim GW, Stanchenfeld NS, Nicholas JA: The influence of flexibility on the economy of walking and jogging. J Orthop Res 1990; 8:814–823.
16. Glick JM: Muscle strains: Prevention and treatment. Physician Sportsmed 8:73–77, 1980.
17. Godges JJ, MacRae H, Engelke KA: Effect of exercise on hip range of motion, trunk muscle performance and gait economy. Phys Ther 73:468–477, 1993.
18. Godges JJ, MacRae H, Longdon C, et al: The effect of two stretching procedures on hip range of motion and gait economy. J Orthop Sports Phys Ther 10:350–357, 1989.
19. Greenfield B, Johanson M: Evaluation of overuse syndromes. In Donatelli RA (ed): The Biomechanics of the Foot and Ankle. 2nd ed. Philadelphia, FA Davis, 1996, pp 191–222.
20. Grimsby O: Scientific-therapeutic-exercise-progressions. J Manual Manipulative Ther 2:94–101, 1994.
21. Hubley CL, Kozey JW, Stanish WD: Can stretching prevent athletic injuries? J Musculoskel Med 1:25–32, 1984.
22. James SL, Bates BT, Osterning LR: Injuries to runners. Am J Sports Med 6:40–49, 1978.
23. Malone TR, Garrett WE jr, Zachazewski JE: Muscle: Deformation, injury, repair. In Zachazewski JE, Magee DJ, Quillen WS (eds): Athletic Injuries and Rehabilitation. WB Saunders, Philadelphia, 1996, pp 71–91.
24. Mann RA: Biomechanics of running. In D'Ambrosia RD, Drez D (eds): Prevention and Treatment of Running Injuries. 2nd ed. Thorofare, NJ, Slack, 1989, pp 1–20.
25. Mc Ardle A, Katch FL, Katch VL: Exercise Physiology: Energy, Nutrition, and Human Performance, 2nd ed. Philadelphia, Lea & Febiger, 1985.
26. Sady S, Wortman M, Blanke D: Flexibility training: Ballistic, static or proprioceptive neuromuscular facilitation? Arch Phys Med Rehabil 63:261–263, 1982.
27. Safran MR, Garrett WE, Seaber AV, et al: The role of warm-up in muscular injury prevention. Am J Sports Med 16:123–129, 1988.
28. Schultz P: Flexibility: Day of the static stretch. Physician Sportsmed 7:109–117, 1979.
29. Slocum DB, James SL: Biomechanics of running. JAMA 205:721–728, 1968.
30. Soderberg GL: Kinesiology: Application to Pathological Motion. Baltimore, Williams & Wilkins, 1986.
31. Taylor DC, Dalton JD Jr, Seaber AV, Garrett WE Jr: Viscoelastic properties of muscle-tendon units: The biomechanical effects of stretching. Am J Sports Med 18:300–309, 1990.
32. Wallin D, Ekblom B, Grahn R, Nordenborg T: Improvement of muscle flexibility: A comparison be-

tween two techniques. Am J Sports Med 13:263–268, 1985.

33. Welsh RP, Clodman J: Clinical survey of achilles tendinitis in athletes. Can Med Assoc J 122:193–196, 1980.

34. Westcott W: Strength Fitness: Physiological Principles and Training Techniques. Madison, WI, Brown and Benchmark, 1995.

35. Wilson GJ, Elliott BC, Wood GA: Stretch shorten cycle performance enhancement through flexibility training. Med Sci Sports Exerc 24:116–123, 1992.

36. Worrell TW, Perrin DH: Hamstring muscle injury: The influence of strength, flexibility, warm-up and fatigue. J Orthop Sports Phys Ther 16:12–18, 1992.

37. Zachazewski JE: Flexibility for the runner: Specific program considerations. Top Acute Care Trauma Rehabil 1:9–27, 1986.

38. Zachazewski JE: Improving flexibility. In Scully RM, Barnes MR (eds): Physical Therapy. Philadelphia, JB Lippincott, 1989, pp 698–738.

39. Zachazewski JE: Flexibility for sports. In Sanders B (ed): Sports Physical Therapy. Norwalk, CT, Appleton & Lange, 1990, pp 201–238.

40. Zebas CJ, Rivera ML: Retention of flexibility in selected joints after cessation of a stretching exercise program. In Dotson CO, Humphrey JH (eds): Exercise Physiology: Current Selected research. New York, AMS Press, 1985.

MARVIN M. ADNER ■ ARTHUR J. SIEGEL

======= CHAPTER NINETEEN

Medical Syndromes in Runners

The 100th running of the Boston marathon was held on the third Monday in April of 1996. It was estimated that there would be 40,000 participants—the largest marathon ever held. (There were 38,000 participants.)

The creation of the medical care plan for Boston 1996 represented a template for the discussion of medical syndromes in runners. The medical problems experienced by the runners in this 26-mile race starting at noon on a spring day in New England are related to (1) the generation and dissipation of metabolic heat, (2) alterations in intracellular and extracellular fluid and electrolyte composition, (3) alterations in vasomotor regulation, and (4) organ dysfunction involving principally the heart, brain, and kidneys. These changes are greatly affected by the environment in which the exercise is taking place.

Running can increase energy consumption 20-fold.[52] Most of this energy is converted into heat. Because alteration in core temperature of as little as 2°C can cause significant impairment of body function, heat dissipation through evaporation, radiation, convection, and conduction is a critical homeostatic process.[53]

HYPOHYDRATION

In runners, the principal means of heat dissipation is by evaporation of sweat. Sweat rates are affected by a number of factors including running speed, state of fitness, and acclimatization. Sweat rates commonly exceed 1 L/hr.[5, 8, 9] The maximal capacity to absorb fluid in the small intestine is about 1.2 L/hr. Although addition of complex carbohydrates and cooling of the ingested fluid may enhance gastric emptying and intestinal absorption, even under ideal conditions a state of negative fluid balance is often obligatory.[10,]

[16, 31] The ionic concentration of sweat is affected by sweat rate and varies inversely with the degree of heat acclimatization. The principal constituents are sodium and chloride, usually in the range of 40 to 60 mEq/L. Development of hyponatremia requires many days of intense exercise.[9] However, a few cases of hyponatremia have been reported to develop in marathon events owing to excess ingestion of hypotonic fluid.[35] Therefore, it has been recommended that in endurance events lasting longer than 3 hours, replacement fluid should contain 20 to 30 mEq/L of sodium and chloride.[16] Potassium concentration in sweat is low, usually 4 to 5 mEq/L. Potassium supplementation is not necessary. Mild hyperkalemia can occur during exercise as a result of breakdown of muscle cells, but this is not usually of clinical significance.[15] Therefore, marathon runners need water, not electrolytes.

The clinical impact of plasma volume depletion (hypohydration) is dramatically demonstrated in the studies performed on Alberto Salazar, who collapsed after winning the 1982 Boston marathon (Fig. 19–1). Salazar was the American marathon record holder and was thought to have a good chance to win an Olympic gold medal in the 1984 Olympics in Los Angeles. This highly trained athlete was found to have an extraordinarily high sweat rate, 2.79 L/hr, considerably higher than other elite athletes performing at the same running speed and heat stress. Even after an intense acclimatization program with optimal fluid ingestion, Salazar lost 8% of his body weight during his Olympic run and did not have a winning performance. Despite the profound hypohydration, his core temperature remained normal.[4]

With as little as 3% reduction in body weight, the performance of marathon runners is impaired. Oxygen delivery is signifi-

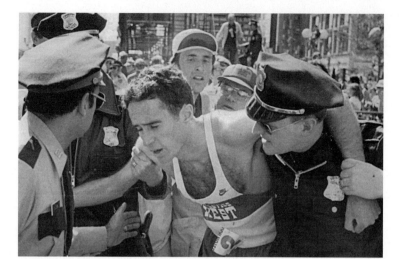

Figure 19–1

Alberto Salazar after completion of the 1982 Boston marathon. (Photograph by Frank O'Brien, Boston Globe, Boston, MA.)

cantly decreased because of a diminished circulating plasma volume due to sweating, with obligatory shunting of blood to the exercising muscles and to the skin. With increasing water deficit, runners become more symptomatic, presenting with anorexia, headache, vertigo, and dyspnea, and experience further deterioration in exercise performance.[43, 44] Hypohydration contributes to the risk of hyperthermia because it limits the amount of blood that can be shunted to the skin for evaporative heat loss.

HEAT ILLNESS

If exercise is performed under conditions of increasing heat stress, the problems of heat dissipation and the development of heat illness are greatly magnified. The impact of environmental heat stress is defined by the wet bulb globe temperature (WBGT).[53] The equation is

WBGT = 0.7 wet bulb temperature
+ 0.2 black globe temperature
+ 0.1 dry bulb temperature

Wet bulb temperature, which is a measure of evaporative cooling, is the major contributor to the heat stress index. The black globe temperature, representing radiant heat, and the dry bulb temperature, representing ambient temperature, contribute considerably less to the WBGT index. The American College of Sports Physicians issued a position statement on the prevention of thermal injuries during distance running; it describes the risk of run-

ning based on the WBGT values (Fig. 19–2).[3] Conditions of low humidity and increased rate of air flow over a runner's body greatly facilitate heat loss by evaporative cooling. On a hot, sunny, windless, humid day, the heat load is maximized and the ability to lose heat by evaporative cooling is diminished, resulting in an increased risk of heat illness. The WBGT heat index does not take into consideration a very important factor—the rate of heat production, which increases linearly with running speed.[53] In races of shorter distance than the marathon, such as a 10 k, the running speed is usually faster than in the marathon, resulting in an increased capacity for rapid heat buildup.

Hypohydration increases the risk of exhaustion for a given degree of heat stress.[46] As heat storage increases with core temperatures exceeding 40°C, the risk of developing heatstroke increases. This life-threatening disorder is characterized by a multiorgan system failure involving the central nervous system (CNS), heart, liver, and kidneys. CNS abnormalities are common, with premonitory symptoms of headache, confusion, and dizziness, which may rapidly progress into delirium and coma. Myocardial failure and cardiac dysrhythmia may cause cardiovascular collapse. What is the mechanism for this medical catastrophe? Disseminated intravascular coagulation with small blood vessel thrombosis may contribute to organ dysfunction.[39] Hubbard and Armstrong believe that to attribute heatstroke to an elevated body temperature per se is a "message without a mechanism."[22] They conceive of an energy depletion model as the underlying basic pathophysiology, with high

The Risk of Heat Injury While Racing in the Heat

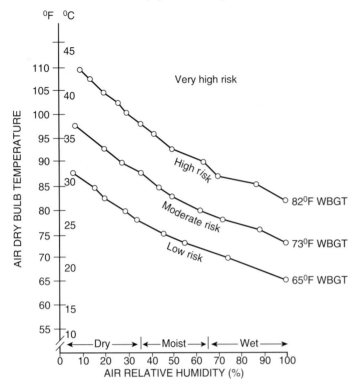

Figure 19–2

The risk of heat injury while racing in the heat. (From Heat Research Division, U.S. Army Research Institute of Environmental Medicine, Natick, MA. From information provided by the American College of Sports Medicine.)

temperature producing energy depletion of the cells, with a decrease in adenosine triphosphate in transport of sodium and potassium with the development of cellular swelling and membrane failure. As the cells fail, a vicious cycle is created, and if it is not interrupted by reparative measures, death of the organism results.

COLD ILLNESS

Hypothermia is an uncommon cause of severe disability among runners participating in the Boston marathon. The lowest ambient temperature recorded was −3°C, in the 1926 race. However, when marathons are held during the winter months in the northern hemisphere, the potential for severe disability due to hypothermia is quite real. Important environmental factors include the ambient temperature and the wind speed, which produce the wind chill index. When the ambient temperature is 10°C and the wind speed is 20 mph, the chill factor results in a temperature of −25°C, creating a dangerous climate for runners. Hypothermia develops when heat loss exceeds heat gain.[20] The heat generated

by exercising muscle is the primary defense mechanism against hypothermia. About 60% of body heat is lost from the head and neck by convection, and the remainder by evaporative cooling from the skin. Therefore, when exercising in the cold, it is necessary to wear garments that optimize heat retention.[17] This can be accomplished by dressing in layers with materials that trap air for insulation and that wick moisture away from the skin. The outer shell garment should be waterproof and fitted so that the wind does not penetrate through openings in the clothing. Inappropriately dressed runners are trapped in a cycle of progressive body heat depletion. As negative heat balance progresses, the capacity for work decreases, running rate slows, heat generation further decreases, and body core temperature falls. Shivering represents a compensatory mechanism to increase body heat generation. However, this requires availability of carbohydrates to fuel the shivering muscles. With glycogen depletion occurring in the muscles secondary to running, the capacity to shiver decreases. Clinical syndromes of hypothermia become manifested with core temperatures of 34°C to 35°C. Circulating blood volume decreases, increasing peripheral resistance and blood viscosity. The oxygen dissociation curve shifts to the left, with decreased oxygen delivery. Cardiac output falls. The risk of cardiac arrhythmia increases. Both metabolic and respiratory acidosis may develop. Cerebral dysfunction occurs, with confusion and delirium progressing to coma.

EXERCISE-RELATED SUDDEN DEATH

Exercise-related sudden death (ERSD) has been a serious concern in endurance sport since Pheidippide's fatal collapse in 490 B.C. (Fig. 19–3), despite only one reported fatality in a century of Boston marathons.[18] The occurrence of three cardiac arrests at the 1994 New York City marathon highlights the dilemma for marathon running in which cardiovascular benefits from training are offset by an increase in the risk for acute cardiac events during the race itself.

The concept of athletic heart syndrome is now a century old, like the Boston marathon itself.[23] The myth of cardioprotection from marathon running evolved in part from that race, with the case report of clear coronary arteries on postmortem examination of Clarence DeMar ("Mr. Marathon"), seven-time Boston Athletic Association champion.[11] Conclusive epidemiologic evidence now exists for both the long-term cardioprotective benefit of endurance exercise training and the triggering effect for acute myocardial infarction (MI) during prolonged, strenuous exertion.[25, 32, 58] Incremental risk during exercise increases from two to six times resting baseline for physically fit and sedentary individuals, respectively.[32]

Current understanding is that acute coronary syndromes without premonitory symptoms may be triggered during exercise in either the presence or the absence of coronary heart disease.[2, 37] Silent myocardial ischemia due to coronary artery spasm may trigger fatal cardiac arrhythmias, proving that painless does not mean harmless during sport as in other clinical circumstances.[30, 34, 36] Plaque rupture during exercise may precipitate acute coronary syndromes in some cases.[7] Ventricular arrhythmias may also be triggered by myocardial hypertrophy, which is the hallmark of athletic cardiomyopathy.[6, 12]

Recommendations exist for determining medical eligibility for competing in endurance events with evidence that such screening can decrease morbidity.[27, 38] Hypertrophic cardiomyopathy as the paradigm of athletic heart syndrome may be indistinguishable from structural cardiovascular conditions and remains the major challenge in assessing risk of ERSD.[28, 57] Medical clearance with exercise stress electrocardiography is also strongly advised for recreational athletes undertaking a marathon, especially if they were previously sedentary or have known cardiovascular risk factors (men older than 40 years and postmenopausal women). Such screening may identify some individuals who have silent myocardial ischemia and who are at high risk for exercise-induced acute cardiac events. Thallium imaging appears to add little predictive information if exercise electrocardiogaphic results are normal.[14] Normal results of such testing provide no guarantees.

Figure 19–3

After running across the Plain of Marathon, Pheidippides delivered his message and died. (Time magazine.)

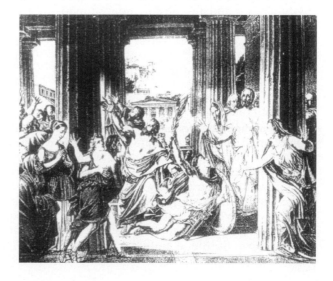

Detection of acute MI in symptomatic runners is problematic in that results of baseline electrocardiograms and postrace serum cardiac markers are frequently abnormal but may be nonspecific. Creatine kinase MB isoenzyme (CK-MB) is widely accepted in clinical practice as the most sensitive marker for acute MI. This isoenzyme is elevated in symptomatic marathon runners after competition owing to exertional release from skeletal muscle biochemically altered by training.[48] Radionuclide imaging techniques to detect acute MI, transient myocardial ischemia, and cardiac cell necrosis all have yielded normal results after competition in asymptomatic runners in whom elevated cardiac markers mimic acute MI.[47–49] Normal results of scanning provide evidence against silent myocardial cell necrosis after marathon competition, despite elevated serum markers including troponin subunits.

These findings confound the diagnostic assessment of runners who have exertional chest pain or syncope or who collapse and who may be overdiagnosed as having acute MI based on nonspecific serum marker elevations.[50] Noninvasive testing such as radionuclide myocardial imaging or two-dimensional echocardiography is necessary to confirm acute MI in such patients. Only runners with corroborative evidence warrant such a diagnosis. Diagnostic advances such as antimyosin antibody cardiac imaging for detection of acute myocarditis and ultrafast computed tomography to visualize coronary artery calcification may identify some conditions that predispose to ERSD in athletes.[13, 19, 24, 59] Genetic findings on the prolonged QT syndrome may serve to circumvent potentially fatal arrhythmias in athletes during nontraumatic sports, just as improved protective chest devices may avert cardiac arrest triggered by blunt chest trauma.[29, 54, 55]

Athletes and race directors must address the reality that marathon running, once touted as cardioprotective, is potentially hazardous and sometimes fatal. Recreational runners contemplating marathon participation should undergo medical clearance to assess cardiovascular risk. Runners should train incrementally, hydrating vigorously at all times, and race within their training. Prevention lies in the education of runners and in providing a medical safety net on race day.

Therefore, in creating the medical care plan for the 1996 Boston marathon, we anticipated the major problems to be hypohydration, often associated with mild hyperthermia, and, less likely, hypothermia. These are not life threatening. With prompt medical attention, runners recuperate more rapidly than if left unattended and delayed complications such as acute renal failure can be avoided. The immediate concerns are the two life-threatening disorders—heatstroke and cardiac arrest.

BOSTON—THE 100TH

Creating the medical care plan for the 100th running of the Boston marathon was not a simple task. Since 1978, the organized medical care team has consisted of physicians, nurses, trainers, therapists, and medical assistants, as well as a team of physiatrists who care for the wheelchair athletes. The field of race participants has included as many as 10,000 runners who have run relatively fast times in a marathon race during the previous year, plus an estimated 3000 unofficial entrants ("bandits") who run the course behind the qualified participants.

In the 100th marathon, 25,000 runners were expected to participate in the qualified group and an open division was chosen principally by lottery and consisted of at least 15,000 individuals whose qualifications were an interest in participating in this historic event. The increased number of runners and the change in the level of fitness due to the addition of the open division entrants who are of uncertain ability and fitness required an expanded medical care plan for the race. The medical care problems of the unofficial runners who have run behind the numbered runners for many years were analyzed. Although their finishing times were slower, they had medical problems similar to those experienced by the qualified runners. On that basis, we assumed that the frequency of the various medical syndromes encountered in previous Boston marathons would occur in the 1996 race as well.

Runners were given prerace instruction on preventing the various medical syndromes both in written materials provided before the race and in educational seminars on race day weekend. Water and sport drinks were available at every mile. The runners were encouraged to drink at least 1 L/hr. It was anticipated that 100 to 200 distressed runners would require ambulance transport to the emergency departments of the five hospitals along the race route, with the collapse rate proportional to the heat stress index. Given the prevalence of silent but severe coronary heart disease in 10% of men older than 40 years, it was predicted that 2000 runners may indeed be at risk for ERSD on race day. Although the chance of a runner's developing serious cardiac arrhythmia or cardiac arrest on the race route was small, based on the experience of the Marine Corps marathon, we planned to place medical personnel supplied with automatic defibrillators along the entire course. At the finish line would be three "code teams" staffed by Medical Team and Boston Emergency Medical Service personnel. At least 85% of the starters were expected to cross the finish line; 5% to 10% were expected to require medical attention. Using data obtained from the finishing times from previous Boston marathons and the 1992 New York City marathon (whose population was expected to closely resemble that of the open division of the 1996 Boston marathon), a computerized projection of minute-to-minute finishing times was created (Fig. 19–4). It indicated that for a period of at least 60 minutes, more than 300 runners per minute would cross the finish line. We estimated that

as many as 2% of these runners would collapse after they crossed the finish line. Most would be treated in a 22,000-square-foot tent located immediately beyond the finish line. The less seriously ill runners who were still ambulatory would be treated at two additional medical facilities, one located 1/4 mile and the other 6/10 mile beyond the finish line. Because a runner's medical condition may rapidly deteriorate, all tents would have the capacity to provide intravenous fluid resuscitation and advanced cardiac life support protocols. Ambulances would be available to take critically ill runners who required hospitalization to one of the major Boston teaching hospitals.

Exercise-associated collapse is a syndrome, not a diagnosis, indicating a runner who is unable to maintain an upright position without assistance. Collapse usually occurs after the cessation of exercise and is associated with postural hypotension.[21] During a marathon, runners can develop significant hypovolemia. Blood flow to the muscles of the lower extremities and to the skin is increased. The pumping action of the leg muscles is the major mechanism used to maintain central blood volume and cardiac output. With cessa-

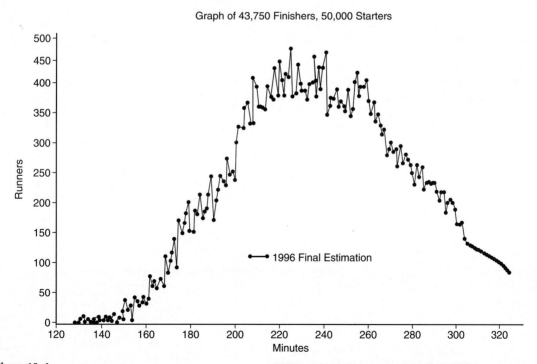

Figure 19–4

Estimating finishing times for 45,000 starters in the 1996 Boston marathon. (From Ciswewski K, Caldwell T, Danubio J, et al: Worcester Polytechnic Institute, Boston Marathon Project.)

tion of exercise, this pumping action ceases. Venous pooling of blood occurs in the lower extremities, and return of the blood to the heart diminishes with decreased cardiac output, which may result in syncope. In addition, neuroregulatory mechanisms controlling heart rate appear to be important in the adaptive response to orthostasis in the postexercise state.[26] Thus, it appears that exercise-associated collapse is often due to hypovolemia, increased venous pooling in the lower extremities, and heart rate variability.

The presence or absence of heat or cold illness is not implicated. To provide appropriate therapy to collapsed runners, it is necessary to measure the core temperature.[40] There is considerable controversy about the best means of estimating core temperature in the field.[41] Conceptually, body heat is distributed between the core and the shell. The core refers to the vital organs such as the heart, liver, brain, and major vessels supplying these organs. The remainder of the body is the shell, whose function it is to regulate the body temperature. Oral thermometry has no role in determining the core temperature of exercising athletes. The cooling effect of hyperventilation on a sublingually placed thermometer results in significant artifact even with attempts to keep the mouth closed for an extended time.[42] Rectal temperature has traditionally been thought to represent a close approximation of the core temperature. Although this may be true in a sedentary individual, rectal temperature measurement has several limitations when used in sensing core temperature of an exercising athlete in a field situation. The rectal temperature lags behind the esophageal temperature during the periods of rapid heat storage and during periods of heat loss (Fig. 19–5).[45] The slow response of the rectal temperature may be related to a relatively low rate of blood flow to the rec-

tum.[33] In addition, in a field situation where large number of heat-related injuries occur, issues of privacy and requirements for universal precaution limit the efficiency and enthusiasm of the medical staff involved in taking rectal temperature measurements.

In a controlled hospital setting, tympanic membrane temperature measured with a thermocouple probe closely correlates with esophageal temperature, the latter considered to be the best measure of core temperature.[56] Hand-held otoscope-like devices have been developed to measure the tympanic membrane temperature using infrared techniques. Other devices measure ear canal temperature. In a field situation, aural temperature is affected by the external environment and reflects the shell temperature. Tympanic membrane temperature measured with an accurate device using proper techniques is probably equivalent to the core temperature, although there is some concern that this method is affected by the external environment as well.[41] Measurements can be made every 5 seconds. Simultaneous measurements of rectal and tympanic membrane temperatures taken in disabled runners participating in the 1989, 1990, and 1991 Boston marathons reveal significant discordance between rectal and tympanic membrane temperatures (Fig. 19–6). A patient's clinical state correlated most closely with tympanic membrane temperature. In those instances in which patients had a high rectal temperature, for example exceeding 40°C, and a normal tympanic membrane temperature of 38°C, the individuals were usually alert and had no significant hypotension, tachycardia, or signs of volume depletion. They responded quickly to modest cooling measures and hydration. When both rectal temperature and tympanic membrane temperature were elevated, the patients were much more ill with CNS symptoms and were

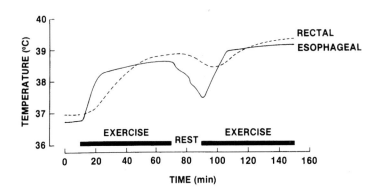

Figure 19–5

Rectal and esophageal temperature response to rest and exercise in the heat. (From Kent M. Pandolf, et al., HUMAN PERFORMANCE PHYSIOLOGY AND ENVIRONMENTAL MEDICINE AT TERRESTRIAL EXTREMES. Copyright © 1988 The McGraw-Hill Companies, Inc. Reprinted by permission. All rights reserved.)

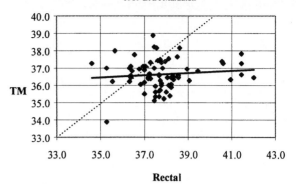

TYMPANIC VS. RECTAL TEMPERATURE FOR 70 RUNNERS
1989 BAA Marathon[2]

Figure 19–6

Tympanic vs. rectal temperatures for 70 runners competing in the 1989 Boston Marathon. (From Pompei F, Pompei M, Adner MM, et al: 1989 Boston Marathon Data.)

clinically judged to be in incipient heatstroke. Therefore, this method may offer a more accurate means of assessing rapid changes in core temperature not reflected by rectal thermometry alone. We currently measure both rectal and tympanic membrane temperature simultaneously in patients with exercise-associated collapse. A high rectal temperature but normal tympanic membrane temperature in a patient who does not appear clinically ill is thought to reflect a situation in which the heat loss mechanism is functioning well, and the patient is at that time not at high risk of developing heat illness. Some patients, however, when lying in a medical tent, may develop an increase in tympanic membrane temperature over a 5- to 10-minute period and therefore must be monitored very carefully. We believe that a high rectal temperature and a high tympanic membrane temperature represent evidence that the heat loss mechanism is ineffective and the patient is at high risk for developing clinical heatstroke. It is necessary to treat heatstroke immediately. To delay treatment until the patient is transported to a hospital facility often results in irreversible organ damage. Cooled intravenous fluids containing glucose and sodium chloride are administered. Ice packs are applied to the scalp, neck, axillae, and groin. The trunk is flushed with ice water. If the tympanic membrane temperature does not decrease during the next few minutes, the runner is placed in an ice water bath to enhance conductive cooling. The skin vasoconstriction response to the cold may also improve venous return and cardiac output. Alternative methods of cooling such as suspending a runner in a hammock and spraying the patient with fine vapor or using a fan to increase airflow over the body are equally effective but are impractical to use in a field situation because of the complexity of the design of the system.

Collapsed runners whose principal problems are hypohydration with only mild heat illness are treated with oral fluids. If patients are unable to drink, they are given intravenous fluids. The average infusion usually is 2 liters given over 30 to 40 minutes. In a study of management of Boston marathon injuries in the years 1984 to 1994, 10% of the runners admitted to the medical tent received intravenous therapy.[1] During the past few years, with changes in triage protocol, the overall population of runners admitted to the medical tent is more seriously ill. In the 1995 Boston marathon, more than 20% of the 600 runners admitted to the medical tent received intravenous therapy.

If a patient is found to be hypothermic, the therapeutic plan is to increase heat production and heat retention. The runner is placed on a cot and wrapped in two heat-retaining layers. A Mylar blanket is placed over the legs and trunk and is covered by a woolen blanket whose edges are tucked under the body to create a nearly airtight system. Carbohydrate-containing warmed oral fluids or, if necessary, warmed intravenous fluids are given to increase the runner's capacity to shiver, to replete plasma volume, and to increase cardiac output. In previous years, runners' warm-up clothes were stored on buses near the medical tent and could be brought to a runner's cot by medical assistants. The wet running clothes were removed. Runners donned their running jacket and pants, which improved the ability to retain heat. In the 1996 race, the buses with the runners' gear were more than a half mile away from the medical tent at the finish line, where most of the severe injuries were treated, and were not readily accessible.

SUMMARY

The 100th Boston marathon was a once-in-a-lifetime experience for the runners and those who volunteered to care for them. A medical care plan was created on the basis of the pathophysiology of the medical syndromes occurring in runners and the collective experiences of many clinicians throughout the world who have treated runners with these syndromes.

REFERENCES

1. Adner MM, Scarlet JJ, Casey J, et al: The Boston Marathon medical care team: Ten years of experience. Physician Sportsmed 16:99, 1988.
2. Alpert JS: Myocardial infarction with angiographically normal coronary arteries: A personal perspective (editorial). Arch Intern Med 154:245, 1994.
3. American College of Sports Medicine: Position statement on the prevention of thermal injuries during distance running. Med Sci Sport Exerc 17:9, 1985.
4. Armstrong LE, Hubbard RW, Jones BH, et al: Preparing Alberto Salazar for the heat of the Olympic marathon. Physician Sportsmed 14:73, 1986.
5. Armstrong LE, Maresh CM: The induction and decay of heat acclimatisation in trained athletes. Sports Med 12:302, 1991.
6. Berder V, Vauthier M, Mabo P, et al: Characteristics and outcome in arrhythmogenic right ventricular dysplasia. Am J Cardiol 75:411, 1995.
7. Ciampricotti R: Coronary syndromes related to sports activities. Prim Cardiol 21:28, 1995.
8. Costill DL: Physiology of marathon running. JAMA 221:1024, 1972.
9. Costill DL: Sweating: Its composition and effects on body fluids. Ann N Y Acad Sci 301:160, 1977.
10. Coyle EF, Montain SJ: Carbohydrate and fluid ingestion during exercise. Med Sci Sports Exerc 24:671, 1992.
11. Currens J, White P: Half a century of running. Clinical, physiologic and autopsy findings in the case of Clarence DeMar ("Mr. Marathon"). N Engl J Med 265:988, 1961.
12. Daliento L, Turrini P, Nava A, et al: Arrhythmogenic right ventricular cardiomyopathy in young versus old patient: Similarities and differences. Am J Cardiol 25:655, 1995.
13. Dec GW, Palacious IF, Yasuda T, et al: Antimyosin antibody cardiac imaging: Its role in the diagnosis of myocarditis. J Am Coll Cardiol 116:97, 1990.
14. Evans M, Christian T: Is thallium imaging for predicting severe coronary artery disease justified? Cardiol Rev 1:19, 1996.
15. Fishbane S: Exercise-induced renal and electrolyte changes. Physician Sportsmed 23:39, 1995.
16. Gisolfi CV, Duchman SM: Guidline for optimal replacement beverages for different athletic events. Med Sci Sports Exerc 24: 679, 1991.
17. Gonzalez RR: Biophysics of heat exchange and clothing: Applications to sports physiology. Med Exerc Nutr Health 4:290, 1995.
18. Green LH, Cohen SI, Kurland G: Fatal myocardial infarction in marathon racing. Ann Intern Med 84:704, 1976.
19. Guidelines for clinical use of cardiac radionuclide imaging: A report of the American College of Cardiology/American Heart Association Task Force on cardiovascular procedures. J Am Coll Cardiol 25:521, 1995.
20. Hamlet MP: Human cold injuries. In Pandolf KB, Sawka MN, Gonzalez RR (eds): Human Performance Physiology and Environmental Medicine at Terrestrial Extremes. Indianapolis, Benchmark Press, 1988, p 435.
21. Holtzhausen L, Noakes T, Kroning B, et al: Clinical and biochemical characteristics of collapsed ultramarathon runners. Med Sci Sports Exerc 26:1095, 1994.
22. Hubbard RW, Armstrong LE: The heat illnesses: Biochemical, ultrastructural and fluid-electrolyte considerations. In Pandolf KB, Sawka MN, Gonzalez RR (eds): Human Performance Physiology and Environmental Medicine at Terrestrial Extremes. Indianapolis, Benchmark Press, 1988, p 305.
23. Huston TP, Puffer JC, Rodney WM: The athletic heart syndrome. N Engl J Med 313:24, 1985.
24. Kaufman RB, Peyser PA, Sheedy PF, et al: Quantification of coronary artery calcium by electron beam computed tomography for determination of severity of angiographic coronary artery disease in younger patients. J Am Coll Cardiol 25:626, 1995.
25. Lee IM, Hsieh C, Paffenbarger R: Exercise intensity and longevity in men. The Harvard almuni health study. JAMA 273:1179, 1995.
26. Markad VK, Fallen EL, McKelvie R: Effects of steady state exercise on the power spectrum of heart rate variability. Med Sci Sports Exerc 23:428, 1991.
27. Maron BJ, Mitchell JH: Recommendations for determining eligibility for competition in athletes with cardiovascular abnormalities. J Am Coll Cardiol 24:845, 1994.
28. Maron BJ, Pellicia A, Spirito P: Cardiac disease in young trained athletes. Circulation 91:1596, 1995.
29. Maron BJ, Poliac LC, Kaplan JA, Mueller FO: Blunt impact to the chest leading to sudden death from cardiac arrest during sports activities. N Engl J Med 333:337, 1995.
30. Marwick TH: Is silent ischemia painless because it is mild? J Am Coll Cardiol 25:1513, 1995.
31. Mitchell JB, Costill DL, Houmard MG, et al: Effects of carbohydrate ingestion on gastric emptying and fluid balance during prolonged exercise. Med Sci Sports Exerc 20:110, 1988.
32. Mittleman MA, Maclure M, Tofler GH, et al: Triggering of acute myocardial infarction by heavy physical exertion. N Engl J Med 329:1677, 1993.
33. Molnar GW, Read RC: Studies during open-heart surgery in the special characteristics of rectal temperature. J Appl Physiol 36:333, 1974.
34. Myerburg R, Kessler K, Mallon S, et al: Life-threatening ventricular arrythmias in patients with silent myocardial ischemia due to coronary artery spasm. N Engl J Med 326:1451, 1992.
35. Nelson PB, Robinson AG, Kapoor W, et al: Hyponatremia in a marathoner. Physician Sportsmed 16:78, 1988.
36. Nihoyannopoulos P, Marsonis A, Joshi J, et al: Mag-

nitude of myocardial dysfunction is greater in painful than in painless myocardial ischemia; an exercise echocardiographic study. J Am Coll Cardiol 25:1507, 1995.
37. Noakes T, Opie L, Beck W: Coronary heart disease in marathon runners. Ann N Y Acad Sci 301:593, 1977.
38. Pellicia A, Maron BJ: Preparticipation cardiovascular evaluation of the competitive athlete: Perspectives from the 30-year Italian experience. Am J Cardiol 75:827, 1995.
39. Perchick J, Winkelstein A, Sadduck R: Disseminated intravascular coagulation in heat stroke. JAMA 231:480, 1975.
40. Roberts WO: Exercise associated collapse in endurance events: A classification system. Physician Sportsmed 17:49, 1989.
41. Roberts WO: Assessing core temperature in collapsed athletes. Physician Sportsmed 22:49, 1994.
42. Rozycki TJ: Oral and rectal temperatures in runners. Physician Sportsmed 12:105, 1984.
43. Sawka MN: Physiological consequences of hypohydration: Exercise performance and thermoregulation. Med Sci Sports Exerc 24:657, 1992.
44. Sawka MN, Francesconi P, Young A, et al: Influence of hydration level and body fluids on exercise performance in the heat. JAMA 252:1165, 1984.
45. Sawka MN, Wenger MN: Physiological responses to acute exercise—heat stress. In Pandolf KB, Sawka KB, Gonzalez RR (eds): Human Performance Physiology and Environmental Medicine at Terrestrial Extremes. Indianapolis, Benchmark Press, 1988, p 97.
46. Sawka MN, Young AJ, Latzka WA, et al: Human tolerance to heat strain during exercise: Influence of hydration. J Appl Physiol 73:368, 1992.
47. Siegel AJ, Lewandrowski KB, Strauss HW, et al: Normal post-race antimyosin myocardial scintigraphy in asymptomatic marathon runners with elevated serum creatinine kinase MB isoenzyme and troponin T levels. Cardiology 86:451, 1995.
48. Siegel AJ, Silverman LM, Evans WJ: Elevated skeletal muscle creatine kinase MB isoenzyme levels in marathon runners. JAMA 250:2835, 1983.
49. Siegel AJ, Silverman LM, Holman BL: Elevated creatine kinase MB isoenzyme levels in marathon runners. Normal myocardial scintigrams suggest noncardiac source. JAMA 246:2049, 1981.
50. Siegel AJ, Silverman LM, Holman BL: Normal results of post-race thallium-201 myocardial perfusion imaging in marathon runners with elevated serum MB creatine kinase levels. Am J Med 79:431, 1985.
51. Siegel AJ, Yang J, Lewandrowski K: Elevated serum cardiac markers in asymptomatic marathon runners after competition. Exertional rhabdomyolysis or silent myocardial injury? (in press).
52. Simon HB: Hyperthermia. N Engl J Med 329:483, 1993.
53. Sutton JR: Heat illness. In Strauss RH (ed): Sports Medicine. Philadelphia, WB Saunders, 1984, p 307.
54. Towbin JA: New revelations about the long-QT syndrome. N Engl J Med 333:384, 1995.
55. VanCamp SP, Bloor CM, Mueller FO, et al: Nontraumatic sports death in high school and college athletes. Med Sci Sports Exerc 27:641, 1995.
56. Webb GE: Comparison of esophageal and tympanic membrane temperature monitored during cardiopulmonary bypass. Journal of International Anesthesia Research Society 52:729, 1973.
57. Wight JN, Salem D: Sudden cardiac death and the "athlete's heart." Arch Intern Med 155:1473, 1995.
58. Willich SN, Lewis M, Lowell H, et al: Physical exertion as a trigger of myocardial infarction. N Engl J Med 329:1684, 1993.
59. Won ND, Louwabunpat D, Vo AN, et al: Coronary calcium and atherosclerosis by ultrafast computer tonography in symptomatic men and women: Relation to age and risk factors. Am Heart J 127:422, 1994.

STUART BERGER

══════ *CHAPTER TWENTY*

The Cardiopulmonary Effects and Consequences of Running in Children—Good or Bad?

Although there exists a large body of literature relative to the cardiovascular effects of aerobic exercise on adults, specifically running, little has been written about this subject in children. As discussed in this chapter, ample evidence shows the beneficial effects of running on the adult cardiopulmonary system. Is the same true for children, and are any untoward or unexpected cardiopulmonary effects expected in children? This chapter attempts to review the information to date and to make some reasonable recommendations for training in the preadolescent and adolescent age group.

BENEFICIAL CARDIOPULMONARY EFFECTS OF RUNNING IN ADULTS

Running is a type of aerobic exercise. Cooper[2] has defined aerobic exercise as that type of exercise that demands large quantities of oxygen for prolonged periods and that ultimately forces the body to improve those systems responsible for the transportation of oxygen. Aerobic exercise has many beneficial effects on the cardiopulmonary system[7]:

1. Myocardial mass increases. The myocardium also becomes better supplied with blood flow via the development of collateral coronary blood vessels.

2. Endurance training results in volume loading of the heart. This effect causes an increase in ventricular chamber volume with no change in wall thickness, and a larger stroke volume both at rest and during exercise. Therefore, a slower heart rate is needed at a given workload to maintain cardiac output. This additionally enhances the perfusion of the cardiac muscle during diastole.

3. High-density lipoprotein (HDL) levels increase, and therefore the total cholesterol/HDL ratio decreases. Studies have shown that this can result in a lower overall risk of atherosclerosis and in fact is thought to have a protective effect.

4. Total blood volume increases, as does hemoglobin concentration. Oxygen transport both at rest and with physical activity is augmented.

5. Running has been associated with increased lung capacity, which has been associated with longer life.

Besides its beneficial effects on the cardiovascular system, running has been shown to be an effective way to lose weight and keep it off. It can also be a means to deal with emotional and physical stress and in fact has been suggested as a treatment for some forms of depression.

In addition to and most likely as a result of the foregoing effects, running and physical activity in general have been shown by numerous studies to result not only in prolongation of life but in an improvement in the quality of life.[1, 5, 8–10]

BENEFICIAL CARDIOPULMONARY EFFECTS OF RUNNING IN CHILDREN

Little research has addressed this subject. A brief review of the existing information is offered.

Raitkari and colleagues[11] reported on the influence of selected coronary heart disease risk factors in a 6-year study of Finnish adolescents and young adults. An important conclusion of their study was that the level of physical activity was closely maintained from adolescence to young adulthood. Equally important was the fact that physical inactivity remained even more constant than did physical activity. Therefore, adolescents who were inactive became inactive adults with a less beneficial coronary risk profile.

Studies by Harsha[4] and DiNubile[3] confirmed that children in the United States today tend to be less fit than children in the United States 20 years ago, as well as less fit than their counterparts in other developed nations. In addition, their studies suggested that U.S. children are adopting a sedentary lifestyle at an earlier age. This is of grave concern because some existing data suggest that the cardiovascular risk factors in children are the same as in adults, although the specific relationship between physical inactivity and risk factors for coronary artery disease in children is not conclusively known. It is known that many cardiovascular risk factors such as obesity, hypertension, and lipid profile do indeed carry over from childhood into adulthood. With this in mind, it seems not unreasonable to recommend running programs as well as other physical activity for youths in order to reduce adult cardiovascular diseases. It is Harsha's[4] suggestion that the positive long-term effects of running are most likely to be successful if lifestyle changes are established early. DiNubile[3] went one step further in recommending parental education about the importance of the benefits derived from parental involvement in fitness-related activities along with their children. This should include the establishment of a healthy balance between sedentary activities such as television and video games and physical activity.

Some data suggest that a child's cardiopulmonary system has a diminished capability of responding to endurance training. Rowland[12] examined the trainability of children. Some information in this study as well as in others[6] has suggested that children may need greater exercise intensity than adults in order to gain the same cardiovascular adaptation to training. The reason for the age-dependent responses to training are not precisely clear, but such responses may be a result of autonomic influences on the heart, myocardial function and mass, or both. Similarly, the influence of growth and maturation in determining a child's performance has not been completely resolved.

To further support the foregoing ideas, Rowland and colleagues[14] investigated the ability of children to improve aerobic fitness after a 12-week period of endurance training. The study did support the concept that $\dot{V}o_2$max can be improved with endurance training during the childhood years. However, the degree of aerobic trainability is limited in healthy, active children.

DETRIMENTAL EFFECTS OF RUNNING IN CHILDREN

The major detrimental effects of running in children are not on the cardiopulmonary system but rather are on the musculoskeletal system. However, with regard to the specific cardiovascular issue, two areas are worth general discussion. These include the topic of screening children for athletic participation and the topic of the athlete's heart syndrome in children.

It is widely believed that children should be screened by their physician before embarking on competitive sports or a semiintense program of physical training. The obvious reason for this practice is to search for any risk factors that might result in the very uncommon event of sudden death or other serious cardiovascular event. These risk factors can be adequately screened for by taking a very careful personal and family history and performing a physical examination. Cardiac abnormalities such as hypertrophic cardiomyopathy, long QT syndrome, and arrhythmogenic right ventricular dysplasia can be familial. Previous symptoms such as syncope or palpitations would also warrant further workup for hypertrophic cardiomyopathy, long QT syndrome, other arrhythmias, or congenital coronary abnormalities. Finally, abnormalities on physical examination such as any marfanoid feature or a pathologic murmur would warrant further studies to rule out Marfan syndrome or any other type of congenital heart disease. Results of the screening history, family history, and physical examination should be very useful in guiding further studies such as echocardiography and electrocardiography. The latter studies, as screening tools themselves, have been shown very conclusively not to be cost-effective.

The athlete heart syndrome is well defined in adults. It is a result of endurance training as well as isometric training and is probably a normal cardiovascular response. It tends to be more common with intense isometric training than with endurance aerobic training. It results in a thickening and increase in mass of the left ventricle. Unfortunately, in some cases, the echocardiographic manifestations of the athlete heart are difficult to differentiate from that of hypertrophic cardiomyopathy. Some features of the athlete heart syndrome are different from hypertrophic cardiomyopathy and are therefore reassuring. Factors that favor the athlete heart syndrome include absence of a family history of hypertrophic cardiomyopathy, concentric as opposed to asymmetric left ventricular hypertrophy, bradycardia, high aerobic capacity, normal diastolic left ventricular function by echocardiography, and hypertrophy that is reversible with deconditioning.

Data regarding the athlete heart syndrome in children are limited. It is believed that this syndrome is much less common in children who undergo endurance training than in adults. Rowland and colleagues[13] studied 10 male prepubertal distance runners. They failed to identify any significant cardiovascular differences in this group when compared with untrained boys. Specifically, no echocardiographic differences were noted in left ventricular wall thickness, left ventricular mass, or left ventricular chamber size. Although the risk of sudden death in individuals with the athlete heart syndrome is debatable, it is at least reassuring to know that this syndrome is very uncommon in children.

CONCLUSION

It is generally believed that the beneficial cardiopulmonary effects of running in children are similar to those in adults. For reasons unclear, however, some data suggest that although beneficial effects can be attained, children may need a greater exercise intensity than adults in order to gain the same adaptation to training. Nonetheless, because it appears that U.S. children of today are less fit than U.S. children of 20 years ago and are heavier and more sedentary than children of other countries, it makes sense to recommend running programs as well as physical activity for youths in order to reduce adult cardiovascular diseases. This approach is logical because many cardiovascular risk factors such as obesity, hypertension, and unfavorable lipid profile not only can be positively influenced by running but also tend to be carried over from childhood into adulthood.

REFERENCES

1. Blair SN, Kohl HW III, Barlow CE, Paffenbarger RS Jr: Changes in physical fitness and all-cause mortality. A prospective study of healthy and unhealthy men. JAMA 273:1093–1098, 1995.
2. Cooper KH: The Aerobics Program for Total Well-Being. New York, Bantam Books, 1982.
3. DiNubile NA: Youth fitness—problems and solutions. Prev Med 22:589–594, 1993.
4. Harsha DW: The benefits of physical activity in childhood. Am J Med Sci. 310 (Suppl 1):S109–113, 1995.
5. Lee IM, Hsieh CC, Paffenbarger RS Jr: Exercise intensity and longevity in men: The Harvard Alumni Health Study. JAMA 273:1179–1184, 1995.
6. Mahon AD, Vaccaro P: Cardiovascular adaptations in 8- to 12-year-old boys following a 14-week running program. Can J Appl Physiol 19:139–150, 1994.
7. Martin DE, Coe PN: Training Distance Runners. Champaign, IL, Leisure Press, 1991.
8. O'Connor GT, Hennekens CH, Willett WC, Goldhaber SZ, et al: Physical exercise and reduced risk of non-fatal myocardial infarction. Am J Epidemiol 142:1147–1156, 1995.
9. Paffenbarger RS Jr, Kampert JB, Lee IM, Hyde RT, et al: Changes in physical activity and other lifeway patterns influencing longevity. Med Sci Sports Exerc 26:857–865, 1994.
10. Paffenbarger RS Jr, Wing AL, Hyde RT: Physical activity as an index of heart attack risk in college alumni. Am J Epidemiol 142:889–903, 1995.
11. Raitkari OT, Porkka KV, Taimela R, Rasanen L, et al: Effects of persistent activity and inactivity on coronary risk factors in children and young adults. The Cardiovascular Risk in Young Finns Study. Am J Epidemiol 140:195–205, 1994.
12. Rowland TW: Trainability of the cardiorespiratory system during childhood. Can J Sports Sci 17:259–263, 1992.
13. Rowland TW, Unnithan VB, MacFarlane NG, Gibson NG, et al: Clinical manifestations of the "athlete's heart" in prepubertal male runners. Int J Sports Med 15:515–519, 1994.
14. Rowland TW, Boyajian: Aerobic response to endurance exercise training in children. Pediatrics 96(4 Pt 1):654–658, 1995.

Note: Page numbers in *italics* refer to illustrations; page numbers followed by (t) refer to tables.